Sex Therapy Manual

Patricia Gillan
MA, PhD

Drawings by Richard Gillan

BLACKWELL SCIENTIFIC PUBLICATIONS
OXFORD LONDON EDINBURGH
BOSTON PALO ALTO MELBOURNE

Dedicated to Richard

Thank you for all your support, advice and understanding, especially over my taking so much time in writing this book. I have always appreciated your creativity and felt good that you've been prepared to work on our relationship and marriage. Having reached our silver wedding anniversary this year it's good to know that you are also my best friend. I must confess I have never found you boring and miss you when we are apart.

Blackwell Scientific Publications
Editorial offices:
Osney Mead, Oxford OX2 0EL
(*Orders*: Tel. 0865 240201)
8 John Street, London WC1N 2ES
23 Ainslie Place, Edinburgh EH3 6AJ
52 Beacon Street, Boston
Massachusetts 02108, USA
667 Lytton Avenue, Palo Alto
California 94301, USA
107 Barry Street, Carlton
Victoria 3053, Australia

First published 1987

Set by V & M Graphics Ltd, Aylesbury
Bucks
Printed and bound in Great Britain by
Redwood Burn Limited
Trowbridge, Wiltshire

DISTRIBUTORS

USA
Year Book Medical Publishers
35 East Wacker Drive
Chicago, Illinois 60601
(*Orders*: Tel. 312 726-9733)

Canada
The C.V. Mosby Company
5240 Finch Avenue East,
Scarborough, Ontario
(*Orders*: Tel. 416-298-1588)

Australia
Blackwell Scientific Publications
(Australia) Pty Ltd
107 Barry Street
Carlton, Victoria 3053
(*Orders*: Tel. (03) 347 0300)

British Library
Cataloguing in Publication Data

Gillan, Patricia
Sex therapy manual.
1. Sex therapy
I. Title
616.6'906 RC556

ISBN 0-632-01938-7
ISBN 0-632-01866-6 (pbk.)

Contents

Acknowledgements

Most of the homework sheet for individual and couples therapy, apart from the stimulation therapy sheets, were devised with the cooperation of Dr Michael Crowe. The physical examination sheets were provided with the help of Dr Willy Monteiro. The homework sheets for the men's therapy groups were devised by Dr Maurice Yaffé and are mainly based on Dr Bernie Zilbergeld's ideas.

Permission has been granted to reproduce all these homework sheets.

Lastly I would like to acknowledge all the cotherapists I have worked with, especially Dr Michael Crowe, Dr Willy Monteiro, Dr Brian Snowden and Dr Antony Fry. Therapists from other cultures who gave me insight into their ways of living and thinking include Dr Harry Czechowicz of Venezuela, Dr Nobel Beharry of Trinidad, Professor Lieh Mak and Dr Emil Ng from Hong Kong, Padmal da Silva from Sri Lanka, Dr Federico Puente from Mexico, Alba Souza from Brazil and Dr David Ndete from Kenya. Working with Dr Susan McMullen, Dr Susan Golombok, Dr Patricia Becker, Dr Keith Stoll and Dr Christine Watson proved to be a happy experience for women's group therapy. Lastly, running the men's sex therapy groups with Dr Maurice Yaffé was a very satisfying experience.

Acknowledgement and thanks also go to Lorna and Phillip Sarrell for allowing me to sit and listen to their therapy sessions at Yale in the USA back in the early seventies.

Introduction

Most sex books on the market are very theoretical. In this book I wanted to be as practical as possible and get down to the 'nitty gritty' of sex therapy, even going so far as to provide dialogues between clients and therapists. This appears to be a good way for a student of sex therapy to learn about clients. Frequently the trainee therapist will be able to identify the illustrated case histories and dialogues with the clients he or she is currently treating.

During the 25 years I have been doing sex therapy I have been very lucky to work with co-therapists who have been helpful and empathic. Dr Michael Crowe and I founded the Maudsley Psychosexual Clinic and I was fortunate to work with a medical man who was willing to try new methods of therapy. Together we devised most of the homework sheets which appear in the Appendix.

Many of my co-therapists have come from other cultures and have given me an insight into different worlds. I have been lucky to visit my co-therapists later and see them operating in their own territories in their own countries and have been fortunate to be able to learn first-hand so much about the Caribbean, India, Africa and the Middle East. Various case histories and dialogues between clients from such countries are included in this book.

The pilgrimage of a sex therapist can be tough. In the seventies sex therapy was not respectable and I had to journey to the USA to undergo my initiation. It ranged from discussing 'Olfaction and Sex' with Masters and Johnson at their sex seminar in St Louis, Missouri to nude participation in Betty Dodson's 'women's sex group' in New York. Who else but a pilgrm sex therapist would have spent a week in San Francisco in a dark room watching SAR videos most of the day and night.

Research on sex therapy is gradually being carried out, but it took a long time to get such projects off the ground. The Maudsley Hospital and Guy's Hospital, London, have both been centres of such investigations and much of this research influenced the treatment methodology in this book. One of the most important research studies was carried out in the Department of Physiology at The Institute of Psychiatry in cooperation with Professor Giles Brindley. The women in our research viewed films, slides, listened to stories, and were vibrated whilst their vaginal blood flow was measured. Results showed that many women were sexually aroused and stimulated by erotica and pornography. Some women became quite annoyed when they learned that although they were saying the nude men in the slides they viewed were disgusting they nevertheless showed an increase of vaginal blood flow! Later these same women admitted that they were secretly interested but did not like to admit this.

This increased my faith in the use of erotica for therapy with clients with low sex interest. Erotic material is, in fact, used in 'stimulation therapy' which is described in this book. Most therapists tend to neglect the patient with the low sex interest but I have found this type of client rewarding in terms of therapy change. In the past many clients who had a partner with a low sex drive made the decision to have an affair with another person with an average sex drive, rather than try to change the partner's sex drive. Recently the author has been inundated with clients who want to remain with a partner who has a low sex drive and to try to change this. This has mainly been due to anxiety caused by the risk of AIDS involved in finding new partners. Several of these male clients have said that they do not like using condoms with irregular partners as this reduces their sensation and decreases their sexual pleasure. They admit that they would now prefer to have sex at home and remain monogamous.

This trend is not restricted to clients with a sexual drive discrepancy as the new trend in therapy is for clients to stay together and try to solve their sexual problems and remain monogamous, rather than seeking new partners. Monogamy is becoming fashionable but this is increasing the number of clients who want therapy for sex or relationship problems. At this rate there are not enough therapists to go round and more will need to be trained.

Group sex therapy has always been an important part of my work and I am sure that the three chapters on group sex therapy methods will help the trainee therapist to deal with some of the typical problems that come up in groups. The methods in this book are eclectic but most emphasis is placed on behavioural methods as I have always been a pragmatist. I am sure the trainee therapist will benefit from some of the suggestions.

The last chapter on forensic sex therapy should be helpful in understanding how some of the clients can respond to sympathetic therapy.

Patricia Gillan

Chapter 1

Sexual Attitudes

What is normal?

Many people are over-concerned with what is normal and consider that there is something wrong with behaviour that is not average practice. Such people are often obsessed with reading Kinsey and other books concerned with sexual surveys. Clients tend to concentrate on the idea that sexual intercourse between two members of the opposite sex is the only desirable goal of human sexuality.

People still associate the 'paraphilias' which were once labelled deviant behaviour with something that is dirty or perverted. Whether a client gets aroused by a member of the opposite sex or a handbag is a matter of sexual conditioning, and this is a matter of chance. In any case, 'average' behaviour or 'average' morality may not be right for everyone, and after all, only fifty years ago there were many who believed masturbation to be both sinful and harmful: nowadays most people believe it to be both pleasurable and 'normal'.

Sexuality is such an individual matter that it is not surprising that when two people come together in a permanent relationship there may be considerable differences in behaviour and preferences. Unfortunately, too, such preferences are not revealed until after the marriage or are only discovered by accident. Transvestites and fetishists are often discovered in this way and such discoveries may cause much hurt and resentment. Several such clients have reported that their partner found a pair of knickers in their cupboard or closet and thought immediately that they must belong to another woman who was having an affair with their husband. Minor differences are usually ironed out in the early part of a relationship but where one partner baulks at joining in some activity that is important for the other it makes for resentment and conflict, and the sad outcome may be that the couple drift apart, each to his or her own, often lonely, sexual scene. Sex therapists may spend a lot of time persuading couples to share activities and fantasies.

In practice, couples who have agreed to cooperate in a partnership might as well agree to cooperate in their sexuality as well, and where the difficulty is caused by the rigid application of old-fashioned standards it is well to remember that standards of behaviour do change from generation to generation.

We are living at present in an era of greater sexual liberality which many people welcome, although the advent of AIDS has put a brake on permissiveness and monogamy is now being promoted as a safe goal. In the last thirty years, male homosexuality between consenting adults has become legal and fairly acceptable in many countries. It is ironic that an American or European homosexual stands a higher chance than a heterosexual of contracting AIDS, just at the time when attitudes towards homosexuality as something abnormal and dirty have changed.

Exhibitionists and transvestites are probably regarded with less fear than by previous generations; perhaps people are beginning to think of them as more sick than dangerous. The general public has never known much about fetishism, but preferences that are known about, such as that of rubber, are regarded with indulgence. It will be fascinating to see what will be considered 'normal' in future. With the way AIDS is spreading maybe mutual masturbation will become more common than sexual intercourse; it seems that wife-swapping and orgies are no longer fashionable nowadays.

The association of sexual behaviour with pain used to attract widespread condemnation. Now the public may perhaps be changing to a more tolerant attitude. Pain and sex are generally referred to as sado-masochism (SM), the sadist being the one who inflicts the pain – the masochist the one receiving it. Sado-masochistic behaviour is an example of an extreme situation, lesser degrees of these tendencies being quite normal. Many people enjoy minor degrees of violence and pain during the sexual act, either giving or receiving. During intercourse either the man or the woman may be the one who does the thrusting while the other lies inert. Either the woman or the man may enjoy the feelings of dominance and power, either may like to act with some force – to embrace with strength, to kiss or bite with such power as to inflict pain and minor damage. Either may enjoy this pain, especially if sexually excited beforehand, and may enjoy the feeling of being used, humiliated or controlled, and the feeling of passivity or servitude.

Such minor degrees of sado-masochism are common. Slightly greater degrees, which involve the deliberate infliction of pain, the use of whips and bondage and so on, can be judged individually. Many clients who have read *The Joy of Sex*[1] are often surprised that Alex Comfort discusses bondage, but when they try it themselves they report that it is fun – but, of course, mutual trust between partners needs to be established before such experiments are tried. Where people are seriously hurt or forced to act against their will, the behaviour becomes abhorrent. *The Story of O*[2] has attracted many shocked comments but quite a lot of clients are aroused by reading the story; the fantasy can be appealing without having to act it out.

In summary, Western society is approaching the view that people should have the opportunity to do what they please, provided the well-being, freedom and dignity of others are unharmed.

There remains a further option – that is, no sex at all. Individuals who have no sexual inclinations are rare but it must be said that there is no reason why a condition of no sex should not be a happy alternative if that is a person's choice.

Sex surveys

Most people get their ideas of what is normal from information about other people's sexual activities but such facts are hard to come by. In the first part of this century, Freud provided information about sexual development based on people undergoing psychoanalysis. It was only when Kinsey[3] carried out his sex survey in 1948 on the sexual behaviour of 6000 men that yardsticks were provided for activities like masturbation, the frequency of sexual intercourse and oral sex.

The Kinsey Report was recently re-analysed by Gebhard and Johnson[4] with the addition of data collected since the original publication. They also excluded those individuals, that Kinsey had included, who were drawn from sources of known sexual bias, like lower-educated individuals from penal institutions or who had criminal records. Men who felt guilty about masturbating must have felt gratified to learn that 94 per cent of the male sample had masturbated to orgasm at some time in their lives.

Data for women shows a change in attitude towards masturbation. In the original Kinsey survey[5] of female sexual behaviour in 1953, 40 per cent of women revealed that they had masturbated to orgasm at some time in their lives but the updated Kinsey survey of 1979 reported a higher figure of 58 per cent.

The Hite Report[6] in 1976, based on 3019 women, threw more light on masturbation and female sexuality. Hite revealed that 82 per cent of her sample masturbated and that 96 per cent were orgasmic during masturbation as opposed to only 30 per cent being orgasmic during sexual intercourse. Half the women in the survey revealed that they had faked orgasm at some time during sexual intercourse. Returning to masturbation, the way some of the women reported their techniques during this activity provided useful sociological information. The principal method was stimulating the clitoris directly, sometimes associated with inserting something in the vagina. 73 per cent of the women came into this category, but only 3 per cent relied on putting objects into the vagina.

Although Shere Hite has been criticised for her sampling, she has revealed some interesting facts about American women which they find reassuring about themselves. The fact that most women in her survey needed direct clitoral stimulation to reach an orgasm was an important revelation and the subject of much media attention. Prior to the Hite Report many women considered themselves abnormal if they needed some clitoral stimulation during sexual intercourse. Another useful purpose of her survey was that it showed how women think about and see their genitals. Various statements made by the informants provide an excellent sociological study of Western women.

In Victorian days masturbation was considered to be abnormal but surveys show it to be an activity practised by the average adult. Nowadays masturbation is no longer believed to cause physical harm like blindness or insanity. It is regarded instead as an important part of sexual development and growing up. For a long time the influence of the Church, which regarded it as sinful, caused people to feel guilty about masturbation. This still holds with some religions, especially for people of other cultures. Nag[7] refers to Hindu, and to some extent the Muslim, belief that semen is a source of strength and should not be wasted.

Some men from the Orient believe that, according to Yin and Yang principles, masturbation is a waste of male or vital Yang essence which should be part of sexual intercourse. In Hong Kong, Lieh Mak and Ng[8] discussed male patients who feared that the loss of semen in intercourse could impair their health and consequently they suffered from ejaculatory impotence. They reported that, even today, sayings such as 'one drop of semen, many drops of blood' and 'deaths due to semen incontinence' are still widely believed and circulated among the Chinese who misinterpret Taoist sex doctrines.

The problem with sex surveys is that they tend to set the standard for what is normal. If people feel they are not up to the national average they begin to think there is something wrong with them.

When Kinsey reported that the average young married couple have coitus two or three times a week many people believed this should be the standard for everyone, regardless of age. In fact, frequency of sexual intercourse is negatively correlated with age. This type of statistical 'average' can be confusing for many as it does not reveal that it includes the complete range, from people who have intercourse twice a day to those who have it once a year.

The main point to emphasise is that people vary considerably and there is no ideal frequency for intercourse. There is also no correlation between quality and quantity.

The frequency of intercourse might be influenced by the hormones which vary according to the time of the woman's menstrual cycle, yet women differ even in this respect. Some peak at the time of ovulation while others reach the time of greatest sexual interest immediately after their period. Pregnancy can also affect the frequency of intercourse, especially towards the end of pregnancy when women are not as interested in sex.

When Kinsey broke down the age range for sexual interest and reported that women reached their peak of sexual responsiveness in their early forties, compared with men in their late teens, many people doubted this information as a traditional stereotype had become established of older women losing interest in sex. Of course, society makes it acceptable for older men to have affairs with young women, but older women are not encouraged to have affairs with younger men.

The Kinsey report also showed the frequency of oral sex, revealing that fellatio occurs less frequently than cunnilingus. Kinsey revealed that only 46 per cent of sexually experienced women accepted cunnilingus but later surveys show a higher frequency, as Chester and Walker[9] discovered in 1979. Kinsey probably helped to establish cunnilingus as a normal and healthy activity, perhaps helping to increase the figures in the later survey.

The prevalence of sexual problems

On the whole, people are not encouraged to hear about other people who have sexual problems. Society expects people to keep a stiff upper lip over sexual problems, especially male difficulties. For many years mental health bore the same stigma; people were not encouraged to talk about their anxiety or depression and mental illness was swept under the carpet.

Few epidemiological studies have been carried out to show the prevalence of sexual problems in our society. Kinsey did show that men are more likely to have erectile problems as they get older. Kinsey was aware that women do have orgasmic problems; his survey showed that among married women the proportion who never experienced orgasm decreased steadily with age, so the women between the ages of 30–50 were more likely to experience an orgasm. Kinsey reported that 78 per cent of women between the age of 16 and 20 can reach orgasm from any source after marriage, compared with 95 per cent of women between 36 to 40 and 94 per cent by the age of 50.

Frank's[10] 1978 study in the United States was based on 100 'normal' couples who were recruited from church and club groups, and were mainly middle class. The criterion for volunteers was that their marriage was working. Nearly half the wives in the sample reported difficulty in getting excited and reaching an orgasm. Most of the wives complained about their inability to relax or too little foreplay, whereas only half of the husbands complained about this. This finding reflected the fact that most of the husbands failed to perceive the difficulties that their partner had. Either women are not as obvious at showing their sexual problems or men fail to notice because they are self-absorbed. 40 per cent of the men reported erecticle or ejaculatory dysfunction.

There is a myth that Scandinavians are better adjusted sexually than Americans and Europeans. Some studies have been reported revealing sexual problems in the Scandinavian population. In Sweden, Nettelbladt and Uddenberg[11] reported that 40 per cent of the 58 married men in their random sample showed a 'tendency toward sexual dysfunction', and 38 per cent of them had experienced premature ejaculation, a finding similar to that of Frank's for American males. Danish women do not fare well when it comes to current sexual problems. In a personal interview survey of a random sample of 225 forty-year-old Danish women, Garde and Lunde[12] found that 35 per cent reported current sexual problems. 42 per cent appeared to lack sexual interest. Two-thirds of the women said they had simulated orgasm, although most of them had experienced orgasm at some time or other.

British studies are few and far between. Golombok *et al.*[13] studied sexual problems encountered in general practice and interviewed a random selection of sixty men and women who were waiting to see their family doctor, asking them to complete a questionnaire. A substantial number were found to experience sexual problems and, like Frank's study in the United States, the women were less satisfied than the men. More of the women (20 per cent) than the men (10 per cent) hardly ever or never became easily sexually aroused. Furthermore, 20 per cent of the women found lovemaking disgusting, compared with only 3 per cent of the men. Complete anorgasmia with their partner occurred in 17 per cent of the women. For men, mild premature ejaculation was quite common in about 20 per cent of the sample but none was completely impotent. This British study reported poor communication about sex although most of the sample declared they were satisfied with their sexual relationships.

Another way of obtaining information about the incidence of sexual dysfunction in the population is to ask family doctors how often they see patients with sexual problems in their surgeries. In the USA Burnap and Golden[14] interviewed physicians in a variety of specialities to survey the frequency with which they saw patients with sexual difficulties. The conclusion was that 15 per cent of patients had sexual problems. Women tended to be anorgasmic during intercourse and men lacked erections. The research also showed that physicians who found it embarrassing to discuss sexual problems reported lower frequencies of sexual problems in their patients.

Another way of finding out about sexual problems in the population is to study referrals to a Family Planning Clinic which Begg[15] researched in Edinburgh, finding that 12.5 per cent of the 759 women who completed their questionnaire indicated that they were suffering from a current sexual problem.

When it comes to direct referrals to sex clinics for sexual dysfunction there is no shortage of referrals. Many clinics have a six-month waiting list. Bancroft and Coles[16] analysed referrals to a sexual problem clinic in Oxford for a three-year period and found that 42 per cent of the men had erectile impotence compared with 23 per cent with premature ejaculation. These figures are similar to those of Masters and Johnson[17] in the USA. The main problem presented by 62 per cent of the women was general unresponsiveness, followed by 18 per cent with orgasmic dysfunction. Masters and Johnson did not include a category of general unresponsiveness so figures cannot be compared.

The effects of sexual problems

It is often difficult to work out whether a sexual problem has occurred as a result of a general relationship problem or whether sexual difficulties caused the general relationship to deteriorate. There is general agreement that sexual problems cause stress and unhappiness for a large number of people.

Often couples with sexual problems have unhappy marriages. The Marriage Guidance Council has reported a high incidence of sexual dysfunction in the population referred to them for marriage guidance, indeed they were so inundated with referrals that they ran courses to train counsellors in sex therapy. The Maudsley[18] finding that it is more difficult to treat people for sex problems if their relationship or marriage is poor is relevant here and maybe explains why some of the Marriage Guidance Council's recent results for sex therapy have not been as successful as those in other UK sex clinics. Sexual dissatisfaction at the beginning of a marriage has been found by Thornes and Collard[19] to increase the risk of the marriage ending in divorce.

Hawton[20] has drawn attention to the fact that many couples with sexual dysfunction cease discussing sex and there is increasing frustration. This can lead to the alienation of affection and the couple can cease to have any physical contact whatsoever, even avoiding kissing or hugging. Some couples drift apart and have affairs with other partners. In a proportion of cases the final outcome is marital breakdown and divorce, sometimes preceded by violence as a result of jealousy.

One consequence of sexual dysfunction is that the whole family can be affected. The children cease to have a 'model of affection and physical contact' in their parents. Stuart[21] has pointed out that the immediate consequence of marital disharmony for children can be very serious.

It is equally bad to have a sexual problem and no help if one is single; this leads to feelings of inadequacy, anxiety and abnormality. In the study of women's sex therapy groups by Gillan *et al.*[22], the researchers found a significant decrease in anxiety for the women who received sex therapy, compared with the waiting list control. Several American reports, including one by Derogatis *et al.*[23], have shown that a relatively high proportion of patients with sex problems experience psychiatric symptoms and suffer from psychiatric disorders. Hawton has pointed out that it is difficult to distinguish cause from effect but depression and anxiety will occur as a reaction to sexual dysfunction, and resolution of the latter will lead to symptom relief.

Behavioural studies of human sexuality

Many people are ignorant of the psychophysiology of human sexual responses and have little idea of what is normal in terms of sexual response. It is unusual to see other couples making love unless this is part of a 'public sex show' where responses would be exaggerated. Usually it is not done to study the sexual performance of couples at home in their bedrooms. Masters and Johnson[24] studied the sexual responses of volunteers in a laboratory situation. They published the results of this research in their book, *Human Sexual Response,* and described in detail the four stages of response. This was an approach founded on objective research and facts which took the scientific world by surprise. People already knew about sexual excitement during foreplay and Masters and Johnson described the body responses of what they called 'the excitement phase' which is initiated by whatever an individual finds sexually arousing. This leads to the plateau phase, which is the goal that has to be reached before orgasm can take place. The other two phases they described in the same painstaking details for both males and females were (a) the orgasmic stage, which is an intense few seconds during which the individual climaxes and (b) the resolution phase, which is the period of recovery during which the couple feel relaxed and loving. In the male there is a further period known as the refractory phase which follows the orgasmic phase and is a time during which a further orgasm is impossible. This refractory time varies for individuals from a few minutes to a whole night.

At last people had an idea of what responses were normal during lovemaking and how other people behaved. Men who could not get an erection after an orgasm realised that there was a wide range of refractory times and that they were not impotent if they could not get an immediate erection after orgasm and had to wait twenty-four hours.

Some women did not fare so well when they learned about some of 'the lucky multi-orgasmic' women in Masters and Johnson's sample. Women who could not identify with these multi-orgasmic women who go straight on to further orgasms after appropriate stimulation sought help as they considered themselves abnormal if they were able to obtain only one orgasm. They needed to be counselled about the wide range of women's responses.

Gender roles

One particular way society influences people's sexuality is by the gender roles process. Children receive messages about sex roles from an early age and are encouraged to behave according to their gender.

Society encourages women to be emotional about sex. Women have feelings, whereas men are encouraged to be matter-of-fact. Women are supposed to be more passive and take a long time to become aroused. In our culture men are seen as more sexually orientated and they appear to be capable of responding very quickly, almost mechanically if they get the chance. Attitudes towards masturbation illustrate this gender role playing as men, not women, are expected to know how to masturbate.

Zilbergeld has already discussed these supposed sexual differences in his book, *Men and Sex*, and described the sexual mystique surrounding women's sexuality[25]. He emphasises that there have actually been more courses on female sexuality and feminism than on male sexuality and, in fact, we know a lot more about women than men. In the book he draws attention to the fact that women seem more willing to admit to having sexual problems. Men try to cover up any problems and exaggerate their conquests, making other men feel that any talk about poor erections or ejaculatory problems would be unmasculine and out of place, because 'real' men perform well. As it is not done for a man to admit to these problems a false impression of confidence is created. A man must appear sexually confident; even if he feels apprehensive or nervous inside he must put on a good front.

One survey that Zilbergeld cites is the *Psychology Today* survey[26] in which the men in the survey guessed that only one per cent of their peers were virgins. This was utterly erroneous, as, in fact, the actual percentage of virgins in that sample was 22. This shows that men readily label other men as sexually experienced and successful.

Sexual attitudes

Attitudes are based on information which may be true or false. It is difficult to change emotions associated with sexual attitudes, particularly when incorrect information has been learned.

Studies in sexual attitudes show, however, that children, adolescents and adults can change. One study in Ohio by Hoch[27] showed attitude change in fifty high school students in a biology class. They were provided with accurate information about anatomy and physiology and birth control. Then they participated in discussion groups concentrating on their problems and concerns over topics like female permissiveness and homosexuality. A control group of fifty students did not receive any such sex education. There was a significant difference between the two groups as the students who participated in the teaching programme changed their attitudes towards birth control and abortion, becoming more liberal towards these topics. They also tended to be less hostile towards homosexuals. An interesting side effect of the study was that these students lowered their anxiety about their own sexual behaviour and felt more confident of making 'correct' decisions in the future.

Talking about topics like masturbation or homosexuality helps to desensitise people as they lower their anxiety. Showing films associated with sexual subjects and discussing them afterwards also lowers anxiety and embarrassment, thereby changing sexual attitudes.

The National Sex Forum[28] in California made some sexually explicit and reassuring films to change people's attitudes towards topics related to masturbation, heterosexuality, homosexuality, group sex, sex and the disabled, sex education and therapy. These SAR or 'Sexual Attitude Restructuring' films are tastefully made and can be shown in groups, following which discussion can take place in smaller groups.

The SAR films were originally made to educate sex therapists and educators about sexual attitudes. Chilgren[29] in the USA reported that the majority of physicians, nurses, medical students and clergy who attended the SAR event considered that it should be part of their training. Evidence that sexual attitudes can be changed has now accumulated on both sides of the Atlantic.

Medical students and also students of human sexuality have benefited from the SAR films. Stanley's[30] study at St George's Hospital and the Royal Free Hospital, London, and the Universities of Edinburgh and Sheffield has shown that the viewing of SAR films interspersed with discussion has helped many of the 329 medical students involved to feel comfortable with the idea of discussing sexual problems with their patients. Stanley stressed that the SAR films differed from blue movies as they were based on warm relationships which were free from guilt.

An SAR day was included in a course on attitudes to human sexuality designed to prepare counsellors to work with sex therapy patients. The course at the University of Southampton was evaluated by Perring and Sketchley[31] who declared that knowledge was not enough and sexual attitudes needed to be explored. They measured attitude and knowledge before and after the course by the SKAT (Sexual Knowledge and Attitude Test) which showed significant attitude change.

Of course, the SAR method is unsuitable for 'budget sex education' in places like the Third World. Indeed, when the author ran an evening course for adults on sexual attitudes at the Extra-mural Department of London University, the SAR films were not available and the group relied on 'role play' which proved to be a successful method for attitude change. Similar courses in the USA and Europe have been objectively assessed and found to be useful in association with changing attitudes towards masturbation and homosexuality. Marshall[32] has described the intensive SAR method of showing 53 films and 114 slides in two days.

The SAR method of showing many films in a set period of time is like the method of 'flooding' sometimes used by psychologists to decrease anxiety. People viewing such material get habituated to it. Originally the San Francisco-situated SAR programme consisted of the 'fuckorama' and this was based on flooding methods. The clients sat around the room on deep cushions watching films projected all over the surrounding walls. These films, eight to twelve at a time, portrayed every conceivable unharmful human sexual activity over a period of twelve hours or so. The effect is partly educative and people's sexual attitudes do change. As they watch how other people behave they learn the range of possible sexual behaviours and become desensitised to sexual activity they previously might have found embarrassing. Indeed, they gain new ideas of how their own and others' sex lives may be expanded. Such films are designed to remove prejudices. The fact that the clients see normal-looking people doing with enjoyment things that they have never done, let alone spoken about, gives some of them the feeling that such behaviour is generally permissible, and the possibility of behaving in new ways is in itself exciting.

Later in the SAR process, films are shown, one at a time to help people structure their attitudes systematically. Each controversial topic is covered by a film showing a group talking about the controversial topic. Topics like female masturbation are covered and the film, *Self Loving*, shows a group of women discussing masturbation. Other films focus on women masturbating, like *Susan* in which a plump woman enjoys masturbating in the bath and later tries some vibrators. The SAR programme is well established and was founded in 1964 by the United Methodist Church and researched by the Rev Ted McIllvenna. Its aim is to help clients and to educate therapists about sexual matters so that they can better understand their own attitudes and the sexuality of others.

Pornography

Society has the political power to dictate what people should read or see when it comes to erotica. Pornography is vaguely defined as 'that which depraves and corrupts', which makes it ambivalent but subject to police raids based on an individual's decision about what is depraved. In the book *Censorship and Obscenity*[33] the chapter 'How our rulers argue about censorship' by Christie Davies sums up political influence and the moralists' stand against pornography in the UK. In fact, society drives a lot of pornography underground and this not only increases the price but gives it a sleazy image that is off-putting to many people.

There is a lot of difference between buying pornography in London and Amsterdam. In London one is made to feel awkward and embarrassed, whereas in Amsterdam the 'porn' shop is welcoming and a normal place for both men and women to browse and enjoy the atmosphere.

Hard-core pornography usually depicts an erect penis associated with foreplay or sexual intercourse and is legally available in many cities in Scandinavia and the Netherlands where people have a more relaxed and healthy attitude to pornography. Kutchinsky[34] has related the sex crime rate in Copenhagen to the availability of sexually explicit materials around the time when the obscenity laws were finally repealed in Denmark in 1969. His finding of a substantial decline in the less serious kinds of sexual offences, like voyeurism and exhibitionism, and a marginal decline in the more serious crimes of rape and attempted rape provide facts about the effects of pornography which counteract the emotive arguments put forward by moralists that pornography causes rape. Indeed, Amir[34], in his study of rape in Philadelphia, makes no mention of sexually explicit materials as a contributory factor in the commission of that crime, whereas alcohol features in over 60 per cent of the cases.

There are, however, many countries where hard-core pornography is illegal and it is difficult or impossible for the average citizen to buy it. The authorities in these countries state that harm will result from the dissemination of hard-core pornography and that they have the right and duty to prevent it. In the USA and the UK individuals like Mrs Mary Whitehouse have formed pressure groups based on religious principles to censor TV or radio programmes which have only a mildly explicit sexual content.

Pornography can be used to expand a person's sexual repertoire and to increase sexual interest. Yaffé[36] in his chapter on 'Therapeutic uses of sexually explicit material' has listed at least ten studies in which people with sexual problems were helped by exposure to sexually explicit material. Many people have difficulties with their sexual interest, especially if one partner is interested in sex and the other partner is not. Sometimes pornography can be used to stimulate sexual interest and reduce this sexual discrepancy between partners. Gillan[37] in her chapter on 'Therapeutic uses of obscenity' points out the therapeutic use of pornography with such clients.

Recently a survey on 'Marriage and Relationships' was carried out by *The Sunday Mirror* and reported on *TV–AM*. When asked about the use of sexy books and movies to produce more sexual excitement over half the sample of 2023 reported the use of this type of material.

Contrary to earlier beliefs, both sexes use pornography. Kinsey's finding that women are more aroused by romantic than erotic stories is no longer applicable. Heiman[38] showed that women respond more to erotic than romantic stories, especially to stories in which they take the sexual initiative themselves. In the USA, Germany and the UK, experimental findings show that women do respond to erotic visual and auditory stimuli. Indeed, on the whole, women respond more to auditory stimuli which are focussed on stories, according to Jacobovits[39], the Danish researcher, because women have more vivid imaginations. Gillan and Frith[40] in their study of British university students found that both male and female students responded to visual erotica.

Schmidt and Sigusch[41] consider that women have been sexually repressed by society. However, since the Second World War the structure of society has changed and women have had not only more opportunity to work but also to control their leisure, buying and browsing through sex magazines if they wish to do so. They have had more opportunity to see erotica since the Kinsey Report and, according to this West German research, women respond to erotica. Bancroft has pointed out that women do respond to and identify with pictures of other women in magazines and see themselves as part of such a fantasy and get aroused. Recently attempts have been made to produce erotic videos for women, in spite of the feminists' protests. It must be pointed out, however, that sex magazines for women like *Playgirl* are not a huge marketing success among women (although they have proved popular amongst gay men). *Forum*, however, has a large female readership.

Sex and the media

Probably the media exercise the most powerful influences on the population. Some people watch television most of the day and night and obviously are affected by what they see, even if it is at a subliminal level. Programmes on sex matters related to sex therapy or sex education are few and far between. The media allocates more space to sexual fantasies than to fact. Radio or television plays about sex can influence people's attitudes a good deal.

Newspaper editors know that stories related to rape and sexual assault sell well, but much more harm can be done by sexually smearing members of society than anonymous porn. Sex scandals about well known people can indeed be titillating but they hurt the people concerned.

People often get their ideas of what constitutes average sexual behaviour from the newspapers, which can be a most unreliable source of information. Also, literature provides people with romances about perfect love and sex; few novelists except Kingsley Amis will write a book (*Jake's Thing*) about a man with low sexual interest. Most novelists' heroes and heroines are receptive and highly sexed. They usually climax together and this increases the readers' expectations for perfect sex.

How do people from other cultures fare when it comes to the media? Some must suffer from culture shock; Indian films, for instance, do not allow shots of kissing and foreplay in their films. Immigrants arriving in the UK or the USA must think these countries are obsessed with sex.

Sometimes the media exaggerates sex research findings, again setting impossible expectations for people; women frantically search for their non-existent 'G-spot'[42] or strive to achieve a second orgasm. At least the pressure is now off women to have what Freud referred to as 'vaginal orgasms', claiming they were immature if they had masturbated and could only achieve a clitoral orgasm.

The way the subject of AIDS has been handled is a good example of British press hysteria. If facts had been presented objectively to the British public and a Dr Ruth Westheimer had revealed the problems associated with AIDS as she did on American television screens, we could have been more objective here. Safe lovemaking techniques and mutual masturbation could have been recommended.

Sex education

Many fallacies and misconceptions persist because of sexual ignorance, yet these could be avoided by a good sex education in schools. Such a sex education could be a prophylactic against sexual problems and dysfunction. But more seems to have been written about abnormal sex and deviations than about normal sexual development. Before Masters and Johnson we knew more about foot fetishists than about the clitoris and normal female sexuality.

Most books on sex education agree that the best way for a child to learn about sex is for the parents to answer his questions as they arise from an early age. Consequently the parents are still seen as 'the best people' for sex education. Watson[43] points out that parents tend not to give education and remarks that in 1974 the Scottish Education Department revealed that 'only a small minority of homes deal with the subject adequately'.

Although sex education has been legislated in various Scandinavian countries this does not apply to the USA or to the UK where the sex education policy is left to the head of the school. It seems incredible that one person should decide on whether sex education is provided. Government officials deny taking responsibility and suggest that it is up to the family to provide such education. Studies by investigators like Farrell[44] who wrote *My Mother Said* show that only 12 per cent of her sample of young people received their first information about sexual intercourse from parents, while 31 per cent received it from teachers and 45 per cent from friends. She discusses the possibility that the taboo on incest implies the inhibition of feelings about sexuality between members of the family and extends to a taboo on talking about it.

Schofield[45] in his book, *The Sexual Behaviour of Young People*, stated that 'Sex education is a basic need, a human right, not a privilege or an optional extra'. Yet it is still a subject which has been avoided as much as possible in the school curriculum and most children still learn about sex from misleading sources. '62 per cent of boys and 44 per cent of girls still learn about conception from friends, usually through smutty and obscene jokes.'

In 1980, British ROSE (Research on Sex Education) was founded and research and several workshops have been organised by the society. A Conference in 1985 on 'Sex Education – Who's Responsible?'[46] provoked much discussion and the conclusion that there was a great need for good sex education and teaching. The introduction was provided by the agony aunt, Deidre Sanders, who organised the *Woman* magazine survey about sexuality. She found that fewer than one in ten parents believed that sex education should be left entirely up to them. The vast majority believed the task should be shared between parents and the school. She mentioned that few parents supported Valerie Riches of Family and Youth Concern over stopping sex education.

One of the ROSE Conference speakers was Carol Lee, the author of *The Ostrich Position*. She pointed out that she tries to find out what the children want to know about and takes it from there, rather than going into the classroom with a set pattern already fixed.

In the UK, objective books such as *Make it Happy* by Jane Cousins[47] are attacked as perverting young people, and made more difficult to obtain. Even Dr Miriam Stoppard's very calm and reasonable book *Talking Sex*[48] was attacked in print and lumped in with hardcore pornographic videos as a threat to any children who might get hold of it. It appears that the description of masturbation is too emotive for some politicians, although children themselves want to know about this subject.

Television seems to be the natural medium for sex education to be communicated, but any discussions on sex education for adolescents are provided late in the evening. Radio is a good source of information and some of the commercial radio stations have phone-in programmes which provide an excellent advice service for the general public. The BBC did provide some excellent sex education radiovision programmes[49] for a target audience of 8-to-10-year-olds called *Merry-go-Round* and *Nature* which were shown in primary schools and proved successful. Most teachers felt that the effect of the programme was positive and helpful.

Sex education for children in primary schools is not usually encouraged, although the figures for child sexual abuse for children in this age group are increasing in the UK compared with such figures in Scandinavia where sex education is compulsory. This would suggest that sex education should be available for every child, not just for a chosen few. Even a very young child has a right to know about sex and details of child molesters should be included.

Adolescents are also in need of sex education although moralists insist that information about contraception will lead to promiscuity. Schofield did state that, in contrast to popular opinion, teenagers usually experienced sex for the first time in a well established relationship. Adolescents should know how to obtain contraceptive devices and advice, with or without the support of their parents, in the area in which they live. An unwanted pregnancy, especially where much blame and recrimination is deployed, can be a traumatic experience all round, and can have a serious effect on later sexual attitudes and experience.

Providing the right methods to back up information about contraception is quite a challenge. Many children do not like reading books as they associate them with school. A community group developed a comic strip pamphlet called *Don't Rush Me*[50] which proved useful when assessed by a research team. The multi-cultural community wanted a comic strip so that their members could identify with and read it in order to understand contraception.

One of the main problems in communicating about contraception has been informing young males effectively that they need to take some responsibility as well as the females. Many young men do not want to bother with a sheath, although it reduces their chance of catching sexually transmitted diseases. The Family Planning Association have made a convincing video called *Danny's Big Night* which does emphasise male responsibility. It is set in a multi-racial inner-city area and is about the relationship between 17-year-old Danny and his girl friend Lorraine. It is particularly suitable for boys aged 16 years or over. The FPA does not recommend it for general use in schools and suggests that a youth club setting is appropriate. Notes for youth workers are included.

Youth clubs appear to be a natural setting for sex education programmes. The advantage is that the setting is more natural and less academic than a school, but the disadvantage is that children who go to youth clubs are sociable and extraverted and fairly well adjusted, whereas those who have developmental problems and need some support and information about sex tend to stay at home.

Young people are not the only group in need of sex education. Many students and adults could benefit from evening classes in sex education. British medical students, compared with American medical students, are sometimes given very brief training in sex education and therapy, although the SAR programmes already referred to are excellent.

As already mentioned in this chapter, the most comprehensive sex education programme comes from San Francisco and is the SAR (Sexual Attitude Restructuring). The bulk of the material comes in the form of films, slides and tapes. The SAR sex education course is programmed to cover 12–14 hours and includes information about reproductive biology, masturbation, heterosexuality, homosexuality, male and female sexuality, special problems related to medical, religious and cultural matters and sex therapy. The material is designed to desensitise students to taboo areas and then to resensitise them with suggestions for improving and enriching their own sex life and that of those whom they help and counsel. Students are encouraged to express feelings and emotions. A full account by Linken *et al.*[51] of this human sexuality programme is available.

It is encouraging that more people are pressing for information about sex. Those who fear moral decline in the young if they are given advice on sex and contraception should remember that: 'People have died, committed suicide, because of a lack of knowledge about sex: nobody has died from knowing too much about it'. (*The Guardian*, 23 February, 1978.)

Sex education needs to include information and advice about sexually transmitted disease, and workers like Yarber[52] have devised excellent programmes to provide such information in the United States. Nowadays information is needed by the general public on such topics.

Some years ago there was widespread publicity about herpes. People suffering from herpes were labelled the new lepers of society. They felt that sex was finished for them, but more positive thinkers amongst them formed a group for herpes victims who could met socially, discuss their problems and form relationships amongst themselves.

With the advent of AIDS, however, publicity about herpes has faded into the background.

AIDS

The 'AIDS plague' has produced more discussion and anxiety than any other sexually transmitted disease, as it can lead to death and there is no cure. AIDS stands for Acquired Immune Deficiency Syndrome which means that the body cannot defend itself against certain illnesses; indeed, many AIDS patients have one or both of the two rare diseases, Kaposi's sarcoma and *pneumocystis carininii* pneumonia.

So far, statistics have shown that three-quarters of all AIDS patients are homosexual and moralists are jumping to conclusions that all gay men are bound to have AIDS. Other victims are patients who have received blood transfusions from infected donors, haemophiliacs, drug addicts and people from Haiti and Central Africa.

Facts about AIDS can be obtained from the Health Education Council[53] and a book by Weber and Ferriman[54] which includes case histories of AIDS patients. Obviously, sex education and publicity should include the connection between anal sex and AIDS. Pamphlets should include information about mutual masturbation being a good and safe sexual alternative. Advice about using condoms to increase safety is already in advertisements.

West Germany is already running a street billboard advertising campaign with the message: 'When everybody protects themselves, AIDS has no chance'. Explicit health education lies at the heart of the matter and a hard-hitting TV campaign should be launched, like Dr Ruth Westheimer's frank American TV campaign, explaining the risks of the disease and how to avoid them.

Many gay men, of course, do not indulge in sexual intercourse. According to Masters and Johnson[55], about half the homosexuals they interviewed practised mutual masturbation only. Promiscuity is associated with gay men but many have realised the danger and changed their life styles.

Perhaps the advent of AIDS will bring about monogamy. Meanwhile, there is widespread hysteria about AIDS which was reinforced by the Thames Television crew who went to film staff of the Terrence Higgins Trust in London but refused to enter the premises and insisted on interviewing the clinic staff in the street.

Sex therapists

Sex therapists usually come from the caring professions. The best qualified to undertake the treatment of sexual problems are usually psychologists specialising in behaviour therapy, or medical workers, often psychiatrists, who have an interest in the treatment of marital and sexual problems. These therapists have usually received training in handling psychotherapeutic interactions and will have discovered during this time whether they have the patience and adjustment to continue with it.

Once equipped with the general theoretical knowledge, the ideal therapist will have undertaken the treatment of patients under the supervision of a more experienced therapist, becoming part of a sex therapy team. Hopefully, recruits for such a training programme will include nurses, social workers and marriage guidance counsellors.

Before anyone undertakes sex therapy they should ask themselves whether they have the personal qualities required. Clearly they must have first-hand experience of personal relationships with a successful sexual adjustment, otherwise the advice they give will be solely theoretical. They should be sexually experienced and enjoy their senses. It does not matter if a therapist has had sexual problems; in fact this can provide empathy. It is best to be able to relate to all types of people, to have no serious personality problems and be able to deal equally with anxiety and hostility without feeling drained and becoming too involved.

Therapist training

Sex therapy training is best done in an established sex clinic. Trainees can join experienced sex therapists working alone or as co-therapists and attend the treatment of a few individuals or couples as an observer.

The research carried out on whether it is better to have co-therapists working together or an individual therapist working alone with a couple shows that both methods are equally effective. It is helpful, however, for a trainee therapist to work with an experienced therapist.

Besides treating patients, many clinics have discussion groups and other teaching activities for the therapists in training. Many training centres prefer trainee therapists to be attached to the centre for a couple of years and gain experience of different types of disorders. During this time, trainee therapists will experience a wide variety of problems and will learn to judge the treatment possibilities inherent in any given case.

Video tapes can also be useful for training purposes and role playing should be a part of a therapist's training to help develop confidence with clients. Trainee therapists can act the parts of therapist and client and reverse roles.

Nowadays there are formal training programmes that result in diplomas of Human Sexuality both in the States and Europe. Usually, student therapists are attached to teaching hospitals and they see clients under the supervision of teaching therapists. These courses include formal lectures, informal seminars and experiential workshops. Sometimes workshops are arranged for trainee therapists and their spouses, aiming to facilitate personal growth and marital enrichment.

It is a pity that more GPs do not have more formal training in sex therapy as family doctors usually know their patients' backgrounds and are usually the first to be approached about a sex problem. Basic sex therapy training should be a part of a medical student's training and attempts are being made to provide opportunities for this type of training in Europe. American sex therapy training programmes have been in existence for longer and there are more courses, but Europeans tend to be more rigorous in measuring the success of their courses, as well as measuring therapeutic success.

References

1. Comfort, Alex. (1972) *The Joy of Sex*. Simon & Schuster.
2. Reage, Pauline. *The Story of O*.
3. Kinsey, A.C. *et al.* (1948) *Sexual Behaviour in the Human Male*. Saunders.
4. Gebhard, P.H. and Johnson, A.B. (1979) *The Kinsey Data*. Saunders.
5. Kinsey, A.C. *et al.* (1953) *Sexual Behaviour in the Human Female*. Saunders.
6. Hite, Shere. (1976) *The Hite Report*. Talmy Franklin, London.
7. Nag, M. (1972) 'Sex, culture and human fertility – India and the United States'. *Current Anthropology*. 13. 231–238.
8. Lieh-Mak, F. and Ng, M.L. (1981) 'Ejaculatory incompetence in Chinese men'. *Am. J. Psychiatry*. 138.5. May.
9. Chester, R. and Walker, C. (1979) 'Sexual experience and attitudes of British women'. In Chester, R. & Peel, J. (eds.) *Changing Patterns of Sexual Behaviour*. Academic Press.
10. Frank, Ellen, Anderson, Carol, Rubinstein, Debra. (1973) 'Frequency of sexual dysfunction in 'normal' couples'. *N. Engl. J. Med.* 299. 111–115.
11. Nettelbladt, P. and Uddenberg, N. (1970) 'Sexual dysfunction and sexual satisfaction in 58 married Swedish men'. *Journal of Psychosomatic Research*. 23, 141–7.
12. Garde, K. and Lunde, I. (1980) 'Female sexual behaviour: a study in a random sample of 40-year-old women'. *Maturitas*. 2. 225–40.
13. Golombok, Susan, Rust, John and Pickard, C. (1984) 'Sexual problems encountered in general practice'. *Brit.Jrnl.Sexual Medicine*. Dec.
14. Burnap, D.W. and Golden, J.S. (1967) 'Sexual problems in medical practice'. *Jrnl. of Medical Education*. 42. 673–80.

15. Begg, A. Dickerson, M. and London, N.B. (1976) 'Frequency of self-reported sexual problems in a family planning clinic'. *Jrnl. of Family Planning Doctors.* 2. 41–8.
16. Bancroft, John and Coles, I. (1976) 'Three years' experience in a sexual problem clinic'. *Brit.Medical Journal.*i, 1575–77.
17. Masters, W.H. and Johnson,V.E.(1970) *Human Sexual Inadequacy.* Churchill.
18. Crowe, M.J., Gillan, P. and Golombok, S. (1980) 'Form and content in the conjoint treatment of sexual dysfunction: A controlled study'. *Behav.Res. & Therap.* Vol.19. 47–54.
19. Thornes, B. and Collard, J. (1979) *Who Divorces?* Routledge & Kegan Paul.
20. Hawton, Keith. (1985) *Sex Therapy: A Practical Guide.* Oxford University Press.
21. Stuart, R.B. (1980) *Helping Couples Change.* Guildford, New York.
22. Gillan, P., Golombok, S. and Becker, P. (1980) 'NHS sex therapy groups for women'. *Brit. Jrnl. Sexual Medicine.* Sept.
23. Derogatis, L.R., Meyer, J.K., and King, K.M. (1981) 'Psychopathology in individuals with sexual dysfunction'. *American Jrnl. Psychiatry.* 138. 759–63.
24. Masters, W.H. and Johnson, V.E. (1966) *Human Sexual Response.* Churchill.
25. Zilbergeld, Bernie. (1980) *Men and Sex.* Souvenier Press.
26. 'Your pursuit of happiness'. *Psychology Today.* August 1976.
27. Hoch, Loren I. (1971) 'Attitude change as a result of sex education'. *Journal of Research in Science Teaching.* Vol.8. No.4. 363–367.
28. Ayres, T. *et al.* (1977) *SAR Guide for a Better Sex Life.* National Sex Forum, San Francisco.
29. Chilgren, Richard and Briggs, Mary. (1973) 'On being explicit: sex education for professionals'. SIECUS Report. i.(5).
30. Stanley, Elizabeth. (1978) 'An introduction to sexuality in the medical curriculum'. *Medical Education.* 12. 441–445.
31. Perring, Michael and Sketchley, John M. (1982) 'Attitudes to human sexuality. The evaluation of an interdisciplinary course at the University of Southampton'. *British Journal of Sexual Medicine.* March.
32. Marshall, Pierre. (1978) 'The use of audiovisual media in sex education for the caring professions: Experience in Europe'. *Proc. III Int.Congr.Med.Sexology.* Rome, Oct.
33. Eds. Dhavan, Rajeev and Davies, C. (1978) *Censorship and Obscenity.* Martin Robertson.
34. Kutchinsky, Berl. (1973) 'The effect of easy availability of pornography on the incidence of sex crimes: the Danish experience'.

In Wilson, W. Cody, and Goldenstein, Michael J. (Eds).: 'Pornography attitudes, use and effect'. *Journal of Social Issues*. 29,(3), 163–81.
35. Amir, M. *Patterns of Forcible Rape*. (1971) Chicago University Press.
36. Yaffé, Maurice. (1982) 'Therapeutic uses of sexually explicit material'. In *The Influence of Pornography on Behaviour*, eds. Yaffé, M. and Nelson, E.C. Academic Press.
37. Gillan, Patricia. 'Therapeutic uses of obscenity'. See above no. 33.
38. Heiman, Julia. (1975) 'Lady's relish'. *Psychology Today*. Vol.1.No.4. June.
39. Jacobovits, L.A. (1965) 'An evaluation of reactions to erotic literature'. *Psychological Reports*. 16, 985–994.
40. Gillan, Patricia and Frith, Christopher. (1979) 'Male-female differences in response to erotica'. In *Love and Attraction*, eds. Cook, Mark and Wilson, Glenn. Pergamon Press.
41. Schmidt, G. and Sigusch, V. (1970) 'Sex differences in response to psychosexual stimulation by films and slides'. *Jrnl. of Sex Research*. 6, 268–283.
42. Ladas, A.K., Whipple, B., and Perry, J.D. (1982) *The G Spot and Other Recent Discoveries about Human Sexuality*. Holt, Rinehart & Winston.
43. Watson, Geoffrey M. (1980) *Sex Education as a Component of Health Education*. The Commonwealth Institute.Dec.
44. Farrell, Christine. (1978) *My Mother Said* ... Routledge & Kegan Paul.
45. Schofield, Michael. (1973) *The Sexual Behaviour of Young Adults*. Allen Lane.
46. 'Sex Education – Who's Responsible?' British ROSE Newsletter. (1985)
47. Cousins, Jane. (1980) *Make It Happy*. Fontana.
48. Stoppard, Miriam. (1982) *Talking Sex*. Piccolo.
49. Lambert, T.J. (1974) 'The contribution of BBC school broadcasts to sex education in primary schools'. In *Sex Education in Schools*. Ed. Nazere, Isam.R. IPPF Publications.
50. *Don't Rush me*. Wandsworth Council for Community Relations.
51. Linken, Arnold, Marshall, Pierre and Thorpe, Darrell. (1980) 'Sensual attitudes factor'. *Nursing Focus*. May.
52. Yarber, William. (1978) 'New directions in venereal disease education'. *The Family Coordinator*. April.
53. *Some Facts about AIDS*. Health Education Council.
54. Weber, Jonathan, and Ferriman, Annabel. (1986) *AIDS Concerns You*. Pagoda Books.
55. Masters, W.H. and Johnson, V.E. (1979) *Homosexuality in Perspective*. Little Brown. Boston.

Chapter 2

Sexual Therapy

Background

In the early history of sex therapy women were given individual therapy in Family Planning Clinics if they were suffering from infertility or painful sexual intercourse. Therapy would have consisted mainly of education and reassurance. Perhaps the use of dilators would have been prescribed if the diagnosis was that of vaginismus. In those days no provision would have been made for helping women with orgasmic difficulties. A woman who did not enjoy sex would have been told to 'lie back and think of England!'. Sex was associated with breeding and although pain was not acceptable, pleasure was not encouraged. Sex tended to be regarded then as a means to an end and was not valued for its own sake.

In those days men would have fared even worse and would only have received advice for problems related to infertility. Premature ejaculation would probably have been regarded as quite normal, provided it did not affect the chance of a woman becoming pregnant. Men, however, were allowed to enjoy sex and the great lovers of olden times were usually male.

Scattered around the place in the late fifties and sixties were psychology and psychiatry departments in some universities or hospitals where therapy was provided and researched. Traditional psychotherapy and psychoanalysis had played a small part in sex therapy, but experts at centres of learning were questioning the validity of such methods. Behaviour therapy had arrived to stay when Wolpe's classic *Psychotherapy by Reciprocal Inhibition*[1] was published. Practitioners were singing the praises of desensitisation and learning theory, saying that treating the symptoms rather than the cause made sense. In any case, Freud's theories were hard to prove and unscientific, whereas the methods of the behaviourists were practical and experimentally proven[2].

In the USA in 1948, Kinsey had led the way in revealing the common man's sexual attitudes and behaviour. Previous accounts of sexual behaviour were in the Kraft-Ebbing[3] or Havelock Ellis[4] medical mould with an emphasis on abnormalities.

In the sixties Masters and Johnson provided an almost revolutionary study of sexual behaviour set in laboratories. Their behaviour therapy was based on their scientific discoveries and the desensitisation model.

The desensitisation approach

Wolpe paved the way for this approach. He suggested that fear and anxiety could be eliminated by relaxing people and gradually exposing them to the things they were afraid of. Wolpe placed a ban on sexual intercourse initially. He suggested that people who had sexual fears should be asked to indulge in foreplay or touch one another until they started to feel insecure or anxious. They should stop their behaviour and relax at this stage, then continue with some slightly easier activity like massage until they felt confident enough to return to the original task. The patient would be requested to repeat these instructions until anxiety was reduced.

Masters and Johnson used similar techniques to Wolpe. Like Wolpe they put a ban on sexual intercourse so as to reassure and relax patients. Masters and Johnson actually based their therapy on desensitisation techniques as patients were asked to massage one another non-sexually. They dressed this task up in the formal language of 'sensate focussing'. When a couple became confident enough to proceed to mutual masturbation, foreplay or what Masters and Johnson called 'genital sensate focussing' they were ready for mutual pleasuring of the genitals, taking it in turns and stopping if they felt anxious.

When Masters and Johnson's book, *Human Sexual Inadequacy*(5) was published in 1970 their therapy techniques were universally discussed and rapidly taken up by sex clinics which mushroomed everywhere. Their principle of the ban on sexual intercourse was debated as though this was a new idea, but historically it goes back to 1786 when John Hunter,[6] instructed his patients who had erectile problems not to make love or 'connect with' a woman for six nights.

There are also similarities between Wolpe's and Masters and Johnson's techniques; one such similarity being the positive aspect of therapy. Patients were being asked to do something relatively easy in which they would succeed. This meant that these types of therapies provided some positive reinforcement for a couple who had previously been very negative about touch or cuddling, perhaps having a long history of avoiding these activities. Individuals were learning new forms of sexual behaviour associated with pleasure. Masters and Johnson were more eclectic than Wolpe as they were interested also in the relationship between the couple. Something new had been discovered for couples which combined learning theory, physiological findings and human relationships.

The disadvantage of therapy for couples is that it is for the chosen few. Therapists counteracted this by treating single clients without partners along behavioural lines. This is very relevant as often a person cannot find a partner because of the actual sexual problem he or she is suffering from. A single man with an erectile problem is often very anxious even about kissing, so a behavioural programme helps to build confidence. It seems a long time since the days of penile splints for such a man with an erectile problem, or methods like testicular diathermy of the thirties.

The state of the art

The question most people ask is 'what methods are used nowadays by sex therapists?'.

Behavioural psychotherapy

Various research studies have been carried out to examine the effective components of what is now called behavioural psychotherapy. Once it was thought that relaxation had to be given in combination with a rigid hierarchy of factors causing anxiety. Researchers showed that desensitisation was a powerful enough component on its own. There was a vogue for 'flooding studies' in which exposure was provided immediately therapy commenced. The patient was exposed to high anxiety and had to remain in the situation until the undesirable response was tolerated or exhausted. Fatigue obviously plays a large part in this theory of extinction or habituation. Most behavioural psychotherapists would agree that some exposure *in vivo* is useful after imagining an anxiety-provoking stimulus.

Therapists eventually realised that tailoring therapy for specific patients was more effective than adhering to a strict therapy formula. Behaviourists were gradually becoming more flexible in their approach to sex therapy. Masters and Johnson were criticised for their rigidity and therapists modified their techniques according to the patient's requirements. Nowadays there are few European clinics which stick rigidly to Masters and Johnson's methods. In any case it is not economically or practically possible for therapists to see patients daily for a fortnight.

Family planning clinics nowadays provide medical help combined with some behavioural techniques for women who are anorgasmic. Most therapists at the FPA are supportive and do give some individual counselling.

Nowadays even the Marriage Guidance Council has become more broad-minded in its therapeutic approach, and counsellors are willing to treat individuals. In the UK, Masters and Johnson therapy has been examined and researched by various clinics in London and Oxford.

Communication

Most clinics offer a modified Masters and Johnson sex therapy approach combined with relationships therapy. Communication is a much emphasised skill in therapy. Couples seeking therapy have often failed to communicate effectively and tell one another what they really want. Maybe an individual client has no relationship because of his or her poor communication, and cannot find a partner. Communication has been the foundation for many self-help groups which teach personal effectiveness to individuals who have previously failed to assert themselves.

Group therapy

Group therapy has become popular in several clinics. It has some advantages like being cost-effective, but often it is difficult to set up and not easy to persuade clients that this is the sort of therapy they need. One big advantage is that members of the group can positively reward one another and create a motivation for homework to be carried out. Group therapy is more popular in the USA where women's sex therapy groups were led by Barbach[7] on the West Coast and Dodson[8] on the East Coast.

Gay clients

The greatest change in the way the medical profession regards therapy has come in their attitude towards therapy for gay clients. In 1967 the American Psychiatric Association ceased to include homosexuality on its list of pathological diagnoses. This was a step forward in the USA. In the UK the Wolfenden Committee recommended a change in English law to make homosexuality legal and in 1967 the law was changed so that men over the age of 21 could choose their life style.

In the UK and many of the USA states the age of consent for homosexuals is 21 compared with 16 for heterosexual acts. In the UK there has been no legislation for lesbianism, as the Victorians did not consider that women could behave in this manner.

Nowadays the attitude towards therapy for homosexuals has changed and the days of aversion therapy are more or less a thing of the past. In the sixties, nausea caused by various drugs and electric shocks were part of this aversion therapy. Nowadays, when a client wants to change his or her orientation, other methods like 'orgasmic reconditioning' are used. Perhaps the gay client needs help in accepting his or her sexual orientation and desensitisation is the best therapy. Since the arrival of AIDS many gay men have been increasingly worried about their behaviour patterns and have sought therapy. Most homosexual men now restrict the number of partners they make love with. Mutual masturbation appears to be the chosen lovemaking pattern, rather than anal intercourse where the risk of contracting AIDS is greatly increased.

Making a choice

Orgasmic reconditioning has been referred to in the context of sexual orientation. In the early days of aversion therapy a homosexual had no choice over his orientation. He received electric shocks in association with his favourite male pin-up or fantasy and later associated his previous sexual pleasure with pain. Sometimes such a client ceased to respond to both men and women and was placed in a kind of 'no-man's land' or state of limbo where he ceased to respond sexually. Orgasmic reconditioning methods are more flexible as at the end of therapy the homosexual can make a decision himself and remain totally homosexual or try bisexuality. He has a *choice.*

The trend today is to give clients a choice. There has been much criticism of sex therapists who insist on women taking more interest in sex or becoming orgasmic. Some behaviourists have been criticised for aversion therapy which provided no choice for a client, but this is now a thing of the past. Perhaps too many people have seen films like *A Clockwork Orange* in which the general public was introduced to an exaggerated form of behaviourism.

Celibacy is also a form of choice that sex therapists should give a client. Celia Hadden[9] has drawn attention to the fact that some therapists raise clients' expectations and almost bulldoze them into sex therapy, but this approach is somewhat naive as most therapists nowadays would give clients a choice of celibacy when appropriate.

One of the big advances made in sex therapy is in stressing the alternatives available in lovemaking. Some clients might enjoy mutual masturbation more than sexual intercourse and it would be foolish to dragoon such people into intercourse. In any case, gay male clients are practising alternative methods of sexual pleasuring and finding mutual masturbation perfectly satisfactory. The problem occurs when one partner wants a type of sexual activity that is unacceptable to the other. Therapy can centre on compromises or a 'give to get' situation in which chosen behaviours can be recommended for mutual satisfaction. Maybe a woman who dislikes giving her partner fellatio would consider doing it if her partner spent more time giving her manual stimulation of the clitoris.

Once sexual intercourse was held up as the only satisfactory way of making love and people were desperate to achieve this, but attitudes are changing rapidly. Nowadays clients are also more willing to consider masturbation as a pleasure in itself.

Some people imagine therapists forcing clients to form relationships and promoting marriage. Many therapists give clients a choice of being single or forming a relationship and the relationship does not have to include marriage. Therapists give partners advice on how to cope with a separation or divorce when appropriate.

Traditional sexual relationships between two partners are probably the choice of most people but others may seek sexual variations like tribadism or going to orgies. The therapist should not enforce his or her moral code on a client. If a therapist does not like treating a client or a type of disorder and feels uncomfortable, that therapist should always have the choice of referring that particular client elsewhere for therapy.

Expectations

Many clients have strange expectations of what sex therapy involves. Some people imagine they have to make love in front of the therapist. Some clients think their therapist might provide a surrogate service. It is always advisable for a therapist to discuss the expectations of clients.

Sometimes issues like multi-orgasms or the G-spot can raise expectations. Such women need to be reassured that responses vary a great deal and not all women can expect 'super sex'. In many ways the media can be blamed for exaggerated claims of sexual achievement. The media have also exaggerated the need for couples to enjoy simultaneous orgasms. Perfect sex is promoted on the screen, where couples rarely have problems. It takes a Woody Allen to humanise a character with a sex problem.

Many clients expect to reach a state of what is regarded as sexually normal. They consider that there is something wrong with behaviour that is not average practice. They want to know how many times a week other couples make love, or how long other people take to reach an orgasm. Sex education and information help to clarify such expectations.

Clients from other cultures need special questioning and support over their expectations. Although the therapist might consider some of their mores to be backward their customs should be respected. Sometimes sex education can rapidly change their outlook. They often tend to be passive about therapy and expect the therapist to make decisions for them in a sort of authoritative manner. Frequently such clients expect some kind of physical treatment for a sexual disorder and find it hard to accept that psychological therapy is the best form of treatment.

Eleven sexual myths

Most expectations clients have about their sexual performance are based on sexual myths. These myths may be put about by newspapers and magazines or even by exaggerated claims of sexual athletes. The trouble with the media is that only extraordinary or abnormal events are reported. Newspaper reports concentrate on sensational sexual events. If one reads certain Sunday newspapers a general pattern of rape and perverted sexual behaviour emerges.

Myth 1: masturbation should be discouraged

This is based on Victorian attitudes in which articles were published stating that masturbation makes habitués blind or insane. Historically, masturbation has been associated with sin. Many people feel afraid and guilty about discussing this topic.

Masturbation is a recognised part of sex therapy and is recommended for clients to practise in order to achieve and recognise sexual arousal. Getting in touch with the genitals can be a good way to learn about pleasuring. Masturbation gives people confidence when alone and helps them to transfer their pleasure to a partner situation later.

Myth 2: sex is tiring

This message stems from sports events before which sexual abstinence is recommended by trainers who believe that their charges will deteriorate if they spend their energy in sexual activity. It would be equally valid to argue that a state of sexual frustration and tension will impair their finer skills and judgement.

Masters and Johnson consider that sexual intercourse takes up as much energy as running fifty yards and that in a healthy person this energy is available many times per day. Where the sexual act has been satisfactory the ensuing feelings should be of relaxation and calm.

Where the sexual act is prolonged or associated with difficulty or anxiety there is a much greater expenditure of energy. If one partner found the act unloving or unsatisfactory this could lead to some depression. Those people who are unfit or run down should let their partner do most of the work and adjust the position accordingly.

Men who come from the East often mention that an ejaculation drains the body of energy. This is a myth which many of them find hard to discard. Some Indian transcendental meditation methods teach men to delay their ejaculation and to last for many hours, but one wonders if their partners enjoy such feats.

Myth 3: oral sex is dirty

If different sexual activities are considered, oral sex is probably the most laden with taboos.

Many people disapprove of oral-genital contact on obscure moral grounds and the practice is illegal still in some American states. Kinsey[10] found that cunnilingus was accepted by 54 per cent of married women who had coital experience compared with 49 per cent for fellatio. It is surprising that so many women are over-fastidious about genital odours and worry about personal genital cleanliness. This could stem from menstruation myths or be due to the fact that the clitoris is more difficult to find and wash thoroughly than the penis. Research on pheromones shows that these odours enhance sexual arousal. If people are still unconvinced that some odours can enhance sex then scented creams could be recommended for smearing on the genitals[11].

Some women find fellatio dirty and disgusting and worry that the penis might make them gag. Linda Lovelace's film *Deep Throat* did not help to dispel this myth and some women were horrified by the 'sword-swallowing activities' they saw on the screen. Some women dislike the taste of semen and worry about swallowing it. A man does not have to ejaculate into his partner's mouth and a tissue can be used.

Oral sex may be a way of transmitting AIDS, although more research needs to be carried out. Oral sex should therefore be recommended as an activity for partners who are in a long-term relationship and know each other well and are not making love with other partners. Oral sex should be treated like sexual intercourse in this context.

Myth 4: sexual intercourse is the goal for good sex

Sexual intercourse is often not the most pleasurable activity for a couple, but may couples are too embarrassed to admit this. Other sexual activities like massage and mutual masturbation can be pleasurable. Oral sex is an exciting alternative to intercourse. When such alternatives are recommended during therapy partners become less anxious as they do not have the same performance pressure. In the past (and, indeed, nowadays) high expectations were often placed on sexual intercourse as something to wait for until marriage. Petting was acceptable and exciting but coitus was forbidden. This led, perhaps, to inexperienced partners having intercourse for the first time on their wedding night, usually exhausted after the wedding day. Many disastrous first sexual encounters have led to sex problems later.

This sacrosanct approach to sexual intercourse has often made couples anxious when they first attempt intromission. They are conditioned to think that sexual intercourse will be the ultimate experience. Often intercourse is a let-down as most women need more foreplay and genital stimulation than men (and men are often anxious that too much foreplay will lead to premature ejaculation). If a woman has enjoyed petting and clitoral stimulation during foreplay it is difficult to transfer to intercourse and obtain the same degree of arousal.

Couples from other cultures, especially Muslims and Hindus, are even more anxious about intercourse as most of them will have had no physical contact with one another before the marriage ceremony. They will have been led to believe that intercourse will be a beautiful experience but the pain and inexperience lead to much disappointment.

The tradition of intercourse as a goal goes back to primitive man. When man first understood that intercourse produced babies his enthusiasm must have been redoubled. Intercourse became a goal-directed activity; the more coitus the more workers to help the family economically, and this remains the case for many couples in the Third World.

Myth 5: women should be orgasmic by penile thrusting and so achieve a no-hands orgasm

Most women are conditioned into believing that they must have orgasms by penile thrusting. Some women say that they are hounded by their partner to be orgasmic by these means and this makes them anxious and depressed. Their partner might say that stimulating the clitoris manually at the same time as penile thrusting is superfluous.

Freud encouraged this attitude by stating that it was mature to have a 'vaginal orgasm' but immature to have what he called a 'clitoral orgasm' by means of masturbation. Freud confused the issue of clitoral v. vaginal orgasm. He believed that the vaginal orgasm was produced by the friction of the penis against the vagina. Masters and Johnson actually showed that there is only one type of orgasm and that it has both clitoral and vaginal components.

The Hite Report[12] drew attention to the fact that only 30 per cent of women in any case achieve an orgasm through sexual intercourse. Hite also found that half the women in her sample had faked orgasm at some point, so as to please a partner.

Once sex therapists encouraged this myth to be propagated and labelled a woman who needs to have extra clitoral stimulation as needing treatment. Attitudes have changed in the past few years and although therapy methods are available to help women achieve this goal they should not be pushed into this situation; they should have a choice. In any case, some women cannot achieve this goal, no matter how much they strive to do so, and they should be encouraged to accept their situation.

Sex therapy provides a good learning setting for changing attitudes. In particular, women from other cultures need a lot of support to change their attitude towards the male's penile contribution to the female orgasm.

Myth 6: women should be sexually passive and not initiate sex

In most cultures women are conditioned at an early age to behave 'like ladies' and not be sexually active. Traditionally men have taken the role of asking a woman to dance or to go on a date. Customarily, the female has to be chosen (or appear to be chosen) by the male and usually the woman expects the man to make the first move sexually. Eastern cultures emphasise womanly virtues even more.

Many women miss out sexually because they think they should be passive and they do not ask for what they want. Many men do not know how a woman likes to have clitoral stimulation and if she does not tell him what she wants he cannot read her mind. Her sexual pleasure is her responsibility and this usually involves telling or guiding a partner how stimulation should be applied. Many women with orgasmic problems find this type of request hard to carry out and some role playing is usually needed.

The curious thing is that experimental studies by American sex researchers like Heiman[13] on Long Island have reported that when women heard stories in which they themselves initiated sex they became more aroused. Men also were more aroused by the stories in which women initiated sex. This totally goes against the myth that men should take charge of asking for sex.

Myth 7: men should always be willing and able to have sex

This myth complements the sex role stereotype of women being passive. One wonders how these myths are spread. Both men and women reinforce the above myths. Clients who complain of occasional poor erections see this as a disorder and are surprised to learn that other men experience the same problem. The trouble is that men tend to compete and boast about their sexual prowess.

Men do not like to admit any sexual problems, whereas women are more willing to discuss their problems with one another. In the UK, when men's and women's sex therapy groups were formed the women tended to befriend one another after the group session, whereas the men disappeared quickly, without talking together afterwards.

Some of the men in the groups have reinforced the myth that they should always be ready to perform. A lot of emphasis is placed on an erect penis. Zilbergeld brought up a similar myth in his book, *Men and Sex*[14]. One of the most important exercises for men in his book is to get them to rehearse saying no to a partner when they do not feel like having sex. Sometimes it can be very difficult actually to say no.

Myth 8: a big erect penis is the key to good sex

There is a saying which dispels this myth: 'It's not what you've got, it's what you do with it that counts'. Some men might have the most fantastic erections but be lousy lovers. Some women say that they get more pleasure from a man's finger than his penis. The penis has been a symbol of virility and potency since ancient days. In some ancient religions the penis or lingam is worshipped in its own right.

Many men complain that their penises are too small. They compare their penis size with other men who are not erect, for instance, when changing for a game of tennis. There is a greater size range for flaccid penises than for erect penises. In fact small flaccid penises increase in size proportionately more than large flaccid ones. The erect penis length is probably fairly constant, though the dimensions of the erect penis have not yet been fully researched.

Another fallacy associated with penile size is the belief that the longer the penis the more sexual satisfaction it will produce for the woman. Masters and Johnson's research ended this fallacy when they reported that only the outer one-third of the vagina possesses the sensitive nerves associated with orgasm; length is quite unimportant.

Myth 9: sex cannot be learned

Many people think that sex should be natural and spontaneous when in fact it is a matter of learning and conditioning. Although sexual behaviour is to some extent biologically determined, a large part of it is learned. Often people with sexual problems have conditioned badly and developed bad sexual habits which can be changed.

Couples sometimes complain that sex therapy is too mechanical and homework exercises are like going back to school. The answer to this type of criticism is for the therapist to say that when left to their own devices the couple have a problem; they are now being guided in the learning of new and desirable habits. The sex therapy programme might lack spontaneity but it has a structure built into it which is predictable and reassuring for many clients.

In any case, a substantial part of sexual behaviour is learned. That is, sexual behaviour in part has to be taught, or discovered by trial and error, or invented. In any event, the individual learns to behave in a certain manner, and the learning takes place piecemeal and comes from diverse sources: friends, films, gossip, newspapers, magazines, and increasingly from sex education.

When clients are asked to view video tapes of sexual behaviour they sometimes object saying that this is a voyeuristic activity and morally wrong. The counteracting argument is that if seeing others making love helps them learn about sex then they are benefiting from such activity which in any case is not occurring spontaneously in their own sexual relationship.

Myth 10: it is wrong to indulge in sexual fantasies

Most people use fantasy and sexual fantasy to some extent, but the richness of the fantasy life will vary from person to person. When a person feels guilty about some sexual behaviour he or she may also feel guilty about fantasising and the fantasy life will be restricted. Many clients are guilty and embarrassed by their sexual fantasies and some deny they have them. The therapist needs to reassure those who are upset by their fantasies. If a client has no sexual fantasies the therapist needs to teach how to generate some: they are a necessary part of a good sex life.

The ability to fantasise sexually is a good and useful ability. Couples who know one another to the point of boredom can use fantasy to enliven parts of the sexual act. These fantasies may be private or shared. Many partners dislike sharing sexual fantasies and they should have the choice of doing this. If shared, the fantasy potential may be doubled. Inventing sexual stories for a loved partner can be creative and fun.

People who are learning to masturbate can benefit from fantasising, as it can help them to get aroused. The therapist can inform clients that most people fantasise when they masturbate – this is quite normal.

The content of sexual fantasy can be extraordinarily diverse. However, there are certain elements that frequently crop up. According to Wilson[15], women fantasise frequently about ordinary sexual intercourse with a loved one in romantic circumstances whereas men tend to fantasise more about different partners and more unusual sexual practices.

Another common element in fantasy is of group sexual activity: a sexual party or orgy in which a meeting with friends begins with games of strip poker or games with certain forfeits and ends with openly sexual activity – group intercourse or group masturbation.

The elements of sado-masochism are extremely common, rape fantasies being enjoyed by men and women equally. The violence may extend to whipping, torture and degradation. Men imagine they can force attractive women to do their bidding, with the free use of manacles and ropes. The idea of humiliating and defiling other human beings while obtaining sexual pleasure is not uncommon in sado-masochistic fantasies. (Of course there has to be a strong element of trust in the relationship between sado-masochistic partners to safeguard against the danger of going too far.)

Masochistic attitudes are more common in women than in men but not confined to them. The idea of being overwhelmed, of being unable to resist, of being swept away, of being raped and of being seduced by attractive and powerful men provides common fantasy material. Often women deny such fantasies, especially feminists who say women do not like being raped. This latter statement is true, but there is a huge difference between imagining being raped and actually being a rape victim. When a woman imagines any fantasy she is in control of the situation as it takes place in her mind. Feminists tend to deny this connection and forget that the first hero of film, Rudolf Valentino, appealed to the masochistic streak in women as he carried them off into the desert, as a sheikh mounted on his white steed. Some women imagine themselves going into dangerous or sinister parts of the town where they surrender themselves to a brutal and insensitive sexual encounter. A man might imagine himself overcome by a group of attractive women who force him to submit to cunnilingus under duress; alternatively they might stimulate him unendurably while helpless. Elements of violence and dominance may occur in 'gang-bang' fantasies, which are imagined by both sexes.

Voyeurism is a common fantasy; people like to imagine watching other people make love. The idea of watching other people who are unaware attracts nearly everyone to some degree. Fantasies associated with exhibitionism are less common.

An element of the forbidden often enters fantasy – breaking the rules of society by enjoying sexual behaviour in forbidden places, in public, on the beach, in churches or in brothels. It may be said that there is no prohibition which is not regularly broken in fantasy, and it would seem with very little harm.

It is extremely unlikely that a well-adjusted person who has forbidden fantasies will act them out; not only have they other outlets but they have much to lose by defying the rules. Clients may need to be reassured that they are not required to act out their fantasies. Therapists should not reject the fantasies of clients no matter how preposterous they seem.

Myth 11: women can become dependent on vibrators for an orgasm and these dangerous machines can become a substitute for a man

Electricity has revolutionised sex therapy. Vibrators were introduced in the seventies into sex therapy for women with orgasmic problems. Thousands of women were delighted that they could achieve an orgasm with the help of a vibrator. Previously vibrators on the market had been of the wrong design, like a plastic phallus with batteries inside. When the batteries ran down and the vibrator no longer operated at an effective frequency the woman would begin to feel she was not responding. The optimal frequency level for such stimulation is 80 cycles per second and the electric vibrators provide this level. The smooth side of an electric toothbrush applied on the clitoris can also be effective.

Some women confess they fear they will become addicted to their vibrator, but research by the Rileys[16] showed no habituation effect.

Research on anorgasmia in the USA by McMullen[17] showed that vibrators played an important part in sex therapy. When vibrators were researched in the UK at Guy's and The Maudsley hospitals[18] it was shown that providing a vibrator for therapeutic use at home was the most effective variable in the therapy, as most of the women who did not experiment with a vibrator failed to become orgasmic.

It is usually men who have a phobia of vibrators but they too can enjoy such a machine. Some men who are threatened by vibrators are macho; they are probably in any case playing a power game and will not cooperate with the idea of clitoral stimulation. Often the partner of a woman with orgasmic problems feels inadequate. It can help a great deal if when the vibrator is applied this results in pleasure. This satisfaction can be transferred to manual stimulation of the clitoris applied by the partner – it is a matter of shaping as far as conditioning goes. Partners can both get some good vibrations and then learn to become more dependent on each other and do without the vibrator.

Individual problems

When couples come for therapy with problems these are often associated with their interaction. Masters and Johnson introduced the principle of couples attending therapy together in order to sort out communication difficulties. British therapists tend to see each partner for some individual therapy rather than relying on conjoint therapy. Often one partner will need some individual therapy consisting of guidance and counselling.

In the early days of sex therapy couples were treated as a unit. Many individual clients wanted help but were turned away from clinics if they did not have a partner. This was like a 'Catch 22' situation: often individuals needed therapy to help them find a partner as they felt a sex problem would handicap them. Gradually the clinics' policy changed and individuals were accepted for therapy.

Single men often need some social skills therapy before their sex problems can be sorted out. They need to learn how to be personally effective. Personal effectiveness training is based on advice and practice. The therapist gives direct advice on how to behave and demonstrates what has been suggested. He might, for example, say to a client: 'You are meeting this friendly woman at a social club and you shake her by the hand when introduced and look at her and smile, like this'. Some single male clients have no confidence about forming relationships with women and do not know how to look at or talk with potential partners because they are shy. Social skills therapy can help this type of man and the occasional woman who lack these skills. Several such men need help in learning to express their emotions effectively, but this does not apply so much to women. Usually this type of therapy is most effective in a group situation but it can be tailored to individual therapy.

Women have more problems in being assertive and various groups have been formed to help women to gain the confidence to say convincingly what they want.

Clients from other cultures suffer more if they are shy. Perhaps the language is unfamiliar and they worry about doing the wrong thing in the alien culture. They usually need more practice in rehearsing the tasks. Sometimes groups are formed for Asian women to learn about Western culture and discuss their sexuality without the presence of men. They often need to learn to be assertive to deal with people in 'the host culture'. Back home many of these women dealt effectively with their servants, but their shopping was done for them and most of their time was spent in the home or visiting other women.

Many clients from other cultures require a great deal of guidance and need to rehearse the behaviour that is expected of them. Often they are involved in sex role stereotyping and need to change their attitudes. The therapist should help them make a compromise between cultures.

The demonstration of behaviour is that of modelling. If a secretary is complaining about her boss's overbearing manner, the female therapist could take the role of the secretary and maintain a more assertive attitude in a mock argument with the boss. When the 'model' of assertion has been given, the client may try it herself in the presence of the therapist. Suggestions can follow.

Clients should always be encouraged and rewarded and never criticised. Even when a client clearly fails in some way, the therapist should only draw attention to some way in which the patient did succeed, however small. Other types of assertive training can take place throughout therapy and, of course, since it is sex therapy there will be more emphasis upon sexual assertiveness[19,20].

Marital therapy background

Personal effectiveness plays a major part in marital therapy. Often the inability of one partner to be assertive may have serious results. The unassertive partner may feel a helpless resentment which may easily develop into passive hostility manifesting itself as a lack of warmth, a lack of enthusiasm, a lack of sexual cooperation and initiative, or perhaps sulking or moodiness. The therapist will quickly discover such behaviour, even if neither partner mentions it. It will become apparent during the early sessions. The more assertive partner will talk more and is more emphatic. He or she will often adopt an aggressive stance, have a louder voice and a more impelling gaze. The more timid partner is more readily squashed.

Role playing can be a useful way of teaching the timid partner to change his or her behaviour and become more effective. One of the most powerful techniques is to get the two partners to change roles for a demonstration of how they appear to each other. Sometimes this can be arranged initially by the therapist taking on the more aggressive role to demonstrate that particular partner's image and personality. Then the timid partner can play the aggressive partner's part, modelled on the way the therapist has demonstrated it. This can be shattering for some clients as usually the overbearing partner is surprised that he or she appears to be so awful. Videos can also play a part in this type of learning.

Another method used in marital therapy to improve relationships is called 'contract therapy'. This is based on looking carefully at areas of friction and concern to see if some simple analysis may suggest a 'give to get' solution. Each partner requests a positive task for their partner to carry out. These tasks remotivate the couple to make certain sacrifices in the interest of greater harmony and increased sexual cooperation.

Contract therapy can also be a valuable lesson in getting the couple to talk to one another. Previous discussions may have failed because the couple could not keep up a dialogue without quarelling. This may be because one partner, or both, begin to feel threatened in some way and retreat into sulking, hostility or pretended indifference. The therapist may suggest ways of overcoming this. One method is to set aside a time each week for marital discussion when it is a rule to keep calm. Another rule could be to break off the discussion at a given time – not to try to solve everything at once. Once communication works, marital and sexual matters can be discussed.

Sex therapists try to appeal to the common sense of a client in explaining the rationale behind contracts. The behavioural approach to marital therapy is practical with interpretations based on simple explanations rather than delving into the client's inner psyche. The therapist can make rational behavioural suggestions why a person is behaving in a certain way if the behaviour is a threat to the marriage or sex therapy: 'You spend all your time watching Dallas or other soap operas as you wish to fantasise yourself as glamorous and successful, perhaps to make up for your other failures'. 'Maybe you wear curlers and plaster thick night cream on your face when you go to bed to avoid contact and homework massage. You refuse to run the risk of rejection or ridicule by making yourself unattractive.'

Explanations and interpretations should be simply expressed. If the client does not understand them the therapist is being too general or is unsure what he or she means – in either case rethinking is needed. Incidentally, it is perfectly reasonable for a therapist to say: 'I don't really know,' or 'I can only speculate', since many behaviours are difficult to explain. The client who expects the therapist to have all the answers will be disappointed.

Marital therapy can play a significant part in helping to solve sex problems, according to research done at The Maudsley Hospital by Crowe *et al.*[21] in London. When comparing couples presenting with sex problems who received a modified Masters and Johnson type of therapy or marital therapy there was no difference in outcome between the two methods. The clients treated had problems like anorgasmia, impotence and low sexual interest. It should be noted, however, that those clients with low sexual interest did improve more with sex therapy but this difference was no longer apparent at follow-up.

SEX THERAPY FORMAT

Once reassurance has been achieved, reorientation aims understood and basic relaxation techniques learned, the therapist can introduce the individual or couple to the sequential stages of therapy.

It is sensible to give an idea of the length of each therapy session time and the expected number of sessions. Expected goals, according to the client and therapist, should be agreed upon.

The first reassurance to be given is that sexual intercourse is not an initial therapy goal; in fact, it is forbidden. Instead, feelings and sensations are first to be explored. The client should be told that weekly tasks will be suggested for homework and these should be carried out and progress reported at the next therapy session.

The homework tasks are outlined in the sections below. The initial massage task forms a foundation for lovemaking and is part of the basic therapy for all clients. Couples are advised that massage relaxes both partners and provides positive feelings. Massage is a good way to start a sexual task and can be recommended as initial foreplay in the future when the treatment has ended. If the client is alone, self-massage can be quite relaxing. The massage instructions in the following section are quite extensive. Not all clients need the instructions about masturbation or self-focussing as many of them will be relaxed and positive about this activity.

The section on stimulation therapy is only for particular clients who find it difficult to become sexually aroused. It is also useful for partners who have become bored with one another as it teaches them to enrich their senses.

The genital sensate focussing section is also part of the basic therapy for all couples. Some homosexual clients will want to stop therapy at this point but some of them will want to continue with the oral sex homework.

The oral sex section is optional and this section will probably produce the most problems and hostility in therapy.

Positions for sexual intercourse often produce some difficulties, especially the first recommended position of 'the woman above' which is the basic position for all dysfunctions and was well researched by Masters and Johnson. As it has been proved that there is a link between anal sex and AIDS the last section on intercourse is aimed at heterosexual couples.

(1) Massage

The first task for homework involves massage. It is a good idea to have a warm bath first; this helps to relax a person. The individual can try massaging himself or herself in the bath or shower, spreading bath oil on various parts of the body or doing this type of masage afterwards.

If a partner is available, mutual stroking, caressing, touching and massage can be tried. Masters and Johnson labelled this type of massage 'sensate focussing'. It is vital to have a warm and comfortable place for this; it does not matter in the least whether this is the bedroom or the lounge.

It should be explained that clients should try to explore new sensations of stroking each other slowly and firmly; of light touch, soft kneading, gentle scratching and deep massage. This massage should exclude all those parts of the body that are closely associated with sexual behaviour and hence with a sense of previous sexual failure. The massage is a fun session and clients should be encouraged to enjoy themselves; the goal is to experience pleasurable feelings and communicate what they like and want.

Massage is obviously more effective between two partners, so the individual client without a partner is at a disadvantage when doing the massage alone. This can be remedied by getting clients in group therapy to do a 'hand or foot massage' on one another, or clients who attend for individual therapy can go to a massage parlour, although this is a 'one way system' in which only the client is massaged.

Some couples have no idea about massage and it is a good idea for the therapist to get them to massage one another's hands and arms during a therapy session, after they have relaxed. This gives the therapist an idea of how they manage and advice can be offered.

Some suggestions need to be made about massage technique, but some excellent books are available[22]. Massage should be given with the fingers and the hands. A deep soothing but gentle kneading massage of the soft parts of the body would be one way of explaining it – this is not a remedial massage for muscle pain. Slow but rhythmic strokes are recommended as a degree of regularity is restful. The partner receiving the massage should make suggestions about what he or she likes best, a gentler or firmer stroke. The passive partner should always try to respond, either verbally or in some way which gives obvious feedback; groans, grunts and sighs carry messages equally well. They are all part of learning to communicate together.

The therapist usually asks both partners to share the initiative in asking one another for a massage. The more passive or shy partner is usually the one who receives a back massage initially and the partners change roles so the receiver becomes the giver. Positions can be changed again for a frontal massage, avoiding the genitals. Both partners should be nude, although sometimes desensitisation is necessary for anxious clients before this can be achieved.

(2) Masturbation

People who are comfortable and experienced over masturbation do not need to go through this stage of therapy. Many clients from other cultures need to go through this stage to gain experience in stimulating themselves before they feel confident enough to put mutual masturbation into practice with a partner.

This section is for clients who have never learned to stimulate themselves sexually, maybe thinking that masturbation is unhealthy or dirty. Other clients may have tried self-stimulation, but perhaps found it unsatisfactory and not continued.

Female self-focussing

More female than male clients need guidance over masturbation. Some women who have never masturbated resist the idea strongly. The therapist may have to use a lot of tact and sympathetic persuasion to get them to try it. Learning to masturbate is particularly useful for women who have not experienced orgasm, or who do so rarely. This will help them to get orgasms during mutual masturbation later.

Before starting the masturbation therapy some women need to be desensitised first and to relax and imagine various stimuli associated with their genitals; they might be asked to imagine looking at their genitals. The woman is asked to set aside some time when she will not be observed or distracted, making sure she is as warm and as relaxed as possible. The first step is to undress in front of a mirror and examine her body carefully from as many angles as possible. In this way she can familiarise herself with her appearance and imagine herself as seen by her partner. This is useful for women who undress and make love in the dark.

The American masturbation programme devised by LoPiccolo and Lobitz[23] is based on a course they devised for anorgasmic women and involves looking at and touching the genitals. Initially the woman is asked to carry out a physical self-examination, looking at her genitals in a hand mirror and identifying the different parts. This is often a problem as many women do not know how to find such parts, particularly the clitoris. Diagrams or rubber moulds of the genitals in a resting and aroused state can help.

Figure 2.1(a) shows the clitoral hood and Fig. 2.1(b) shows how the hood can be pulled back to reveal the glans clitoridis which is the most sensitive part.

The next step is for the woman to touch the various genital parts. A lubricant or massage oil can be recommended. She should lie back into a comfortable position and begin to rub her genitals gently, finding out if there is any special area which seems best. The actual movements will vary from one woman to another. Most women use either the index or middle finger or both in a to-and-fro motion along the shaft of the clitoris, including the clitoral hood and glans when ready. Alternatively a circular movement can be tried.

Rest pauses, fantasising and enjoying the sensations are all subjects the therapist should discuss, along with guilt feelings. A vibrator is an alternative method of stimulation.

Male self-focussing

Most men have learned to masturbate, but the therapist must tell those who have not how to proceed for their homework. Most men need some reassurance about the size or shape of their penises. Figures 2.2(a) and (b) show a flaccid and an erect penis of the same man. Most textbooks show only diagrams and this type of drawing is useful for the client.

The client should explore his genitalia in private and find out which parts give him sexual feelings to whatever degree. The touching should include the testes and all parts of the penis. He should also

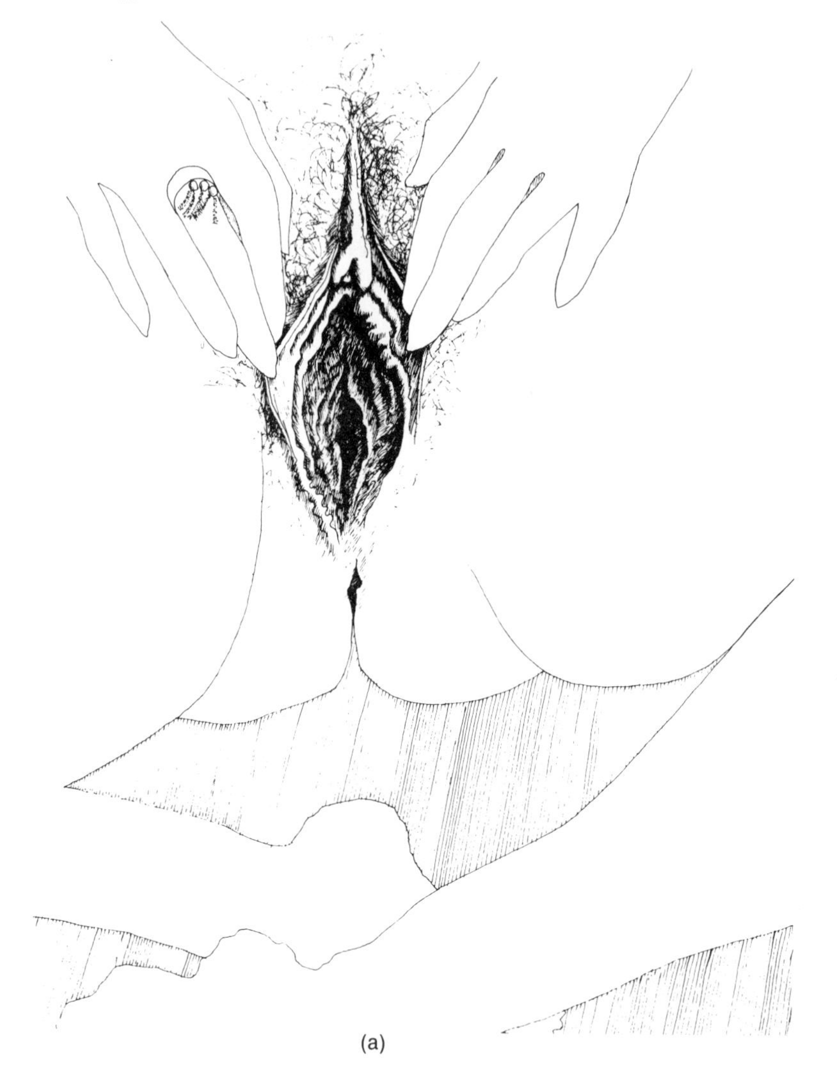

Fig. 2.1 (a) Clitoris in relaxed state. (b) Clitoris in aroused state. Glans clitoridis exposed. (*Drawings by Richard Gillan.*)

touch the underside of the penis along the urethra towards the basal parts adjacent to the anus. The frenulum and the glans are generally the most sensitive parts and are best stimulated gently until some degree of sexual excitement is felt. The therapist may have to tell the man how to move the foreskin backwards and forwards. The commonest method of stimulation is to grasp the erect penis fairly firmly with the fingers and thumb and rub it up and down its length in imitation of the thrusting of the penis in the vagina.

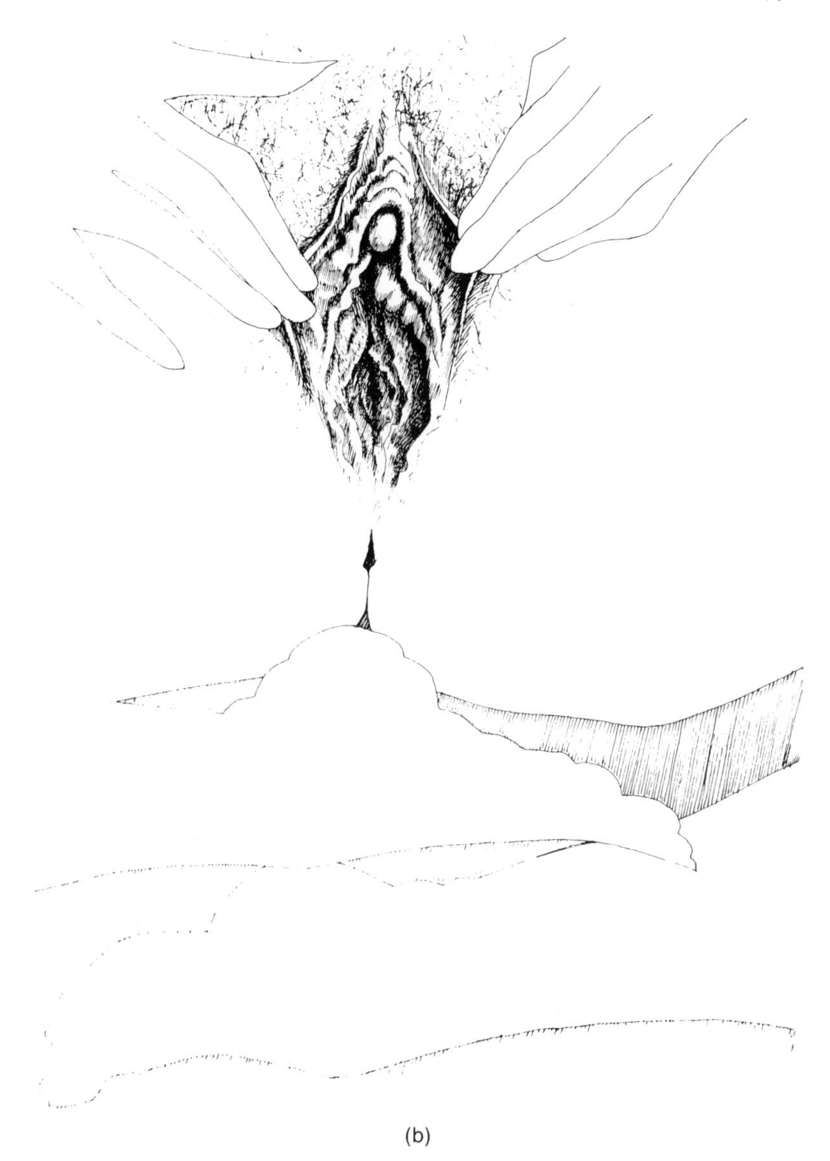

(b)

Time should be spent reassuring the client and getting him to relax and fantasise.

(3) Stimulation therapy

Some clients need to be told how to fantasise so that they can get sufficiently stimulated to enjoy their masturbation. Couples who have

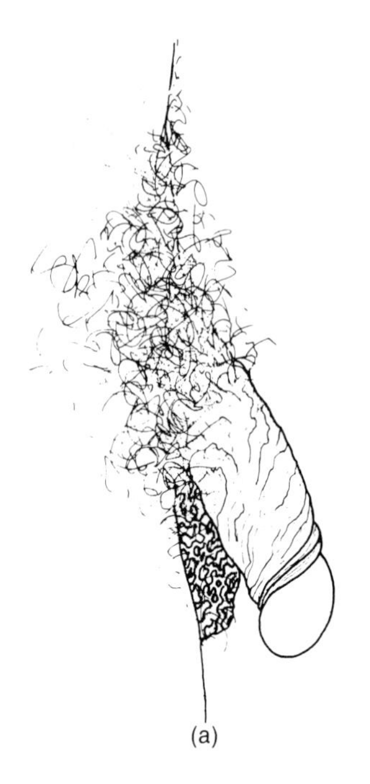

Fig. 2.2 (a) Flaccid penis. (b) Erect penis. (*Drawings by Richard Gillan.*)

become sexually bored can use fantasy to stimulate their sex lives[11].

Books, magazines and erotic audio cassette tapes and videos can be recommended. Erotic prints like Fig. 2.3 can be discussed with a client and used as a stimulus for masturbation at home later. Fantasies can be shaped by getting clients to read books about women's fantasies like Nancy Friday's *My Secret Garden*[24] or *Forbidden Flowers*[25]. They might find such fantasies outrageous at first but the therapist can be supportive and tell the client that there is a whole range of fantasies available in these books and the client can select one or two fantasies to work on and forget about the rest. Anne Dickson's *The Mirror Within*[26] contains some more subtle sexual fantasies of British clients and is a good book to read in itself.

The senses should be explored fully and the therapist can recommend tactile stimulation tasks in which the client is asked to explore touching different textures and objects with various hot/cold, wet/dry, smooth/rough, hard/soft dimensions. Some clients need to be encouraged to do something mildly sensuous together, like cookery. The massage they will have done already will have helped them tune into touch.

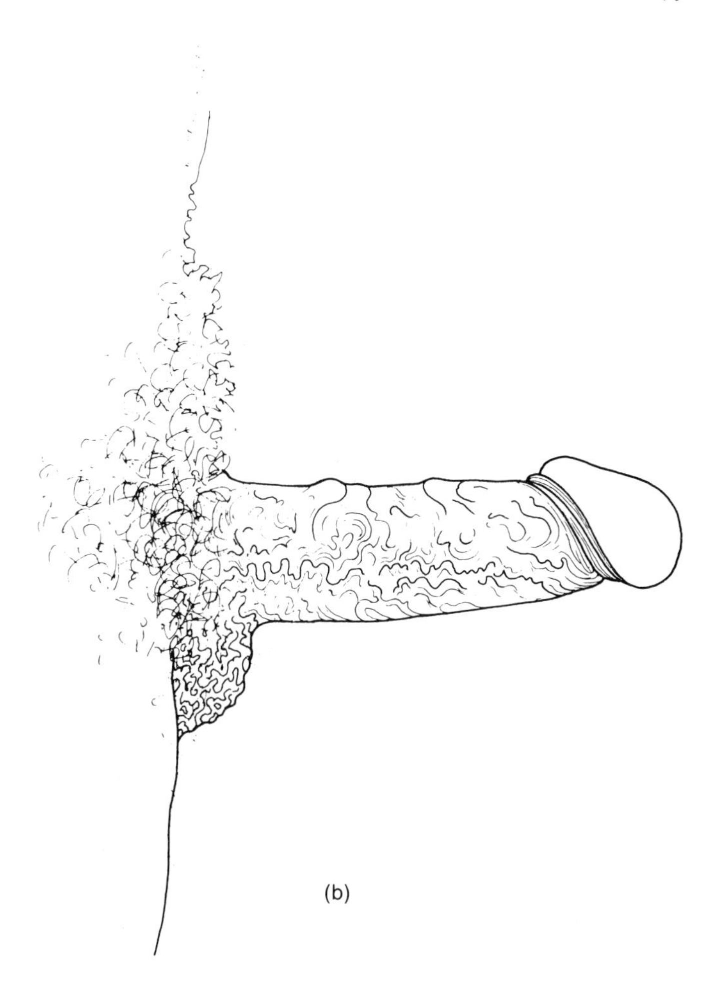

(b)

(4) Genital sensate focussing

It is a matter for the therapist to decide whether the genital manipulations should begin as individual self-focussing or as mutual genital sensate focussing shared by the couple. It will depend on the masturbatory experience of each individual client.

A session of genital sensate focussing should be a continuation of massage or sensate focussing. It is easy to lead on to touching the genitals from massaging the whole body. Nipples and breasts may be stimulated. Some men are surprised that they get aroused when this area is focussed on but in fact 50 per cent of men respond sexually to such stimulation.

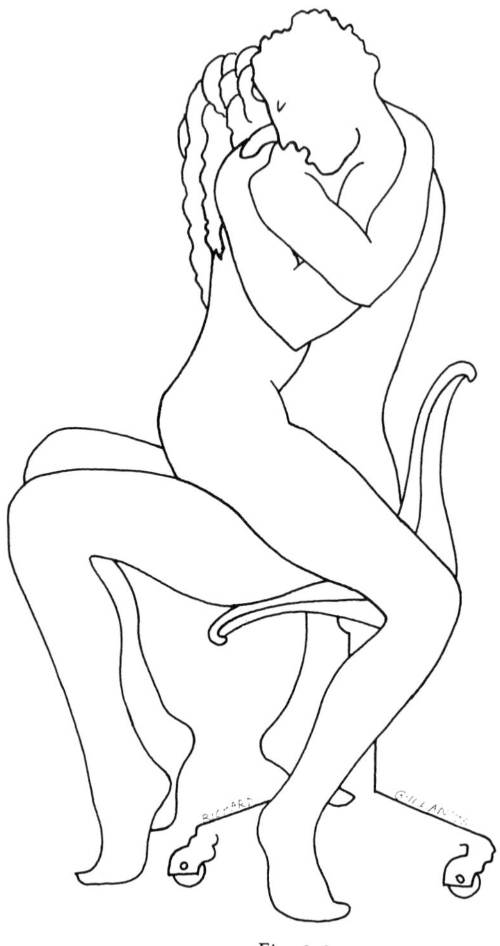

Fig. 2.3

Female pleasuring

Figure 2.4 shows a suitable position for the man to stimulate the woman. He can easily touch her breasts and genitals. She can look down and watch the stimulation, guiding his hands as she wishes. She can indicate where to start, the most desirable motion, the speed and pressure to be employed. Gentle stroking with a circular to-and-fro motion can be advised at the onset, with not too much pressure. The glans clitoridis is the most sensitive area and some women do not like to be stimulated directly there, only gently brushed. The clitoral shaft and hood may be rhythmically rubbed and stroked. She should guide his hand in order to get the right technique as her satisfaction is her responsibility.

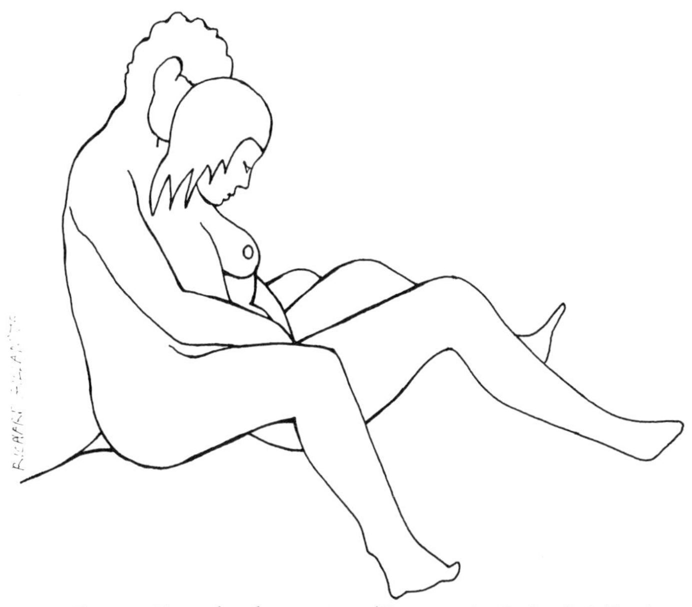

Fig. 2.4 Female pleasuring. (*Drawing by Richard Gillan.*)

The therapist should explain that the genital stimulation may be varied at will. The man should not be afraid to stop for rests, especially where the woman may have maintained a plateau of excitement for some time, or where the orgasm will not quite come. He can tease her by almost bringing her to orgasm and then letting the stimulation subside. The therapist should also stress that the goal is for pleasure and not actually to strive for an orgasm. The woman might be told to exaggerate any anxiety she has over this type of masturbation, like breathing loudly or moving a great deal.

Male pleasuring

The man's turn can be next and the position shown in Fig. 2.5 is recommended. The woman can begin by stroking his thighs. She can start with gentle tickling, stroking, pinching and scratching. She can ask the man what he likes in an exploration of the testicles. Next the penile shaft can be held, squeezed and gently masturbated.

The therapist should explain to the man that he should tell and show his partner how he likes to be stimulated. He should feel relaxed and fantasise. She should tease him and deliberately give him rest pauses so he loses his erection if he has one, and then stimulate him again. The goal is fun rather than getting an erection.

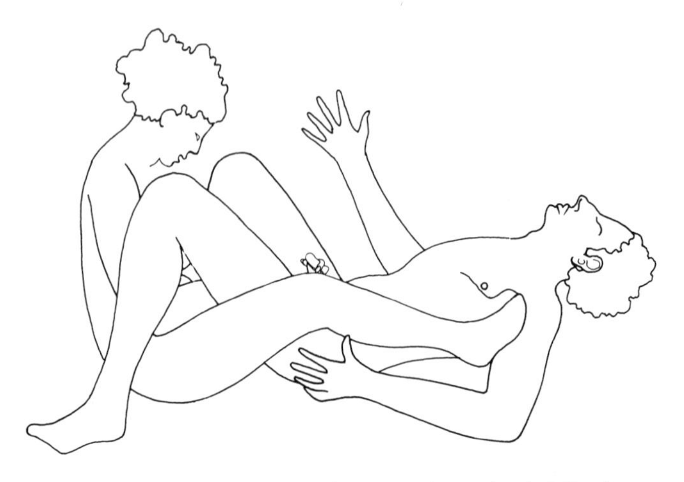

Fig. 2.5 Male pleasuring. (*Drawing by Richard Gillan.*)

(5) Oral sex

When the therapist brings up the topic of oral sex during therapy clients often respond negatively to this idea. In fact, oral sex has been practised from ancient times, when it was widely recommended for potency problems. For people who are interested in sexual conduct, Vatsayana, the author of the *Kama Sutra*, refers approvingly to the pleasures of oral sex.

Often couples have tried *soixante neuf* or *69* in which they have tried to lick or kiss each other genitally at the same time but this has not worked out as it is difficult to achieve simultaneously and comfortably.

Cunnilingus

The couple should begin with some sexual massage until there is arousal. The woman should try lying on her back with her legs open. She may half turn sideways until her thigh rests on the bed forming a pillow for the man's shoulder and head. He can then gently lick the clitorial region with his tongue. If she is excited he can increase the speed and pressure of the stimulation with his tongue and lips. This might result in orgasm but the goal is enjoyment.

Fellatio

The therapist should point out to the couple that if one partner prefers to give rather than receive this is all right. No one is forced to give or receive oral sex.

Some women dislike the idea of fellatio but if it is tactfully explained by the therapist that there is no need for her to take the whole penis

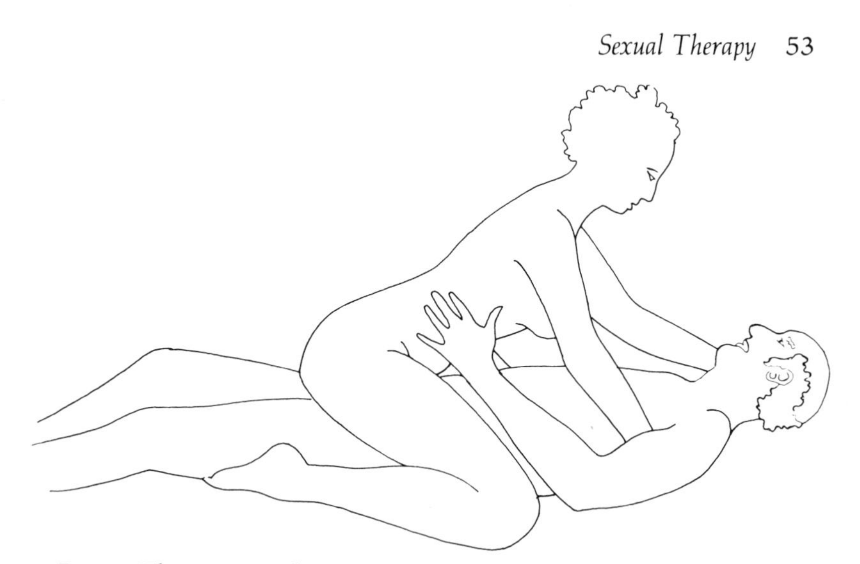

Fig. 2.6 The woman above position. (*Drawing by Richard Gillan.*)

in her mouth or to swallow the sperm many women feel reassured. Indeed, if a woman is prepared to lick and kiss the shaft and glans this can be exciting for the man. It is usually possible for most women to suck the glans, pushing it gently in and out of her mouth while encircling it with her lips. The couple can decide how to deal with the ejaculate if the man comes to orgasm. Again the goal is to have fun.

(6) Positions

The woman above position

The best known and most commonly used position for sexual intercourse is the so-called 'missionary' position with the man lying on top of the woman. This position gives the woman little freedom, which may be the reason for its popularity in a male-dominated society. Women have mixed feelings about this position and it does have some disadvantages. Practically, the weight of the partner makes it difficult for the woman to move her pelvis during intercourse. Psychologically, the missionary position is associated with failure for most clients.

Figure 2.6 shows an alternative, the 'woman above position' which Masters and Johnson recommended as the first step of sexual intercourse for all the sexual disorders they treated. Their choice appears to be successful as the woman can move much more freely and

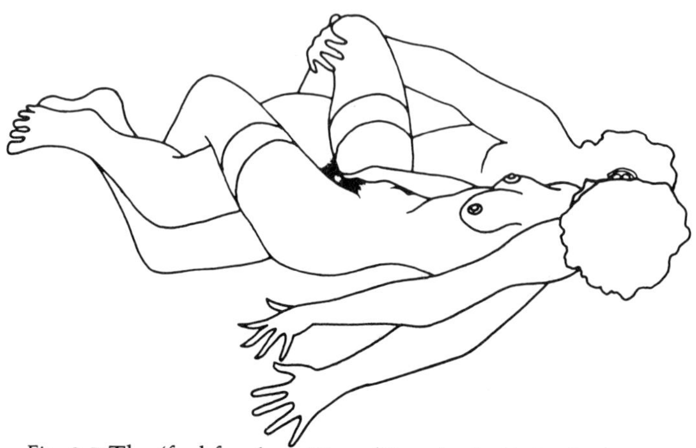

Fig. 2.7 The 'feel free' position. (*Drawing by Richard Gillan.*)

take more responsibility. She can decide if the man is erect enough for insertion and he can lie back and enjoy her kneeling over him as she guides his penis into her. If her partner is getting over-excited she can easily stop moving. If he needs extra stimulation she can move more.

This position gives the woman full control over depth of penetration and is an excellent way for a woman who has suffered from pain in the past to experiment with coitus. The position is intimate and the couple can kiss and caress easily, showing affection.

The feel free position

This is an important position for therapy for orgasmic dysfunction. In this position (Fig. 2.7) the woman is free to enjoy some manual stimulation, provided by herself or her partner, and training instructions for orgasmic dysfunction can be practised.

When the woman has stimulated herself or has been stimulated to a point just prior to orgasm the man can insert his penis and thrust vigorously as she comes to orgasm. At later stages in the treatment the man makes his entry and the masturbation is stopped progressively earlier.

The other therapy method is just as easy to carry out in the feel free position and consists of penile entry followed by manual stimulation to orgasm. Little by little, the manual stimulation is stopped earlier, at first just prior to orgasm and then earlier and earlier until such manual stimulation is unnecessary.

American therapists like Kaplan[27] recommend this method for women who cannot obtain orgasms by the penile thrusting of their partner. However, opinion is changing over whether this type of

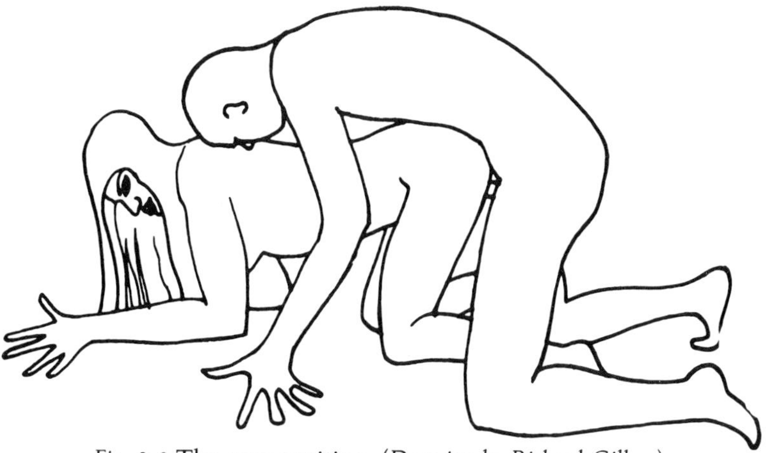

Fig. 2.8 The rear position. (*Drawing by Richard Gillan.*)

therapy is necessary and many couples prefer to combine both penile insertion and manual stimulation of the clitoris in this easy and convenient position. The feel free position is pleasant for undertaking both types of stimulation.

The rear position

This is not a manual of sexual plumbing so this will be the last position discussed as often the therapist finds it awkward to inform clients about this position. Some clients will say that this is like an animal or 'doggy position' and it is dirty or defiling, but the therapist can counteract this by saying that animals have a healthy approach to sex. The position is normal and natural.

Penetration is quite easy once the woman is kneeling and the man can watch the penis sliding in and out which is exciting for him. It is a position allowing deep penetration and one which emphasises masculine control.

Clitoral stimulation by the penis and pubis of the man is not very good. Manual clitoral stimulation is possible either for the woman or the man, though not easy. The man is able to caress the body, buttocks, breasts and thighs of his partner easily. The position does not allow much face-to-face intimacy.

This rear position is often recommended for use in pregnancy as the woman bears no weight and her uterus sinks into the body cavity away from the thrust of the penis. The depth of penetration can be controlled by the man not going the whole way if his partner dislikes this.

References

1. Wolpe, Joseph. (1958) *Psychotherapy by Reciprocal Inhibition.* Stanford University Press.
2. Eysenck, H.J. and Wilson, G.D. (1973) *The Experimental Study of Freudian Theories.* Methuen.
3. Kraft-Ebbing, R. Von. *Psychopathia Sexualis.* (1965) Translation by Klaf, F.S. Stern & Day, New York.
4. Ellis, Havelock. (1910) *Studies in the Psychology of Sex.* F.A. Davis & Co., Philadelphia.
5. Masters, W.H. and Johnson, V. (1970) *Human Sexual Inadequacy.* Churchill, London.
6. Hunter, R. and MacAlpine, I. (1963) *Three Hundred Years of Psychiatry.* Oxford University Press.
7. Barbach, Lonnie. G. (1975) *For Yourself: The Fulfillment of Female Sexuality.* Doubleday.
8. Dodson, Betty. (1976) *Liberating Masturbation.* Box 1933, New York 10001.
9. Hadden, Celia. (1982) *The Limits of Sex.* Michael Joseph.
10. Kinsey, A.C. *et al.* (1953) *Sexual Behaviour in the Human Female.* Saunders.
11. Gillan, Patricia and Richard. (1976) *Sex Therapy Today.* Open Books.
12. Hite, Shere. (1976) *The Hite Report.* Dell, New York.
13. Heiman, Julia. R. (1977) 'A psychophysiological exploration of sexual arousal patterns in females and males'. *Psychophysiology.* 14,266–274.
14. Zilbergeld, Bernie. (1980) *Men and Sex.* Souvenir Press.
15. Wilson, Glenn. (1978) *The Secrets of Sexual Fantasy.* Dent.
16. Riley, A.J. and Riley, E.J. (1978) 'A controlled study to evaluate

directed masturbation in the management of primary orgasmic failure in women'. *Brit.Jrnl. Psychiatry*. 133,404–9.
17. McMullen, Susan and Rosen, Raymond. C. (1979) 'Self-administered masturbation training in the treatment of primary orgasmic dysfunction'. *Jrnl. of Consulting and Clinical Psychology*. 47, 912–18.
18. Gillan, P., Golombok, S. and Becker, P. (1980) 'NHS Sex Therapy Groups for Women'. *Brit.Jrnl. Sexual Medicine*. Sept.
19. Gillan, P. 'Sex therapy for single people'. *Psychology Today*.
20. Yaffé, Maurice and Fenwick, Elizabeth. (1986) *Sexual Happiness*. Dorling Kindersley.
21. Crowe, M.J., Gillan, P.W. and Golombok, S. (1980) 'Form and content in the conjoint treatment of sexual dysfunction: A controlled study'. *Behav.Res. and Therapy*. Vol.19. 47–54.
22. Downing, George. (1972) *The Massage Book*. Random House.
23. LoPiccolo, J. and Lobitz, W.C. (1972) 'The role of masturbation in the treatment of orgasmic dysfunction'. *Archives of Sexual Behaviour*. 2, 163–7.
24. Friday, Nancy. (1975) *My Secret Garden*. Virago/Quartet.
25. Friday, Nancy. (1975) *Forbidden Flowers*. Pocket Books.
26. Dickson, Anne. (1985) *The Mirror Within*. Quartet.
27. Kaplan, Helen. (1974) *The New Sex Therapy*. Brunner-Mazel, New York.

Chapter 3

Referrals

Source of referrals

Referrals can come from widely different sources and the actual problem can frequently be obscured or covered up by other symptoms. The therapist will also need to refer clients with suspected organic problems to other specialists if inadequate screening has been done at referral. Nowadays, however, it is much easier to get referred to a sex clinic than it was fifteen years ago. More sex clinics have opened and there is increasing publicity about sexual difficulties.

The majority of clients with sexual problems ask for help from their family doctor. Such doctors can handle these problems directly if they are not severe. Other clients may want help over sexual problems but may be too embarrassed to seek help and discuss their symptoms. They might present with backache which could be a cover-up for orgasmic problems, or claustrophobia might be a cover-up for erectile problems.

Many family doctors are too busy to probe for possible sexual problems but others are so skilled that they can immediately detect what lies behind a psychosomatic complaint. Much depends on the doctor's willingness to enquire about the client's sex life. Most family doctors will have had almost no training in sexual disorders. They often feel helpless when confronted with psychological problems and prefer to deal with organic problems which are easily defined and for which treatment is clear cut.

Several family doctors have discussed the issue of presentation and have concluded that it is easier to pick up a sexual problem when it is presented in the context of a gynaecological complaint, like repeated concern about normal vaginal discharge, requests to change the contraceptive pill, or infertility (Hawton[1]).

Some clients go to Family Planning Clinics and complain about pain during intercourse and the doctor might discover a vaginismus problem on examination. Similarly, a case of infertility might be referred but the real problem could again be vaginismus or maybe an erectile disorder.

Other referral sources are the Marriage Guidance Clinics. In the UK a referral study was carried out by the Marriage Guidance Council[2] where sex therapy was available and many of their clients took advantage of this. One of the findings of this research was that those clients with severe marital problems do not respond as well to sex therapy as clients with mild relationship problems.

Psychiatry out-patients clinics can be another referral source. One never knows what to expect and the variety of problems from such a source can range from erectile impotence in alcoholics to depressed clients who have gone off sex. The Maudsley finding[3] of a negative correlation between severity of psychiatric disorder and response to sex therapy should always be remembered. Schizophrenics probably have the worst prognosis, followed by depressives.

Social skills groups often lead to sex therapy. Once the clients have conquered their social fears and anxiety they want to experiment with sex but often are too anxious to do this, being inexperienced and worried about their sexual performance. This can lead to sex therapy. Often this type of client does not have a terribly good prognosis.

The best prognosis for a sex problem is one that is referred early on rather than waiting until the problem is chronic. Outcome may also depend on previous good sexual adjustment. Hawton found that the more disturbed a couple's sexual relationship is at the outset of therapy, the more difficult it may be to help them. There is also an expected correlation between how attractive the couple find one another and how successful their therapy is.

Another factor in prognosis is related to how quickly clients progress with the early stage of therapy, especially the first three therapy sessions.

Obviously, motivation is another relevant prognostic factor, especially the motivation of the male partner who can easily sabotage sex therapy. Hawton has suggested that the model of sex therapy is more acceptable to women than men.

SCREENING REFERRALS

Before accepting a client for sex therapy, physical or organic causes of the sexual disorder need to be investigated and ruled out.

Sexual arousal problems

Usually men with erectile problems are investigated before they are referred to a sex clinic. One simple routine investigation is checking the urine for sugar to investigate for diabetes mellitus which is associated with erectile dysfunction in approximately half the cases[4].

With the advent of sleep laboratories where 'nocturnal penile tumescence' can be recorded various organic factors can be ruled out if the man gets erect during sleep or on waking. This technique has proved useful in making decisions whether a penile implant or vascular surgery may be required. The man spends the night in the laboratory and wears a penile cuff which inflates when he is erect. Such responses should be recorded for several nights to get reliable readings since responses may be inhibited on the first night of recording[5].

Karacan was the first to recommend this technique for distinguishing between organic and psychological causes of impotence. If organic factors are involved the basic mechanisms of erection are affected and sleep erections do not occur. If the problem is psychological the man's anxiety is reduced during sleep and erections occur. Further research is needed with this diagnostic technique especially when surgical decisions are based on it.

Arterial disease needs to be ruled out as interference with the blood supply to the pelvic organs can lead to erectile problems. This is more common in older men. Ebbehoi and Wagner[6] have recently investigated arterio-venous 'leaks' causing erectile failure. Arteriography of the internal pudendal artery and its branches is being used at various centres to investigate impotence thought to be associated with peripheral arterial disease. Bancroft[7] points out that these procedures are not without risk, as they require an anaesthetic and usually arterial catheterisation.

Bancroft talks about 'non-invasive measurement of penile blood pressure' such as penile plethysmography and points out that as yet there is little evidence available of the level of penile blood pressure in men with psychogenic impotence and without that it is difficult to judge the diagnostic value of this measure. It is good to have these pitfalls pointed out as too many people are blinded by science.

Recently various studies have been carried out in laboratories to measure sexual arousal in both men and women. Women's sexual arousal can also be measured by blood flow devices and a probe is inserted into the vagina to measure blood flow. Admittedly the method of producing sexual arousal by getting clients to view sexual films is artificial but it is useful to see whether woman reporting low sexual arousal respond. Wagner and Semmens[8] have used measures of vaginal blood flow to demonstrate the impaired response of post-menopausal, oestrogen-defective women, who improved in response after treatment with oestrogens.

Obviously men or women who report that they do not get aroused because sex is painful need to be carefully investigated by a urologist or gynaecologist. Often a foreskin that is too tight can be associated with pain and surgery can put this right. Sometimes women who complain of painful intercourse fail to lubricate during foreplay and then the penis rubs against the vaginal walls causing irritation and soreness. Post-menopausal women are particularly vulnerable but oestrogen therapy can help them.

Vasocongestion in the female is similar to that in the male. Both men and women can have their arousal impaired by neurological defiencies. In fact, Bancroft states that any condition which interferes with the nerve supply to the erectile tissues, whether a pathological process, trauma or the consequences of surgery, can interfere with arousal.

Orgasmic and ejaculatory problems

Retrograde ejaculation can occur as an early symptom of diabetes.

Whitelaw and Smithwick[9] described the sexual effects of sympathectomy, finding permanent loss of ejaculation in roughly half of the men in which the first three lumbar roots had been removed. They did not investigate orgasms in the same men.

Various reports have shown that certain anti-adrenergic hypotensive drugs can affect ejaculation. Other drugs can affect orgasms more directly, presumably by a central mechanism. Most antidepressants and monoamine oxidase inhibitors sometimes produce failure of orgasms and ejaculation as a side-effect. The irony is that these drugs have actually been used to treat premature ejaculation.

Premature ejaculation is not associated with drugs or organic dysfunction. It is more related to sexual immaturity and psychological issues like anxiety.

Little research has been carried out on the female orgasm. There is conflicting evidence about the effect of diabetes on female orgasm, although like men the opiates may have a direct inhibitory effect on it.

If a woman comes too quickly this would not be classified as a problem. On the other hand, pain associated with orgasm can be a problem, but more work needs to be done on this. Bancroft[7] has mentioned that occasionally head pains of a migrainous kind may follow orgasm, presumably due to some vasomotor effect. Some research has been reported in which orgasms reduce menstrual pain.

Drugs

The side effects of some therapeutic drugs have already been mentioned, although most of the research has been confined to men. Women are neglected in this field and are generally not asked about their symptoms. Of course, impotence in men is a clear symptom but perhaps there is also a tendency for the predominantly male medical profession to ignore the possibility of female sexual side effects.

Drugs used for the treatment of hypertension have been closely examined in association with ejaculatory failure, rather than erectile failures. On the whole, however, it is agreed that erectile dysfunction is usually psychological.

Tranquillisers like the phenothiazines and butyrophenones have received a lot of attention. Impairment of sexual interest has been noted with some reports of erectile failure.

Antidepressants also have side effects. The MAOIs have already been mentioned in association with ejaculatory failure and again some reports of decreased sexual arousal have been noted, particularly when patients on these drugs are less depressed and seem much better but show no interest in sex.

Anticonvulsants used to treat epilepsy have sometimes been shown to impair sexual interest.

It is not always drugs associated with psychiatric disorders that affect people sexually. Excessive alcohol can impair sexual response and lead to erectile failure. Again little attention has been paid to women and alcohol in relation to sexual response.

Some people believe that marijuana acts like an aphrodisiac but this is not the case. Kolodny[10] reported that men and women marijuana users did not increase their sexual desire but experienced an increased sense of touch and greater degree of relaxation. Long-term marijuana users show a high incidence of impotence according to Kolodny.

Heroin and morphine have a marked inhibiting effect on sexuality in both men and women.

Cocaine and LSD are associated with sexually enhancing effects but not enough evidence is available. In any case, where addiction occurs sexual drive will be reduced. An interesting effect of some of these drugs is that the patient thinks certain things are going on, like producing a good erection, when in fact this is not the case.

Hormone investigation

Many male clients, especially those from Asian countries, would like the cause of their sexual disorder to be hormonal. They understand that an imbalance of hormones can easily be corrected and rather than consider surgery or sex therapy they see an injection or pills as an easy remedy.

Unfortunately for such clients, few suffer from hormonal disturbances. However, most physicians like to organise blood tests for sex hormone levels for men with erectile dysfunction, impaired sexual interest or ejaculatory failure. It has long been hoped that even where no deficiency exists, the prescription of an excess would increase sexual performance and interest.

Sometimes women on the pill complain about low sexual interest and a change of pill can be effective, otherwise they could come off it and try some other means of contraception.

PSYCHOLOGICAL DYSFUNCTION

The majority of clients need to be referred because of psychological dysfunction.

(1) Bad habits

Sexual behaviour once learned becomes established in the form of a habit – a sequence of events, which is, in a way, almost automatic. In the sexual act appropriate foreplay leads to sexual excitement which leads to intercourse which leads to orgasm. The step from excitement to orgasm may depend on a series of acts which, however often repeated, still produce the same results. A useful habit has been learned. When a woman either does not want to respond or is not given the necessary pleasure to respond, a sequence of acts during intercourse may lead to no orgasm – and this can develop into a habit.

Here the bad habit consists in not responding with orgasm. Some men have the bad habit of premature ejaculation.

Clients are often referred simply because of such bad habits but this might seem too simplistic an approach. The good thing about bad habits, however, is that they can be replaced by appropriate behaviour which can be learned.

(2) Fear and anxiety

Clients are often referred because they have a fear of sex. The woman with dyspareunia or vaginismus is afraid of pain in the vagina, usually associated with the penis but this often generalises to the finger. The partner of such a woman is afraid of hurting her and this often makes him anxious, causing premature ejaculation outside her and loss of his erection, thus making penetration impossible.

Sometimes there may be a direct link between some sexual event which was punished and anxiety. Sexual intercourse for the first time is fraught with anxiety especially for the male in our culture. Perhaps initially he was nervous; maybe there was a chance that discovery was likely or possible; perhaps the noise of intercourse may have been obvious and felt as embarrassing; perhaps he was ridiculed to 'get on with it'; perhaps he was having to perform in front of his 'gang'. Any of these situations could produce anxiety with resulting loss of erection or premature ejaculation. Later on, sex can be connected with anxiety and a similar pattern of losing an erection or coming too quickly results.

Fortunately, anxiety and fear are easy emotions to replace with relaxation and pleasurable feelings provided by successful sex therapy, which usually involves an initial ban on sexual foreplay and intercourse.

(3) Upbringing

Many clients are referred because of strict upbringing over sexual matters. The character and personality of the mother or father will largely determine the attitude towards sex which pervades in the home. Parents with an inhibited and guilty attitude towards sex will react quite differently from parents who are unashamed and free. Some parents punish their children from an early age if they are seen touching the genitals.

Parents also act as a sexual model for children while they are learning about sex. The child watches how the parents behave towards each other, how loving and affectionate they are, how they embrace, how embarrassed they are.

Children also learn about gender roles from their parents. Girls who have seen their mothers dominated and exploited may find it difficult to assert themselves in the sexual situation in later life. Boys, on the contrary, may develop selfish attitudes towards sex.

Sometimes traumatic early sexual experiences might result in a referral for sex therapy as this has conditioned anxiety and fear in sexual situations. Surprisingly many clients have been involved in incestuous situations in which they were terrorised 'not to tell'. Not all children are badly affected, however, and some clients when reporting past events refer to 'the man in the park' with humour, even though he might have been the local exhibitionist and regarded as dangerous by adults.

Sex education is part of upbringing and in homes with a repressive sexual atmosphere the child's natural curiosity may be stifled. Simple questions about birth and sexual activity may be avoided or turned aside with inevitable harm. Such a child may enter adolescence quite unprepared and ignorant. Parents, of course, are not the only influence. Farrell[11] has pointed out that children receive most sexual information from their peers. Some children have learned about sex through dirty jokes; no wonder so many sexual fallacies exist.

Sex education in schools varies enormously. Some schools include information about sexual relationships, contraception and abortion in the curriculum, but these schools are rare. Fortunately many such attitudes are changing and future generations will be better informed. However, ignorance about sexual matters can lead to the need for referral as it has led to sexual dysfunction, especially ignorance about orgasms in women. The clitoris is like some forbidden fruit for many women and men.

(4) Particular experiences leading to referral

Sometimes the first sexual experience can be traumatic but usually the person will go on to try other experiences and find another sexual partner. Non-consummation of a marriage, on the other hand, leads the couple to seek help.

Childbirth can be a time when problems come to the surface as sometimes a woman's sexual interest decreases mainly due to fatigue and stress. Her partner gets frustrated and puts pressure on her to have sex. Several therapists have noticed that this pattern tends to occur after the birth of the second baby, especially when the gap between the first and second child is small.

Some women feel depressed about their body image after childbirth, they feel sore and have probably examined their episiotomy scar in a mirror and were shocked. Also, the frequently reported decrease in vaginal lubrication does not help.

Infidelity might occur at this or at some other time and can cause depression in the partner, leading to a loss of interest in sex. The unfaithful partner might feel little sexual interest in his or her regular partner and this could result in guilt as often sex with the new partner is better than with the established partner. Eventually, if the old partners get together again there may well be recrimination on the part of the one who was let down, who also may have lost sexual interest in the unfaithful partner. or perhaps has sought revenge by having an affair with someone else who has turned out to be more satisfying in any case.

The relationship itself might easily go wrong for other reasons. Communication could be a problem. If there is a discrepancy between the sexual interest of partners and the couple fail to discuss this sexual jealousy could develop and the sexually interested partner may accuse the other of having an affair. Perhaps one partner fails to tell the other about pain and this results in sexual avoidance.

Chloe and Ray: A case of poor communication

Chloe had reached the stage of the menopause and was worried about her sexual response. She felt that at 47 she should still respond normally but felt awful during sex. Her vagina felt sore and she failed to get an orgasm even by masturbating if Ray was with her. Friends at work had mentioned a clinic for hormone replacement therapy but she had laughed that off, thinking she could not take time off from her computer job. Chloe thought it could not be the change of life as she still had very occasional periods, but the gap between them had widened considerably.

Ray did not know what was going on. He was quite a fit and athletic man and had aged well for his 51 years. He still had a healthy sex drive but found that Chloe ceased to initiate sex and he began to think there could be something wrong with him. He had enjoyed occasional affairs with women in the office where he worked but had never told Chloe about them. He had always been quite jealous of her interaction with men in the computer world but as far as he knew she had remained faithful to him.

At first Ray noticed that when they had foreplay she no longer wanted him to stimulate her clitoris and this made him suspicious as he has always done that to her previously and she had appreciated it. Later he noticed that her vagina had become less well lubricated. He said nothing and thought she must have another man.

The atmosphere at home became worse, with many quarrels over trivial matters. The whole thing came to a climax when Chloe was made redundant. That night she crashed the car and was taken to casualty. During convalescence she became friends with another woman patient who told her about the sex clinic at the hospital.

Chloe managed to get a referral and the therapist immediately realised how badly the couple communicated their fears. She had hormone replacement therapy and they built up a better relationship and learned to talk about doubts they had.

Sexual assault

The last and most unpleasant experience leading to referral is sexual assault or rape. Usually the victim of rape is dealt with sympathetically but this is not always so in some societies where the victim is ostracised and the husband refuses to have anything to do with her. Usually in countries where there are rape crisis centres there is a good support system and an understanding attitude.

Some clients have reported a sexual phobia after being raped. They avoid touching and sexual activity with a partner, but masturbate and want affection. Others have simply decreased their sexual interest.

Obviously, the quicker the referral is made the better it is for the woman. Some of them may have suffered humiliating experiences in reporting the incident to the police and feel dirty and ashamed. When referred, such women need to talk about the actual rape experience and the investigation and become desensitised to stimuli involving both these events. They need to be desensitised to being touched and taking part in foreplay activities.

Sexually transmitted diseases

Another type of referral is made through clinics specialising in sexually transmitted diseases. The clients referred have usually been treated but have remained anxious or phobic although they have been cleared by the clinic and there is nothing wrong with them.

Awkward situations can arise for clients living together when the diagnosis is made if they have been with other partners and want to keep this a secret. Hiding such information can lead to tension in the relationship as the other partner becomes suspicious because sex is avoided during treatment and there is usually no explanation for this. When treatment is over and they can have sex there is tension and guilt to be dealt with. Even if both partners know about the diagnosis and have been treated together there is stress.

Other illnesses

Various physical illnesses or operations can lead to referral for sex therapy. Probably the most common operation which may lead to sexual difficulties is a prostatectomy. This can often cause retrograde ejaculation. Sometimes erectile dysfunction can follow the more radical perineal prostatectomy. But it is the psychological reaction to the operation that is really important. Often the surgeon says nothing about sexual performance after the operation; the patient is anxious that his potency might be affected and is even more anxious when he attempts intercourse later with his partner. Maybe something will go wrong? He almost wills a 'performance anxiety state' on himself and probably will lose his erection. He then gets referred to a sex therapy clinic but if the surgeon had given him some confidence and reassurance he would have been perfectly all right.

A heart attack can lead to sexual problems.

Mr X: Sexual phobia after a heart attack

Mr X is a surgeon in his late fifties who had a heart attack when he was at his lover's residence. He did not want his wife to know about his affair and there were various complications over arrangements made to take him to hospital. He was very anxious about the whole business especially as he was familiar with the Japanese study of men having heart attacks when they are being unfaithful. He had suffered a lot of guilt in any case over his affair and his religious beliefs were quite strong. He knew that his wife did not want sex and probably would not stop him from having a mistress but he did not want to spell it out and avoided telling her.

The irony of the situation was that when he recovered from his heart attack he was worried about having sex again with his mistress and persuaded his wife to come for sex therapy. She was willing to attend but not at all interested in the homework. When she confided to the therapist that she would much rather he found someone to have an affair with, the therapist decided to discuss this with him. Mr X could hardly believe that she had actually said this.

During the next session the topic of an affair was deliberately brought up by the therapist and Mrs X repeated her words. She said she felt too old to have sex and that she would be relieved if he could find a girlfriend. She looked her age, admittedly, but her clothes were strict and tailored and her grey hair was scraped back into a chignon which made her look like a spinster. She emphasised that she would not want him to get emotionally involved with such a woman and leave home, nor would she want him to have children with such a woman. He agreed with her terms and they decided to discuss the conditions at home before they gave up the sex therapy.

Mrs X phoned the therapist and said she would not be attending the clinic any longer but suggested that Mr X should report back. What finally happened was that Mr X returned for therapy with the woman he had been making love to when he had suffered the heart attack. Interestingly, she was only a year younger than Mrs X but looked at least twenty years younger. She was lively and attractive. Her tinted auburn hair hung loosely around her shoulders giving her quite a voluptuous look. Mr X found her very attractive sexually but associated her with his heart attack.

Therapy took place and he was reassured and desensitised. It was suggested that they should make love in the woman above position as this would not tire him too much. He was also attending a gymnasium and getting fit and he had reduced weight.

Therapy worked well in this new position which had no previous associations for him and he lost his phobia.

A stroke can produce similar anxiety or fears, especially if this results in paraplegia and occurred when sexual intercourse was taking place. Such men are suitable clients for sex therapy as they can be re-educated about suitable sexual positions. Hawton[1] points out that approximately half do not resume sexual relationships and that dominant hemisphere lesions may often cause impaired sexual interest. Obviously, some men who have had strokes respond to sex therapy based on desensitisation and relaxation and go on to sexual intercourse, finding that the woman above position is the most relaxing and rewarding position. Some men prefer to make a choice of successful mutual masturbation with an understanding partner.

The Indian man who was shot in the back

Accidents can occur in which lesions of the spinal cord cause erectile dysfunction and failure of ejaculation. An Indian man of 34 attended the clinic with his wife. He had been shot in the back five years before, when they had been married for six months only. They were bitterly disappointed that they were not able to have sex and children. When his wife was on holiday in England she read about sex therapy for paraplegics and electro-ejaculation for infertile men.

This Indian lady of 26 came to the clinic and she was extremely gentle and kind; when she talked about not having children tears came into her eyes. It seemed that children were her main ambition. When her frustration was discussed it became apparent that she masturbated and felt guilty that she was excluding her husband. She explained that she had a healthy sexual appetite, but that in India such matters were not discussed with the man. She had never mentioned this to him and he had never referred to sex since he had had the shooting accident and told her that his doctor had informed him that he would no longer be able to perform.

When the therapist suggested that they did some massage together he immediately became very worried, remarking that his wife might get aroused and that would be unfair. The possibility of masturbation at a later date was discussed and he said he had not thought of this before.

By the time electro-ejaculation was carried out the couple were quite relaxed about the procedure and she was ready, standing by to receive the phial of sperm. They now have three much wanted children and are very happy.

Referring accident victims with spinal injuries to a sex therapist can often help individuals and couples a great deal. It is good for a nurse or doctor to discuss sexual matters with such patients immediately after the accident. They can explain to men with complete cord lesions who have recovered from the initial phase of 'spinal shock' that some reflex erection is to be expected, providing that the sacral segments of the cord are not destroyed. Bancroft[7] points out that psychic erections are more likely to continue with lower lesions, and with incomplete rather than with complete lesions, although usually they are also associated with reflexive responses. On the whole, women with spinal injuries seem to fare better than men in re-establishing good sexual relationships.

Too many people are unimaginative and conventional in their attitude towards sex, thinking that sexual intercourse is the main aim and that there are no substitutes.

References

1. Hawton, Keith. (1985) *Sex Therapy*. Oxford University Press.
2. Heisler, J. (1983) *Sexual Therapy in the National Marriage Guidance Council*. MGC, Rugby.
3. Crowe, M.J., Gillan, P.W. and Golombok, S. (1981) 'Form and content in the conjoint treatment of sexual dysfunction, a controlled study'. *Behav.Res. and Ther*. 19,47–54.
4. McCulloch, D.K., Campbell, I.W., Wu, F.C., Prescott, R.J. and Clarke, B.F. (1980) 'The prevalence of diabetic impotence'. *Diabetologia*. 18, 279–83.
5. Karacan, I, Salis, P.J., Thornby, J.I. and Williams, R.L. (1976) 'The ontogeny of nocturnal penile tumescence'. *Waking & Sleeping*. I. 27–44.
6. Ebbehoi, J. and Wagner, G. (1979) 'Insufficient penile erection due to abnormal drainage of cavernous bodies'. *Urology*. 13. 507–10.
7. Bancroft, John. (1983) *Human Sexuality and its Problems*. Churchill Livingstone.
8. Wagner, G. and Semmens, J.P. (1981) 'Effect of estrogen on vaginal function in menopausal women'. Paper at *5th World Congress of Sexology*, Jerusalem. June.
9. Whitelaw, G.P. and Smithwick, R.H. (1951) 'Some secondary effects of sympathectomy, with particular reference to disturbance of sexual function'. *New England Jrn. of Medine*. 245. 121–130.
10. Kolodny, R.C., Masters, W.H. and Johnson, V.E. (1979) *Textbook of Sexual Medicine*. Little, Brown & Co. Boston.
11. Farrell, Christine. (1978) *My Mother Said …* Routledge & Kegan Paul.

Chapter 4

Taking a Case History

Ideally, by the time clients arrive at the clinic they should have been adequately screened for all the problems referred to in the last chapter. This is, however, rarely the case in the UK, so the therapist should always be on the look out for clues leading to non-psychological diagnoses.

Before clients attend a clinic they will usually have been sent a short questionnaire to fill in about themselves. This is quite a good introduction to the questions they will be asked in the clinic and is the first step in the sex therapy saga. By the time they arrive in the therapist's office they will probably have been anxiously waiting in a hall full of other clients. Sometimes, in a general psychiatric out-patients clinic, they may have been accosted by the occasional dement, which obviously can be quite disturbing. Masters and Johnson's clients and most other American clients have usually had the luxury of privacy and isolation when waiting for assessment and therapy.

Initial assessment

Initially the therapist should explain to the client that the treatment of sexual disorders is in the nature of a contract between the client and the therapist. Before such a contract can be agreed upon, the client or couple must know what is offered and the therapist must have a clear idea of the problem and symptoms. It is also useful to have some idea of causal factors and how these will influence the client's attitude to therapy.

The complete account of the problem; the story of the relationships which have been made; the current relationship, if there is an on-going commitment; the attitudes and personalities of the client and partner; the life style; details of leisure and work; enrichment of the senses and fantasy life. These are all important elements and together constitute the client's history.

In the case of couples therapy there are really two partly overlapping histories to consider: the personal history of each partner and the history of the relationship, be it marriage or otherwise. The partners should always be interviewed separately to allow for confidentiality. This confidentiality might be related to uncomplimentary facts about the partner, affairs or guilt about sexual development and experience before marriage. The therapist should be reassuring about confidentiality:

THERAPIST: 'When I see each of you in turn I will of course want to ask you some private things about yourselves that maybe you have never told each other and would not wish to discuss together. I will, of course, respect your wishes throughout therapy and not reveal anything to either of you that you do not wish to be known.'

Before beginning the assessment the therapist should explain its aims to the client or partners. It is also a good idea to reassure the client that no sexual behaviour is expected in the clinic, that any recommended sexual tasks will be carried out at home.

THERAPIST: 'The idea of this assessment is to get an idea of your personality, background and how you have developed sexually. By the way, in case you are worried about this being a sex clinic and having to do something sexual in front of me, please forget about that. Nothing of this nature will happen here; all the work involving sexual tasks will be given as homework.'

Usually the client or partners look relieved when given this information. Later on clients have often admitted that they had all sorts of strange ideas about what goes on in sex clinics and how they might be expected to have sex with the therapist.

Usually the therapist sees the partner who sought help first. If co-therapists are working together they usually see the same sexed partner first as this is usually easier.

The benefits of this arrangement appear obvious. Both clients may find it easier to discuss embarrassing matters with someone of their own sex. Women may initially prefer to talk about masturbation and orgasm with another woman who has shared such intimate problems, and similarly, men may find wet dreams and masturbation methods easier to describe with another man. Then each partner has an interview with the other co-therapist to assess briefly the other partner's reactions and attitudes towards each other and their relationship. When the 'changeover' takes place, the potentially embarrassing material, the difficult admissions, have hopefully already been made and the material is available for the second encounter. A general description of the sexual problem is obviously the first thing to be assessed. Clients may wrongly label themselves as abnormal, perhaps claiming they are impotent because they cannot obtain another erection one hour after ejaculating. It is essential to find out exactly what the client means when he or she initially presents a 'labelled disorder'.

Communication

All therapists should be familiar with the sexual vocabulary in current use and that of previous generations. It goes without saying that therapists should not show embarrassment when hearing the common colloquialisms such as 'screw' or 'fuck'; nor should they show surprise if some words are not understood. If the client looks blank, the term should be explained or a synonym used: for example, masturbation may be better understood as self-stimulation, self-relief, wanking, tossing- or jerking-off, or the pejorative 'self-abuse'. Of course, colloquial terms are often imprecise and couples may be uncomfortable using them in a clinical setting. On the whole it is easier to teach clients the medical terms, to provide common ground for therapy so that therapists and clients can communicate more effectively.

If the inexperienced therapist finds it difficult to take a case history initially, some role play with an experienced therapist or other trainees is useful for desensitisation and gaining confidence.

Communication with the client also provides a lot of non-verbal information. The client's demeanour is revealing, whether he or she is confident and assertive or uncertain and timid. The way in which he or she looks at the therapist will also indicate not only social skills and attitudes but also the areas where there is some embarrassment. Many people are embarrassed by discussing their sexual behaviour and they will show this in various ways: their glance may drop; their voice falter; they may become restless; the hands may fidget or be constantly touching their face, nose or lips.

Body language helps to communicate a client's sexual attitudes. The way people sit is probably significant too: some sit bolt upright, suggesting alert preparedness; others lounge with apparent ease;

some cross their legs which may suggest a defensive attitude; others seem unaware of their sexual parts, behaving as though they did not exist; some seem to flaunt their bodies in a manner of challenge. The interview is the time to study and be studied – a two-way communication is taking place.

The client's clothes carry sexual signals associated with emphasis or exposure or the body. The client walks in as a self-advertisement which may proclaim, at a single glance, what might take hours to discover over a telephone. The game of reading people is slightly complicated by those who wear uniforms or very formal dress; but even bankers and politicians manage to find ways of advertising themselves as individuals.

Signs of nervousness should be noted, like sweating. Nervous people may tremble in the hands or in the voice and may blink frequently. Blushing and red mottling of the skin can be common signs of embarrassment and tension, as are dry mouths and lips. Breathing is another 'giveaway' which the nervous person cannot easily conceal.

Anger or suspicion may also produce similar reactions and here the facial expressions will often give the clue. Frowning or an intimidatory gaze may warn of anger. The person who is continually smiling may be signalling that they wish to placate, allure or charm the therapist whom they fear. Therapists have to face the fact that most clients will respond to them as sexual beings and that while they are reading the clients the clients are reading them. Occasionally sexual signals will be exchanged and sexual arousal will occur, but sexual behaviour between clients and therapists is, of course, taboo. However, the therapist must be warm and easy – to put down a client's sexuality is no part of the scheme.

To call the first interview the assessment and history-taking session is only to name its most obvious function. At many points the therapist is already giving therapy by reassurance, by opening up different areas, by demonstrating that certain subjects are not the danger they were supposed to be, by being relaxed about things that cause the client tension. Sometimes the therapist might provide sexual information in response to anxiety expressed about some form of sexual behaviour which is taboo to the client, such as masturbation. Occasionally a client may be so reassured after assessment that he or she might feel that therapy is no longer necessary.

The sexual problem

It is useful to get the client to reveal the nature of the problem.

THERAPIST: 'Can you tell me how the problem began?'

It is also useful for the therapist to see how the problem affects the partner.

THERAPIST: 'Does your partner's problem affect you in any way, or does it make little or no difference to you?'

Allowing the clients to phrase the problem in their own words avoids a kind of 'inquisition' effect in which the therapist fires endless questions. At this stage it is preferable for the partner with the presenting problem to continue the discussion with the therapist while the other partner waits for his or her turn or simultaneously sees the other co-therapist.

Once the client has started to describe how the problem began, a process of desensitisation takes place and it becomes easier to discuss things with a stranger who is warm and permissive and does not pass value judgments. A discussion should take place about how the problem developed and what factors make it worse, like fatigue or stress at work or holidays when sex is expected. Factors which lead to improvement, like masturbating, extended foreplay or viewing sex videos should also be discussed.

The therapist should try to be absolutely clear about the nature of the problem and should also enquire about arousal, orgasm and sexual interest. The same questions should be asked of the partner.

Sexual development

This part of the history is naturally taken in a lot of detail. It should be established first how the client learned the facts of life: were they picked up piecemeal from other children or was some sex education given either by the school or by the parents? What were the attitudes of the family to sex? Was sex discussed in the home? Were the parents affectionate towards each other, towards the client? Were the early sexual associations good or bad; associated with pleasure or guilt?

The age of puberty should be roughly worked out and whether this was the average age for the client's peer group. Attitudes to sexual development should be worked out.

A woman should be asked about the onset of menstruation. How old was she? Was she prepared? Did she understand what was happening? Who told her? Was she frightened or embarrassed? Details should be taken of her early periods: were they painful, frequent or irregular? How did she feel emotionally about her periods – happy that she was a woman and could have children, or just inconvenienced and embarrassed by them?

A man may be asked to describe his early experiences of erection. Did he have wet dreams? How did he feel about it and did he understand at all? Was he punished or made to feel guilt in association with these early experiences?

Clients should be asked how they 'made out' with the opposite sex. Did they have opposite-sexed friends or mainly same-sexed?

All clients should be asked if they were pleased to be the sex they were and also if their parents were pleased. Masculine and feminine attitudes depend to some extent on parental attitudes. Ask what roles they liked in children's games and whether such roles were consonant with their sex. Did they play any sexual games with or without dolls: for example, games relating to babies or love; games involving fantasies of doctors or nurses; sexual games with pets and so on? Were they ever punished for doing this? Did they spend much time dressing up in opposite-sexed clothes or in their parents' underwear?

It is useful to find out details of the family unit in which the client was reared. Find out how old the parents were when the client was born. Are they still alive? What kind of relationship did they have (loving, distant, formal, quarrelsome, warm, and so forth)? Estimate their social circumstances and attitude towards leisure, money and friends. Did the client have brothers and sisters? If so, how did they relate together? Did sex ever come into it? Did the client believe his parents had a good sex life? For some people it is difficult to imagine their parents in sexual activity of any kind, which is probably due to the blanket of silence which they have thrown over the subject.

Ask what the relationship with each parent was like – was it loving and affectionate? Were the parents strict? Ask whether religion was important in the family or at school, and get an idea of the moral values prevailing.

In the next part of the interview masturbation should be brought up. As this is quite a delicate issue, an actual interview will be illustrated.

Ann: the partner of a man with problems

Ann is a 43-year-old housewife; her partner Mark is a 45-year-old carpenter suffering from a combination of premature ejaculation and erectile impotence. Ann has come from quite a poor but very affectionate family but sex was a taboo subject and never discussed at home. Her sister, who was two years older than she, told her about her periods and the facts of life, so she was reasonably prepared for her first period which came at 13, the average age for her friends.

Ann dressed in rather a dull manner, usually wearing rather old-fashioned blouses and skirts. Later on in therapy she surprised the therapists by turning up in a very smart track suit that transformed her. She was quite tense but had so far discussed her sexual development quite readily.

FEMALE THERAPIST: 'When did you find out about masturbation?'
ANN: 'I'm not sure what you mean.'
FEMALE THERAPIST: 'Touching your clitoris. Some people call it "playing with yourself".'
ANN: 'Oh that. My sister told me it was nice to touch yourself down there.'
FEMALE THERAPIST: 'How old were you when your sister told you?'
ANN: 'I can't remember.'
FEMALE THERAPIST: 'Just approximately, was it at the same time or after she told you about your periods?'
ANN: 'After. I think I was about 14 and we shared a bed and I woke up when she was doing it to herself. She told me how to do it but not to tell Mum.'
FEMALE THERAPIST: 'Did you try it?'
ANN: 'Yes.'
FEMALE THERAPIST: 'Did you enjoy it?'
ANN: 'It was all right.'
FEMALE THERAPIST: 'Did you have fantasies?'
ANN: 'What do you mean?'
FEMALE THERAPIST: 'Did you think of exciting things connected with sex or boys when you masturbated?'
ANN: 'No. I don't see why you are asking me these questions. It's Mark who is ill not me.'
FEMALE THERAPIST: 'As you are going to help him get right again it's helpful for us to know how you developed sexually. For example, you said you were a Presbyterian. We have found that many Roman Catholic people feel guilty about sex and need to be reassured.'
ANN: 'Yes, I feel bad that I touched myself down there, it's not right.'
FEMALE THERAPIST: 'Most people regard it as a normal part of sexual development and consider it healthy.'
ANN: 'Really?'
FEMALE THERAPIST: 'When you masturbated initially you shared a bed with your sister. Did you try and keep very still and silent when you masturbated?'

ANN: 'Yes. How do you know that?'
FEMALE THERAPIST: 'Because I have met a lot of women like you who are afraid of being discovered. Did anyone ever catch or punish you for this?'
ANN: 'No. Not then. Later on, Mark caught me once. He woke up and was very angry that I was touching myself down there.'
FEMALE THERAPIST: 'Did you tell him there was nothing wrong with that, it's normal?'
ANN: 'No, because he said I was doing it as he could not do it to me because he's impotent.'
FEMALE THERAPIST: 'How long does it take you to get an orgasm during masturbation?'
ANN: 'I don't do it now, but it takes about 15 minutes or so.'
FEMALE THERAPIST: 'When did you last masturbate?'
ANN: 'About a year ago.'
FEMALE THERAPIST: 'Do you ever use a vibrator or something else?'
ANN: 'No, certainly not.'

Obviously Ann is very uptight about masturbation but she did at least admit to having done it. It is obviously an issue that her husband has objected to. At this stage the therapist thought it worthwhile pursuing the subject of mutual masturbation.

FEMALE THERAPIST: 'Do you and Mark enjoy touching each other or masturbating one another mutually?'
ANN: 'No, we don't do that.'
FEMALE THERAPIST: 'What about foreplay?'
ANN: 'I don't touch him there as he comes too quickly.'
FEMALE THERAPIST: 'Does he touch you?'
ANN: 'No.'
FEMALE THERAPIST: 'Would you like him to?'
ANN: 'I don't know.'

The next step is to enquire about the client's sexual development during adolescence.

FEMALE THERAPIST: 'Did you have much contact with boys when you were about 13 or 14?'
ANN: 'Yes. My brother was a year older than me and he used to bring friends home but they thought they were too important to speak to or play with me.'
FEMALE THERAPIST: 'How old were you when you first kissed?'
ANN: 'I remember that I was 16 and it was Christmas. My first

boyfriend kissed me under the mistletoe at first and we kissed in the kitchen after that. It was nice. I remember it quite well.'
FEMALE THERAPIST: 'What about petting?'
ANN: 'Yes, we did that later. We used to go out every Saturday night. My brother didn't like him but Mum and Dad did.'
FEMALE THERAPIST: 'Did you have an orgasm when you petted?'
ANN: 'No. I was worried someone might find out. I did have once, though, in the country when we were lying in a field and he touched me down below. Later we had sex, but I would not want Mark to know about that. He thought I was a virgin when we married.'
FEMALE THERAPIST: 'Was sex with your boyfriend nice?'
ANN: 'No, it was disappointing; we were rushed and outside and afraid of being caught.'
FEMALE THERAPIST: 'Did it hurt?'
ANN: 'Yes. He didn't mean to be rough but he was clumsy and that made it hurt.'

Sometimes it is useful to pursue whether contact with the opposite sex was easy, frequent, pleasurable or full of anxiety and embarrassment. Obviously, Ann did not want to talk much about her first sexual experience, which was not up to her expectations. However, more information was needed about her progress over sexual intercourse.

FEMALE THERAPIST: 'Did you have other boyfriends later?'
ANN: 'Yes. I had one other boy'
FEMALE THERAPIST: 'Was he romantic and did he also want sex?'
ANN: 'He was romantic and quite sexy too. We courted for a couple of years and sex was good. It didn't hurt with him. I had orgasms; he used to touch me in the right place down below. But I don't want Mark to know; he is very strict about other men.'
FEMALE THERAPIST: 'But Mark must have had some experience with other women before he met you.'
ANN: 'That's all right for men but not for girls, is it?'
FEMALE THERAPIST: 'I don't think like that but we can talk more about that during another session.'

It turned out that Ann had enjoyed sexual intercourse in the missionary position at her boyfriend's house when his parents went away on holiday, but had preferred the foreplay that her boyfriend had been quite skilled at when he took her home after the Saturday night dance and they petted standing up in a dark alley. Otherwise she had not enjoyed any further experience.

For other clients who have had more experience it is useful to find out more about how they reacted to it. Did they talk to their partner about sex during the act? Did their behaviour depart from the entirely conventional? Was the light usually left on? Did they ever have sex in the open? Usually dressed or undressed? Ask either sex how many orgasms were aimed at or obtained. Ann volunteered the information that she had an orgasm only when her friend stimulated her, but some clients need to be asked whether they came to orgasm during penetration alone or was some clitoral stimulation necessary? Did the partner do this, or did she do it herself? Did she consider it permissible?

Either partner may have had several sexual partners. Discuss how sex differed in each relationship. Ask what qualities seemed to attract the client and ask if such qualities still retain their power? Find out if the client had any difficulty in finding partners for sexual or social activity. Were they ever engaged to another person or were they married previously? Describe these relationships. Are there children from a previous marriage?

It turned out that Ann never got engaged to her steady boyfriend.

ANN: 'He moved from our town with his parents. He could have stayed. I was bitterly disappointed and felt let down.'
FEMALE THERAPIST: 'How long did it take you to meet someone else?'
ANN: 'I met Mark at a friend's house a month later.'

Obviously Ann had met Mark on the rebound and had not wanted to let him know she had been let down.

The therapist knew it would probably be difficult to broach the subject of intimacy with a person of the same sex but realised that this must be done as part of the case history.

FEMALE THERAPIST: 'Have you had any sexual contact with another girl or woman?'
ANN: 'Goodness me, no.'
FEMALE THERAPIST: 'Do you ever imagine what it would be like making love with another woman?'
ANN: 'No. I would not want to think about things like that, it would be wrong.'
FEMALE THERAPIST: 'A lot of people are bisexual. Some among them give expression to this entirely natural tendency. It's quite common.'
ANN: 'Well I am not like that.'

Ann was obviously defensive. If she had experienced some homosexual contact it would have been useful to enquire whether her first sexual or genital contact with the same sex involved an older or younger person.

The next part of the interview involves asking about other unusual sexual outlets such as transvestism, exhibitionism and voyeurism, sexual activities that can bring people in conflict with the law.

THERAPIST: 'As a matter of routine I should ask you if you ever get excited by other sexual activities, like exhibitionism, which might be considered illegal?'
ANN: 'You ask some difficult questions. No I haven't. I'd think men would do that more.'
THERAPIST: 'Have you ever been persuaded to have sex against your will, or been sexually assaulted?'
ANN: 'No. My brother played games once with me and stuck his finger inside me, and showed me his thing, but that was all.'
THERAPIST: 'I'd say that was a normal thing to do, part of growing up and exploring one another.'
ANN: 'Do you think so? I've never told anyone about it before. I've always considered it dirty. I'm glad you don't think it wrong.'

Taking a sex history can indeed be therapeutic. People like Ann are not that uncommon, especially if the clinic's catchment area includes many working class people. Working class women are often more permissive in their attitude, however, than working class men.

The current relationship

In this part of the enquiry the nature of relationship and the qualities of the partner can be examined. Usually people are more forthcoming during this part of the interview.

It is useful to ask about the partner's appearance and personality. Ann had known Mark for 24 years, since she was 19. It turned out that Ann was not very attracted to Mark initially, but he was persistent.

FEMALE THERAPIST: 'What attracted you to Mark eventually? What did you like about him?'
ANN: 'He was a kind man.'
FEMALE THERAPIST: 'Is he still like that?'
ANN: 'Yes, he is.'
FEMALE THERAPIST: 'Is there anything you did not like about him at the time you met?'
ANN: 'Yes. I did not like the way he smoked.'
FEMALE THERAPIST: 'Does he still smoke?'

ANN: 'Yes, but not in the house any more.'

Some clients fall in love at first sight and need to be questioned about infatuation. Many couples report the transition from passion and infatuation to a more companionable existence but Ann had always lacked that sort of passion. Other clients, like Ann, are more attracted to the qualities of mind shown by the partner, or to qualities of personality. Opposites can attract at first and grow to dislike the differences between them. It turned out that Mark was the dominant and assertive partner in the marriage and had always been, especially with the children. Mark had always been more confident until Ann came into her own and got a job at a local newsagent where she was respected and looked up to because she was a good organiser. This resulted in an offer of another job leading to another one, until she was running the local grocery store. Mark had slightly changed his attitude to her then. She effectively dealt with a whole range of people and was liked.

Clients should be asked to what degree either of them is anxious, neurotic or insecure? Ann said that sometimes she had headaches but that was on a Sunday when she and Mark were home together all day.

Most therapists find it revealing to go into how much the relationship has changed over sexual matters and personality. Usually partners do not have much opportunity to know each other before settling down together, unless they are already living together. What way have the partners changed during the relationship? Have they remained physically healthy and attractive or not? Have they developed bad habits such as smoking, drinking and gambling? Ann remarked that they had both put on a bit of weight and got breathless if they had to run anywhere as normally they both travelled to work in their own cars.

The nature of the contract between the couple should be enquired into, and whether the partners believe this contract is being observed by them both. Is the contract ever negotiated in any sense? Are they free to alter the agreement if they wish? Contracts vary, of course, but whether within marriage or without, there usually exists a complex of understandings which regulate the behaviour of each partner but which may be broken or disregarded unless regularly redefined.

The sexual relationship

If the details of early sexual behaviour between the couple have not already been elicited they should now be obtained.

Ann described how they had waited until marriage to have sex and had gone on their honeymoon exhausted after their big white wedding. She had actually felt guilty to be married in white but had gone through with it. Mark insisted on doing it on the first night and Ann was quite relieved that he was quite quick as she was tired and unaroused. Mark was always aroused and quick to make love throughout their sexual history; it was only when he started losing his erections that the main problem started. Ann no longer had any expectations of sexual satisfaction; she was resigned to no arousal and no orgasm.

It is essential to sum up the present sexual state of the couple.

FEMALE THERAPIST: 'How often do you make love nowadays?'
ANN: 'About twice a week.'
FEMALE THERAPIST: 'Who takes the initiative usually?'
ANN: 'Mark always does. He certainly would not like me to.'
FEMALE THERAPIST: 'Have you ever tried?'
ANN: 'No.'
FEMALE THERAPIST: 'Do you usually make love at the same time, or expect to do so?'
ANN: 'We make love at night, and always on a Saturday night.'
FEMALE THERAPIST: 'Do you ever make love spontaneously?'
ANN: 'Goodness, no.'
FEMALE THERAPIST: 'Are you usually too busy to make love?'
ANN: 'I suppose you could say that. I make myself busy and he watches the telly.'
FEMALE THERAPIST: 'Where do you usually make love – in bed?'
ANN: 'Of course.'
FEMALE THERAPIST: 'Some people make love in the lounge or elsewhere.'
ANN: 'Well we wouldn't. We do have children, you know.'
FEMALE THERAPIST: 'Do you use a particular position for sexual intercourse?'
ANN: 'Yes. The natural position, you know, with my husband on top.'
FEMALE THERAPIST: 'Do you ever depart from this position?'
ANN: 'No. Mark likes it like that.'
FEMALE THERAPIST: 'What about you?'
ANN: 'It's all the same to me.'

The usual next question the therapist should ask about experimenting with unusual positions was left out as it was obviously out of place. The therapist wondered what sort of foreplay the couple enjoyed:

FEMALE THERAPIST: 'How do you touch one another before you have sexual intercourse? What sort of foreplay do you like?'

ANN: 'If I touch him he comes, even if he is not erect.'
FEMALE THERAPIST: 'What about him touching you?'
ANN: 'He has never been much good at that. I find it easier to get a move on than ask for things.'
FEMALE THERAPIST: 'You must feel very frustrated.'
ANN: 'Not really. I am used to it.'

The next questions about how the partners handled each other and whether this is satisfactory or could be improved were left out for obvious reasons. Questions about asking the partner for special favours were included:

ANN: 'I never ask for special favours. It's not that I'm a shy person. Mark is not very good at making love and I'd rather go without than go through all that.'
FEMALE THERAPIST: 'How would you like to be stimulated?'
ANN: 'Down below, but he is not any good at that. Look, I don't mind, it does not worry me. The sex thing is his problem.'
FEMALE THERAPIST: 'Do you talk to one another during sexual play?'
ANN: 'No, of course not. That's not the time for talking, is it?'
FEMALE THERAPIST: 'Some couples find this arousing.'
ANN: 'Well, I think it's out of place to talk when you are doing it.'
FEMALE THERAPIST: 'Do you ever have oral sex?'
ANN: 'No. It's not very hygienic.'
FEMALE THERAPIST: 'Have you ever tried it?'
ANN: 'No. We would not want to.'

There was little opportunity to explore sex play when Ann was so negative about everything. It was useless asking whether these activities were enjoyable when they were not taking place. The therapist imagined asking Ann the next listed question about fellatio. How does the woman deal with the ejaculate: swallow it; some of it; none of it? The therapist could imagine Ann spitting it out fast. Many therapists find asking about oral sex too intimate at this stage and prefer to leave these questions until oral sex is discussed in therapy. Other therapists prefer to go through all the sexual behaviours; even if they prove very embarrassing this can reveal a lot about the client.

The next questions about the manner of intercourse and the length of time necessary for insertion before orgasm were tricky, as Ann was already showing signs of annoyance. Obviously she did not have orgasms so it would be a waste of time to ask things like: do both of you come to orgasm during intercourse? does one of you come before the other? do you delay your pleasure until your partner has come? how many orgasms do each of you achieve? Instead the therapist tactfully stated:

FEMALE THERAPIST: 'I suppose Mark ejaculates outside you when he is not even erect and that's the end of the lovemaking session.'
ANN: 'That's exactly how it is. He goes to sleep immediately afterwards and snores.'

The questions covering how satisfied and relaxed the client is afterwards had already been answered by Ann. Other female clients would be asked if the male assists the female manually if necessary or whether the couple go on to another round of sexual intercourse. How long after the first? How long may sexual activity continue? Does either partner ever wake the other for sexual purposes and how does the awakened one respond?

In long-standing relationships people have usually established a characteristic sexual or orgasmic frequency; find out what it is. Also, is there any disparity between the needs of each partner? Does it cause conflict? Orgasm frequency may, of course, include orgasm induced by masturbation. Ann was willing to cooperate with Mark for intercourse twice a week, but if she was to choose her ideal frequency she admitted it would be rare, maybe twice a year.

Careful enquiries should be made as to the sexual taste of each partner. One partner may have asked for some activity – perhaps dressing-up or role-playing – and has been rebuffed. This had happened to Mark:

ANN: 'Yes, he once asked me to wear black stockings and suspenders. I felt a real tart and I refused ever to do it again. It disgusted me.'

So much for Ann's statement that Mark was the dominant partner. She called the tune in the bedroom!

FEMALE THERAPIST: 'Is there any sexual activity you have wanted or fantasised, for which you have not dared to ask or which you have been denied?'
ANN: 'I can't think of anything.'
FEMALE THERAPIST: 'Excuse my asking you this – it's a routine question – have either of you had affairs during the marriage?'
ANN: 'No, we have not. It's a happy marriage.'
FEMALE THERAPIST: 'Have you ever been involved in group sex or an orgy or something like that?'

ANN: 'Certainly not. We have always been faithful to one another. Sex is a private thing, you know.'
FEMALE THERAPIST: 'Have you ever tried tying one another up? Some people like bondage.'
ANN: 'I wouldn't go in for anything kinky like that.'

At some point in the discussion of sexuality the nature and occurrence of fantasy should be examined. What is the subject of fantasy? When is the fantasy used? People use fantasy idly – during masturbation and during intercourse. Fantasies which are used during intercourse are sometimes used throughout the act all the way to orgasm. They may be attended to so closely that the partner is forgotten – is this so? Inhibited people rarely tell their partners of their fantasy. Does this particular client to do so? Again, some people have no fantasies at all. This indeed applied to Ann.

FEMALE THERAPIST: 'Do you ever have sexual dreams?'
ANN: 'Yes and they are wrong. Sometimes I dream that one of the young lads at the shop touches me up when I bend over. I think that's wrong.'
FEMALE THERAPIST: 'Most people have forbidden dreams. I wouldn't worry about it.'

Home and social life

At this point it is helpful to find out how the couple get on in the home. How are the household tasks apportioned? In the case of Ann and Mark there was sex role stereotyping as she did most of the household activities and he maintained the garden and the cars. Are the finances discussed and agreed? Does either partner feel any major injustice exists? Ann handled the finances which they both agreed to. How many children are there? Were they planned? Did they agree? If there are none, why? Is the couple trying to have children at present? The therapist should ask carefully about each child and its relationship with each parent. There may be disagreements over the upbringing practice. Parents sometimes use the children as pawns in their own conflicts. Two of Ann and Mark's children lived at home and the eldest daughter had gone to live and work in France, which disappointed the couple as they hardly saw her, except at Christmas and when they visited her.

Contraceptive practices should be investigated, especially if these have caused problems. In any case they should be asked about since a fear of pregnancy or a failure of fertility may underlie some problems. Ann had no worries about pregnancy as she had been fitted with a coil.

The social life of the couple should be discussed. Do they share it with mutual friends? Do they have some social activity which they do alone? Does either insist on always being together every day and evening of the year? Ask whether they are possessive or jealous to any degree. At a party or social event do they keep together? Would they mind if their spouse was flirting with another person or dancing intimately with that person?

ANN: 'I would not stand for that. Mark and I do respect each other's feelings. He is quite jealous of me although I am not the attractive young woman I once was.'

Work should also be discussed and whether the partners are stressed or strained by the amount of work they do. Are they too exhausted to have sex?

Lastly, the couple may have decided to part. Has this been discussed? Does one partner feel trapped? Are there options? Ann wanted to stay married as their non-sexual relationship was happy.

The senses

The last part of the interview is an attempt to assess the sensuality of the couple and how ready they are to respond to sensation in whatever form it may present. What sensations do they commonly seek out? How responsive are they? Estimate their ability to change by finding out how flexible they are.

The female therapist predicted that Ann would not be very aware of her senses, but in fact Ann's sense of smell was highly developed. The male therapist concluded that Mark was very conventional and unemotional. He was surprised when Mark confessed he would like Ann to wear kinky gear.

Many people are not fully aware of the effect of the senses on sexual arousal. Indeed, many people are unaware of the wide range of sexual stimuli which their senses can provide them. The process is probably at its most powerful when the individual is sexually developing and makes the initial association between sexual excitement and whatever event or stimulus happened to be around at the time.

Every person has different switches: the stimulus which turns one person on leaves another indifferent. What is it that arouses the client sexually? Is it touching, caressing, kissing, looking or listening? While some people seem to respond mainly to visual cues, others respond mainly to voices and sounds, others still to warmth and closeness. Each of the senses needs to be explored.

Looking

This is easy to explain to a client who finds it easy to describe what is visually exciting. Particular parts of the body or clothes may be described. Some people prefer colour or pattern to texture, some like diaphanous material or nylon and lace. Black materials with a sheen are very popular. Many people like pictures of the opposite sex – pictures of sexual arousal or sexual activity. Such people would prefer the stimuli to be either alive or at least moving in films. Would the couple like to see a live sex show?

Both men and women occasionaly reveal the anxiety that they become sexually aroused by the sight of a person of the same sex and question whether they are homosexual. They can rest easy; it is quite normal to have a degree of homosexual interest – in fact, the more things there are that turn a person on the luckier they are!

Do the partners watch each other during sexual arousal? Do they like to do so? What excites them most of all? Does one partner like the other to dress in any special way during foreplay or intercourse?

Hearing

The partners should next be questioned about the sounds of sex. Do they like to utter or hear verbal caresses? Do they like to discuss sex as it goes along? Are they switched on by sexual sounds – breathing, sighing, giggling, groaning or screaming? Do the partners allow themselves to be noisy during orgasms? Does this excite them in itself? What sort of voice do they like? What kind of music do they find sexually exciting? Some strong rhythms, particularly drumming, have a sexually arousing effect. Do they listen to music when making love? Some people have reported being carried away making love to Ravel's 'Bolero' or to an Indian evening raga or to reggae or soca music. Ann preferred silence whilst making love but had got turned on in the past by the tango.

Other people find the spoken word very exciting and can get sexually aroused by listening to excerpts from erotic literature or to their partner uttering dirty words. Other people prefer to listen to erotic tapes of people making love.

Many people are stimulated by stories in which there are detailed descriptions of sexual behaviour. They may prefer this to films, because they can use their imagination in a freer way. Perhaps these people prefer to listen to tapes of stories or have their partner read to them? Ann occasionally liked to read sexy stories.

Touch

The sense of touch is much more alive in some than in others, but is often neglected. Women are probably conditioned into being more sensitive to touch than men. Children are less self-conscious than adults and will approach a piece of sculpture in an art gallery and immediately explore it by touching it. The need to be stroked, tickled, held, caressed or massaged during sexual contact is very strong in some people. Partners should be asked how they like to be touched in return. Ann and Mark never massaged one another, although Ann liked to be touched. They never experimented with massaging with creams or lotions.

Certain materials like fur, rubber or satin may be associated with sex. Ann liked the feel of cotton sheets and she associated angora sweaters with sex.

Smell

The sense of smell comes last, though a partner with no sense of smell is unthinkable.

Ann remarked that Mark always took a bath after work but he smelled of cigarette smoke and this was a turn-off. She liked the smell of tweed on a man and generally used perfume herself. Surprisingly, she liked a heavy, intoxicating perfume.

Conditioning can have a powerful influence over scents. A man might, for example, associate a certain scent with a particular woman who jilted him, and this might make him dislike another woman who wore the same perfume. Some clients prefer body odours to perfume. Others are excited by body odours. It is interesting to know whether the specific smells of the genitalia excite clients. Some like them at any time; others not at all; some only when sexually aroused. Do sexual smells disgust the partners?

At the end of this enquiry on sensation the therapist will know how sensual the partners are and whether they need to be taught the pleasures of the senses.

Questionnaires

Most clients dislike filling in questionnaires, but they can form a useful part of the diagnosis and treatment policy.

The trend in the UK has been for questionnaires to be developed for couples. The most effective and best known questionnaire which covers the sexual adjustment of a couple is the GRISS which stands for The Golombok Rust Inventory of Sexual Satisfaction, published by

Windsor, NFER (1985). The GRISS assesses the quality of a sexual relationship and of a person's functioning within it. It is designed for heterosexual couples or individuals who have a current heterosexual relationship. The male and female fill in separate forms and profiles are obtained from these.

The sexual adjustment of the couple is obtained from the scores of the two people and their interaction can be assessed. The questionnaire covers the present state of the relationship.

The blueprint of the GRISS was drawn up by a 'think tank' of sex therapists at The Maudsley Sexual Dysfunction Clinic. They concluded that many factors are involved in a satisfactory sexual relationship. These include motivational, behavioural, attitudinal and communicative aspects as well as specific problems. The questionnaire was standardised using a sample of 88 sex therapy clients from clinics throughout the UK.

The final scales provide scores for impotence, premature ejaculation, vaginismus, anorgasmia, male and female non-sensuality, male and female avoidance, male and female dissatisfaction and non-communication and infrequency.

The GRIMS (The Golombok Rust Inventory of Marital State) assesses the quality of a couple's relationship and is the companion to the GRISS. It provides useful information about the relationship in areas of interests shared and degree of independence; communication; sex; warmth, love and hostility; trust and respect; roles, expectations and goals; decision making; coping with problems and crisis. Questions covering beliefs and understanding, behaviour and attitudes and motivation for change are also included.

These questionnaires are useful for a quick diagnosis and for preliminary screening but a case history should still always be taken, face to face with clients.

Chapter 5

Easy Cases to Treat

Some cases are easier to treat than others. In a clinic where trainee therapists are working it is advisable to get them to work with a suitable client initially so that they get some positive feedback and success. It is obvious that certain characteristics provide a good prognosis: a good marriage apart from sexual disharmony; a stable personality. Research on prognosis also points out that if a client with a problem seeks help almost immediately the prognosis is better than for a long-standing problem.

It is useful for general practitioners to know what type of disorder can be successfully treated in the surgery and what type of client is better sent elsewhere for more specialised therapy. It causes bad morale in a client if he or she has failed in a too simplified type of therapy, only then to be referred elsewhere. The new therapist can be confronted with a sigh and words like: 'Sensate focussing again – that did nothing for us last time'.

Masters and Johnson reported an extremely high success rate for premature ejaculation and for vaginismus. Other therapists in the USA and Europe have not usually achieved as high a degree of success as Masters and Johnson[1] who selected their clients extremely carefully and weeded out any clients with psychiatric symptoms. Measures of success were not objective and there were no controls.

Most therapists would agree that primary anorgasmia is easier to treat than secondary or situational anorgasmia. (Primary anorgasmia is the term used for women who have never experienced an orgasm, whereas situational anorgasmia is when a woman can experience an orgasm only in certain situations as, for instance, when masturbating.) Male clients who have never been potent, on the other hand, are more difficult to help than those who have secondary impotence. Men who have retarded ejaculation are more like women with anorgasmia and they are difficult to treat compared with premature ejaculators.

Premature ejaculation

There is no satisfactory definition of premature ejaculation. It can be described as that condition wherein orgasm and ejaculation persistently occur before or immediately after penetration of the female during coitus. Masters and Johnson consider a man to be a premature ejaculator if he cannot delay ejaculation long enough for his partner to reach orgasm at least 50 per cent of the occasions. This is still an unsatisfactory definition as the woman herself might have a problem, but at least it moves away from the stopwatch concepts which had previously been used.

Kinsey[2] questioned the abnormality of this condition. He stated that in the USA it is usual for males of lower educational levels to try to achieve an orgasm as soon as possible once they have entered their female partner. Upper class males more often attempted to delay orgasm. Rapid ejaculation is also quite normal for young men and control usually develops as age increases. Kinsey went on to say that three-quarters of the males interviewed reached orgasm within 2 minutes after insertion. He examined other mammals in which the male ejaculates almost instantly on intromission and remarked that this is true of man's closest relative among the primates. The chimpanzee takes 20 seconds to effect ejaculation.

Physical causes are probably very rare but should be considered in a man who becomes premature after a history of good ejaculatory control. Helen Kaplan[3] cites cases caused by inflammation of the male urethra or prostate. Again, where there is a loss of urinary or defecatory control of neurological origin, the same may bring about ejaculatory incontinence. This may be found in disseminated sclerosis and other diseases causing degeneration in the central nervous system.

Psychological factors like anxiety and stress can contribute to the cause of premature ejaculation. Performance anxiety is quite a common precipitating factor. Absence from a partner can also be a contributing factor for a man who attempts coitus again after an interval of time. This is a normal reaction. It is only when a man starts to worry about his performance the next time that he psychologically conditions himself into a state of anxiety.

A man with premature ejaculation

This 27-year-old Italian travel agent working in London was keen to have therapy. He had a fairly long history of premature ejaculation which had started when he had visited a prostitute in Naples for his first sexual experience. He had been extremely nervous and she was unsympathetic and in a hurry. He had not explained to her that this was his first time, but in any case it sounded as though it would have made little difference to her.

Mario was extremely presentable, dark and handsome with very lively eyes. It was hardly surprising that he was attractive to women, especially Scandinavian tourists in Italy who appreciated his gentle manner. He hardly conformed to the Italian stereotype of the bottom-pinching male. He found it easy to get women who wanted to go to bed with him but always felt a failure as he considered he was too quick.

Eventually he met a very charming 25-year-old Dutch woman while he was working for a travel agency in Venice. She was a blue-eyed, blonde courier who had a happy and reassuring personality. She spoke fluent Italian and they became engaged much to the envy of all his friends. Little did they know about his premature ejaculation. Ingrid did not complain about it as she asked him to stimulate her clitoris manually.

It is preferable for a couple to attend therapy together but in the case of Mario and Ingrid it was not possible to arrange this initially as she was still working in Venice. She could come over later, however, for a holiday.

It was decided that Mario could start therapy on his own by learning the 'stop-start' technique. He was to masturbate with a dry hand and to stop if he felt aroused. The goal was to last for 15 minutes on three successive occasions. He was also given a relaxation tape to teach himself self-control. When he returned a week later his progress was discussed.

THERAPIST: 'How did you get on with the homework, Mario?'
MARIO: 'Not too well.'
THERAPIST: 'Did you try masturbating three times?'
MARIO: 'No times.'
THERAPIST: 'Did you not understand the homework?'
MARIO: 'I had friends staying so I couldn't do it.'
THERAPIST: 'I thought you lived in quite a big flat. Did you have to share your bedroom, then?'
MARIO: 'No.'

At this stage he looked angry.

THERAPIST: 'Are you angry about it?'
MARIO: 'Yes. I get angry when I try to masturbate. I don't like it; it's not like a man.'
THERAPIST: 'Yes we did talk about that last time and we did agree that masturbation was only a short-term or temporary thing for you to do so as to help you gain control. Did you listen to your tape?'
MARIO: 'No. How can I relax when I feel angry?'
THERAPIST: 'I agree. What about getting a pillow and hitting it hard to start with before you even relax? I can understand your anger, it's quite normal. Let's talk a bit more about your anger now.'

Although premature ejaculation is usually an easy disorder to treat, the present case of Mario started off badly. Mario's reaction to masturbation was unexpected. When his case history was taken he had been quite easy-going and relaxed about having masturbated previously. He had also played down his anger when he had first been premature with the prostitute. He had rather bottled up his emotions which were now coming out in therapy. The therapist's attitude was to remain calm and understanding but to be firm about the necessity of masturbation as a way of helping to solve the problem. At the end of his first session there was a long discussion about his anger.

After five sessions Mario was learning to control his premature ejaculation when he masturbated. He had progressed to the 'wet hand technique' and had passed the test of lasting on three successive occasions. Ingrid was unable to take a holiday in London to help him with the next stage of therapy where he would ask her to masturbate him with a dry hand. Initially the therapist was rather suspicious and thought he was perhaps avoiding this part of therapy but he phoned the next week to postpone his next appointment as he had managed to arrange a trip to Venice.

When he returned to London after his trip which had lasted two weeks his angry look had returned.

MARIO: 'You are not going to be too pleased with me. I broke the rule of no coitus and did it with Ingrid.'
THERAPIST: 'Yes. I expect from what you have told me before that you find her very attractive and like being with her and couldn't help it.'
MARIO: 'Yes. You don't look angry with me.'
THERAPIST: 'What was it like? How did you get on?'
MARIO: 'It was no good.'

THERAPIST: 'That is hardly surprising as you were only asked to do a limited number of exercises.'
MARIO: 'True. I came more quickly than ever. I came outside and that has happened before once only.'
THERAPIST: 'What was Ingrid's reaction?'
MARIO: 'Oh, she did not mind. She never does.'
THERAPIST: 'That's good. At least she did not blame you.'
MARIO: 'No. I blame myself.'
THERAPIST: 'Let's talk about the exercises you did initially with Ingrid. How did you get on with the dry hand technique when she stimulated you? Could you last out?'
MARIO: 'Oh that. Yes, it was all right. She wanted to do it every night, so we went on to the wet hand technique quite fast.'
THERAPIST: 'That's really good. How did the second lot of homework go, Mario?'
MARIO: 'It was all right. We did it several times.'
THERAPIST: 'But that's fantastic. You have done really well.'
MARIO: 'No. I wanted to come inside her and I did not.'
THERAPIST: 'That's all right. It's easy enough to get that right later. What is important is that you succeeded over the other stages. That's really good. You have done well.'

Here the strategy of therapy was to concentrate on the success that Mario had enjoyed, rather than reprimanding him for breaking the rules and failing.

Mario had another session where future homework was discussed for Ingrid's Easter visit to London. There was then a gap in therapy after which they attended for Mario's sixth session. Ingrid was just as Mario had described her. She was affectionate towards him and sensible. She was relaxed when discussing sex and remarked that she had tried to encourage him to listen to the relaxation tape by actually doing it with him.

When Ingrid was seen for an individual session she brought up Mario's anger when he had failed after breaking the rules. She had calmed him down, but she said it had bothered her that he did not enter her although she had not told him this. She said that she had never obtained an orgasm only by penile thrusting but she did like the feel of an erect penis inside her. She said it was quite easy for her to climax with manual stimulation and that Mario rubbed her clitoris the way she liked it. She also revealed that the only time she had felt annoyed with Mario was when she had first met him and he was trying to control his premature ejaculation by reciting train time tables out loud, during foreplay.

When instructions were given for the next stage, Mario was quite relaxed. Ingrid had been practising the wet hand technique with him and he had not broken the rules. The advantages of the woman above position had been discussed with him and they had rehearsed the position with Ingrid sitting on top of him, without any penile stroking or containment.

MARIO: 'It was nice with Ingrid sitting on top of me. I did not really think of coitus.'
THERAPIST: 'Yes, you told me previously that you always like to have coitus with you lying on top. That is why I want to break previous associations. The next stage involves the wet hand technique for five minutes. Ingrid, for your homework I would like you to stimulate Mario's penis and stop stroking when he says he is getting aroused and wants to stop to have a rest pause for a while.'
INGRID: 'Just like we have been doing, Mario.'
THERAPIST: 'Then, Ingrid, you get on top of Mario. Mario, you lie still. Ingrid, you then put Mario's penis inside you and you both lie still together.'
MARIO: 'What if I ejaculate then?'
THERAPIST: 'You must not think about that; try to relax. You will have learnt to control yourself if you stick to the rules. Try moving a little but as soon as you feel you are getting excited stop and relax. The goal is for you to last 15 minutes stopping and starting; then you are allowed to ejaculate.'
MARIO: 'Okay.'
THERAPIST: 'Is there anything you do not understand, Mario?'
MARIO: 'It's okay, but 15 minutes can be a long time. I'll try.'
THERAPIST: 'Ingrid, are you happy with the instructions?'
IINGRID: 'Yes, they seem quite straightforward.'
THERAPIST: 'Mario, please could you go over exactly what you both have to do.'

The last strategy of getting a client to repeat instructions can be rather tedious but if the client is the rule-breaker type it is better to go over the instructions and clear up any misunderstandings before they go home and do the homework. Mario actually spoke reasonable English but other foreign clients sometimes do not understand everything and are too polite to reveal this.

When they returned a week later they were both delighted that the sessions had worked and Mario could thrust a little and then stop, controlling his ejaculation. They had done this for 15 minutes on several occasions and Mario had been able to last, much to his surprise.

They later experimented with other positions. The most difficult position for Mario to maintain control was the man above position.

Usually the 'stop and start' technique is quite straightforward and most clients respond well to it. If this is not the case the 'squeeze technique' described in the Appendix at the end of the book can be suggested. The 'squeeze technique' is more difficult to carry out and needs the full cooperation of the partner. Most men can train themselves to squeeze the penis. When sexual intercourse becomes possible the upright rear entry position (with the woman kneeling) is the best. This position leaves the hands free to manipulate the penis. The squeeze can be applied either before entry or in the middle of intercourse by a quick withdrawal, squeeze and reinsertion.

Good communication between partners is essential if one has to practise self control during pleasuring. If a partner is resentful, this attitude can be expressed in sabotaging therapy and this would have to be dealt with tactfully in a discussion of attitudes, preferably in an individual session. A number of reasons could be suggested as to why there was such poor cooperation and these could be:

(1) A wish to leave the partner and not to help him.
(2) No desire to give the partner pleasure.
(3) A hostile attitude towards the partner.
(4) Resentment that he never gets it right.
(5) The homework is too anxiety-provoking.
(6) Time is wasted on therapy and homework.
(7) Stroking the penis is 'disgusting' and it's 'dirty' doing that.
(8) It's the partner's own problem so he should be the one having therapy and getting it right on his own.

Many women report that they do not feel confident about stimulating a man's penis and feel embarrassed by such a task. The man needs to provide guidance. Often it is easier to counsel clients who are homosexuals as there is rarely any question of not knowing how to provide satisfactory mutual masturbation. Gay men are rarely worried about something like 'the squeeze' technique as they are not afraid of hurting the penis when they squeeze. Women, on the other hand, see the penis as a much more delicate object.

Primary anorgasmia

The failure to achieve an orgasm can be primary, that is, it has always been impossible to climax, either in intercourse or in masturbation.

Some women do get climaxes in their sleep but might fail to acknowledge this. Other women might experience an actual orgasm, but the contractions are very slight and expectations associated with an orgasm might be totally different to what is experienced. Subsequently they deny having had an orgasm.

There is a small number of women who are totally anorgasmic, ranging from those women who experience low sexual arousal with little or no lubrication to women who get very close to an orgasm but cannot let themselves go to experience it. Most women can achieve an orgasm if they masturbate alone or with a partner's help. Probably 90 per cent of women are orgasmic at some point of their lives. According to the Hite report only 30 per cent of women are ever orgasmic during coitus.

In the old days the word 'frigid' was used to describe a woman with a sexual problem. This is an insulting word which is not used these days; in any case it covered a multitude of disorders like low sexual interest, anorgasmia, and vaginismus and was vague in meaning.

Why are some women anorgasmic? Probably a basic underlying cause is a lack of sex education, but guilt and anxiety spring to mind. Most therapists believe the commonest cause to be psychological, although there is a current belief that slack pubococcygeal muscles may make an orgasm more difficult. Inadequate self-stimulation or that applied by an ignorant or heavy-handed partner is another factor. Strict or repressive upbringing can also be a causative factor. Masters and Johnson reported the influence of religion on many of their cases, in which sex was equated with sin and punishment.

A case of primary anorgasmia

Usually women who have never masturbated before are not difficult to treat once their attitude towards masturbation changes. The breaking of the initial barrier is probably the hardest step in therapy.

Sylvia, a 25-year-old Irish model, was extremely shy about discussing sex. She was Roman Catholic and had attended a convent where no sex education was provided. She was a well-developed girl for the age of 11 when her periods started. She was shocked and upset by the sight of blood on her knickers and thought she must be suffering from some disease. When she told her best friend they both were frightened about the menstrual blood but her friend reported it to a practical nun who reassured Sylvia and provided her with sanitary towels but with no adequate information about growing up.

Sylvia went home for the holidays to a large farm where her father bred racehorses and her mother was busy enjoying the social rounds. They had little time for Sylvia, but her younger brother had all the time in the world for her. He was only a year younger than his exquisite sister but the gods had not been kind to him as he had suffered from polio as a child and this resulted in a misshapen body. He moved slowly and took advantage of his invalid role. The adults did not supect that this pathetic boy was absorbed with sex and Sylvia. The children were left to their own devices and played mother and father games in the fields. Sylvia lost her virginity at the age of 11. Sylvia's guilt was intolerable. She carried her own burden as she felt too ashamed to tell the priest. She was too kind to stop her brother from fondling her as she felt sorry for him and thought he would get into trouble if the adults found out.

The guilt that Sylvia experienced was associated with the pleasant feelings she had when she was caressed. Her brother showed her a book on sex he had bought which both shocked and fascinated her. At least she knew the facts of life at the age of 13 and knew when she got pregnant one year later. Her pregnancy terrified her and she arranged a riding accident for herself to solve the problem. She succeeded in aborting but broke her collar bone. At this stage she confided in the local family doctor. He knew what the awful consequences would be if her parents were informed and instead dealt with the brother, severely threatening him that the parents would be informed if he touched Sylvia again. The doctor also recommended some vacation trips abroad for Sylvia, including visits to a female cousin in Virginia every summer, so there was no time for her little brother to indulge. Her cousin's friend ran a model agency in New York and at the age of 16 Sylvia started a successful career in modelling.

When Sylvia came to the clinic she was happily married to an English businessman and had two beautiful children. She had read an article about orgasm therapy and wanted to know more about it. She had never experienced an orgasm, nor had she masturbated. During the first session we discussed her attitude towards masturbation and she had looked uncomfortable. When she returned the next week she discussed her homework.

SYLVIA: 'It was nice taking the bath. I usually use an oil and I liked taking time putting it on my body.'
THERAPIST: 'What about looking at your genitals in a hand mirror later?'
SYLVIA: 'Yes, I did that but I did not enjoy it.'
THERAPIST: 'The idea was to identify the different parts of your sexual anatomy. Were you able to find your clitoris?'

SYLVIA: 'Yes, but I could not find the glans.'
THERAPIST: 'Did you pull back the hood which covers it?'
SYLVIA: 'No. I could not find it.'
THERAPIST: 'It can be tricky to find. A lot of women are not used to touching themselves in that region and feel anxious. I expect you felt a bit tense.'
SYLVIA: 'Yes, I did. I know we talked about the way I grew up in my last interview and you were very understanding, but I feel sick when I look down there and it's even worse if I touch.'
THERAPIST: 'Obviously, many women need time to do this. There is no rush. I think it would be useful if you used this relaxation tape I have here before you try again, and imagine doing the task in advance of actually doing it. If you feel too tense when you do it, stop and try relaxing again.'

The tactics used were meant to be reassuring. The therapist guessed that Sylvia had not done the homework as she disliked touching herself and this was correct. The therapist went on to show Sylvia some models of female genitalia to desensitise her. Sylvia held the models as she examined them and appeared to be relaxed.

The next homework planned was not too ambitious and involved repeating the instructions. This actually worked well as when she returned a fortnight later she was more relaxed and had successfully touched her genitals for a short time whilst identifying them. We talked about her sexual development and her brother's behaviour as there was still a lot of guilt to deal with in this area. She had never talked with anyone about her guilt about becoming pregnant, let alone deliberately aborting herself. At the end of the session she went away in a happy mood, ready to try touching her clitoris a little longer and using various pressures.

Sylvia returned for her third therapy session looking upset. She had found it difficult to touch herself for a longer period of time. Most of the therapy session involved talking about stimulation.

SYLVIA: 'You did not say it was masturbation.'
THERAPIST: 'I agree that I did not use that word as too many people have bad associations with it. But there is nothing wrong with it. It's a good step to learn about your own sexuality.'
SYLVIA: 'I don't like the idea.'
THERAPIST: 'Nor do a lot of women, but they usually like the feeling when someone else does it. I have asked you to touch yourself so you can get confident before your husband touches you. You also said at

the beginning of therapy that you did not like the idea of anyone touching you down there.'
SYLVIA: 'No, because I think of my brother. You see, I must tell you I did like it and could not stop him and that was wrong.'
THERAPIST: 'It was unfortunate that your brother was the one to initiate you in these things when you were developing sexually. Try and forget about it. It's not that abnormal; it can happen in families and you had a bad time, but try and think of how nice it is when you touch yourself and think of nice things.'
SYLVIA: 'I am willing to try. I want to forget the past.'

Eventually Sylvia became orgasmic after her sixth session. She accepted masturbation and fantasising. It was not difficult to transfer her knowledge to enjoying sex with her husband. She was orgasmic with him during penile thrusting but needed quite a lot of genital stimulation prior to this, which she enjoyed. The first part of therapy had been very difficult but, once her attitude to masturbation changed, therapy was straightforward.

Vaginismus

Vaginismus is a spasm of the perivaginal muscles surrounding the vaginal introitus, making sexual intercourse either impossible or extremely painful. Women with vaginismus are often seen in fertility clinics as they want children but fear penetration. Vaginismus is a dramatic and compelling reason for sex therapy as it is a major cause of marital non-consummation.

Vaginismus may either be primary – that is, there has been no period of normal penetration beforehand – or secondary, in which case it develops in a woman who up to that time was able to allow normal penetration. This secondary development can be described as psychosomatic and could occur after recurrent vaginal infections or as a result of a poorly repaired episiotomy. It can be psychological, resulting from rape or other unpleasant experiences or psychic trauma. The anticipation of pain becomes a conditioned fear response producing the spasm of the perineal muscles whenever penetration is attempted. Careful history-taking will elicit previous dyspareunia.

Most cases of vaginismus are primary in nature and often caused by a repressive sexual upbringing. Obviously such women are difficult to examine physically. The attempt to insert a finger or fingers into the vagina in the usual manner will be almost impossible and certainly inadvisable. The woman may back away and take avoiding action as the finger approaches. When the condition is less severe a finger may be allowed entrance, but encounters an increased resistance. During the examination the woman is usually very anxious.

Most women with vaginismus are phobic about childbirth. They imagine the vagina is very small and the process will cause pain. Whether tampons are used is significant in the diagnosis. If a woman has used or uses tampons, the prognosis is better.

Usually women with vaginismus are interested in sex and they enjoy petting and are orgasmic by clitoral stimulation, but turn off their sexual interest and become phobic when threatened with penetration. Such women are inclined to choose unassertive partners, and often the partner is a premature ejaculator or becomes impotent as well.

An account of a couple in therapy

Jasmin and Ali looked out of place in the hospital waiting room. Jasmin was 22 years old and colourfully dressed in peacock blue Pakistani trousers and a long scarlet and blue tunic. She wore a lot of gold bangles and a pair of long gold earrings. Jasmin looked over-decorated. Ali contrasted with her and looked sombre and old for his 40 years. He was dressed in a dark grey, well cut suit in European style, with a dark grey tie. Their families had arranged the marriage and he had found Jasmin young at 18 but not as beautiful as he would have liked.

The marriage had been arranged by their families back home in Pakistan. Ali had taken leave from his job as an engineer to return to his homeland to find a wife. Jasmin's family approved of Ali and she had been forced to interrupt her art school course where she was studying textile design. She liked the idea of marriage and was promised that she could continue with her studies in England. The Muslim marriage ceremony was impressive and was followed by a sumptuous wedding feast. Associated with this public event was the consummation of the marriage. Of course, this was done in private but the families expected evidence that Jasmin's virginity had been lost. The embarrassing thing was that Jasmin had vaginismus. She actually was a virgin, but the deflowering was not helped by the fact that Ali got over-excited and ejaculated outside her.

The unfortunate couple quickly made a pact to keep silent about their failure as they both thought they would succeed if they were given more time. They told their relatives that all was well and that they were very happy. But time did not heal and when they returned to England the problem persisted for three years. Ali began to get highly anxious when his erections gradually got worse. The expected baby did not arrive to satisfy both their families. Jasmin's father was a heart surgeon and he arranged for her to be seen by a female colleague of his who ran a fertility clinic. When she became hysterical at the clinic and refused to be examined the woman doctor realised the extent of the problem and referred her to the sex clinic.

Jasmin was extremely anxious and the first thing she asked was:

JASMIN: 'Doctor, are you going to examine me now?'
THERAPIST: 'Not today. There is no rush. I will wait until you are ready for an examination.'
ALI: 'Jasmin, you should be pleased that the doctor is a lady. We were worried that the hospital would not arrange this, as we had requested a lady doctor.'
THERAPIST: 'Yes, I believe that is your custom in Pakistan. I will try to make allowances for your culture as much as I can in therapy.'

At this stage they both looked more at ease. Clients from Eastern cultures need the understanding that their culture will be respected[4,5]. Most Eastern men do not like their partner to be interviewed alone with a male therapist, and certainly not to be physically examined by a male doctor. Women who have vaginismus need to be reassured that the physical examination will occur only when she is prepared for it to happen.

Both their case histories were taken. Ali was very much the 'father figure' to Jasmin. When asked about the age gap she did not seem perturbed, explaining that several of her friends had similar arrangements but they had become pregnant. She liked him physically and thought he was good-looking and kind. He never forced her to do anything she did not want to do and was consistently considerate. Ali's consideration came out when we discussed penetration:

ALI: 'I would not want to hurt her. She is very young, only 22. Pain is a terrible thing isn't it?'
THERAPIST: 'How far have you got in penetrating Jasmin?'
ALI: 'Not too far.'
THERAPIST: 'Can you insert your finger?'
ALI: 'Oh no. That would hurt her, wouldn't it?'
THERAPIST: 'Not if you were gentle and did it slowly. How many times have you tried?'
ALI: 'Only twice. You see, she cries with the pain.'

Obviously Jasmin was very much in control of the situation as she had actually stopped her husband from attempting finger insertion which was obviously a step to penile insertion. Her fear of pain was extreme and she revealed that the idea of childbirth was very frightening. Her older sister had suffered and this had upset Jasmin.

The fortunate thing about Jasmin was that although she refused any penetration she was quite happy for Ali to stimulate her clitoris and touch her. Apparently, she provided him with a very satisfying massage and then he masturbated to a climax. They enjoyed a lot of kissing and affection. Their non-sexual relationship was good and, contrary to many Eastern husbands, Ali encouraged his wife to attend an art college where she was doing well, almost ready to graduate and get a job. Although he was well off he liked the idea of his wife working at something she enjoyed.

The first therapy session was quite helpful for both Jasmin and Ali. They learned to relax deeply together and then individual therapy was given to each of them. As Jasmin seemed to be the least relaxed she was seen first and a discussion took place about the idea she had of what a vagina is actually like:

THERAPIST: 'Jasmin, pretend you are a mini-person only one inch high and you are climbing up a woman's thigh like a mountaineer, climbing up towards the vagina. What can you see?'
JASMIN (initially she giggled): 'I can see a lot of black hair – it's thick and rough. Now I am going further into this sort of forest and its cold and dark. I have come to a strong door of a vault that is padlocked.'
THERAPIST: 'That is a very good description. Is it wet or dry inside?'
JASMIN: 'It's wet but I can't see. I don't think I like it.'

This fantasy exercise acts as a trigger for the expression of attitudes and feelings. Obviously Jasmine disliked her trip. It was interesting the way she saw the vaginal entrance as a padlocked door. This led to a discussion of the PC or pubococcygeal muscles and how she could learn to control the entrance to her vagina by contracting or relaxing these muscles. She agreed that she should practise the PC exercises (see Appendix) during the week. Jasmin suddenly interrupted the session:

JASMIN: 'I suppose you think me very silly, but if you really want to know, I think my vagina is cold, slimy and horrible. I don't like it.'
THERAPIST: 'You don't need to worry about these feelings; you just have bad associations which will gradually change during your therapy. You will, of course, have to do the exercises to change yourself.'

JASMIN: 'But what if I have to put things in myself?'
THERAPIST: 'What do you mean?'
JASMIN: 'One of my friends went to the Family Planning Clinic and was given a glass penis to put inside herself to be stretched.'
THERAPIST: 'Yes, some people have that sort of therapy. But the therapy here is based on your own resources. When you come to the stage where are ready for it you can learn to put your own finger inside your vagina. There is no need to use artificial things like dilators.'
JASMIN: 'Is that what they are called?'
THERAPIST: 'Yes, but it is not going to apply to you. Does that make you feel any happier?'
JASMIN: 'Yes, thank you.'

Obviously Jasmin had been worried about what was expected of her and she revealed her fear. Usually such matters are discussed at a later session, but she needed reassurance at this stage.

Ali was more relaxed and said he was pleased the therapist was female as he would not have liked to have told a male doctor about his impotence. It turned out that he felt his masculinity was suffering as he valued his erections. He became so worried about hurting Jasmin that his sexual interest waned during foreplay. He said the initial problem was that of premature ejaculation and when the homework for the 'stop start method' was described he was eager to attempt this. He asked a relevant question:

ALI: 'I suppose there is no injection available to help me?'
THERAPIST:: 'Not really. It would be nice if an aphrodisiac pill were available to produce an instant erection.'

Many clients from the Middle or Far East request an injection to solve their problem. They do not like an explanation that the cause of the problem is psychological as they consider an organic cause to be more acceptable.

The couple then had a joint session and the homework was discussed. Very limited homework was outlined initially so that they could be sure to succeed. They were asked to put a ban on any attempt at sexual intercourse, which was a relief to Jasmin as she had feared that perhaps she might be forced to have sex. Relaxing together daily and some non-sexual massage was recommended. They appeared to be happy about things and it was pleasant to see Ali put his arm around Jasmin when they left the consulting room.

When they returned a week later they had relaxed together and enjoyed some massage. Their individual homework was discussed in private. Ali had carried out the dry hand technique of the 'stop start method' effectively. Jasmin had practised her PC exercises.

JASMIN: 'I must say I find it easier to squeeze those PC muscles than to relax there.'
THERAPIST: 'That is quite normal. You see, you have built up anxious associations there which are connected with tension. I would like you to try practising them several times a day. Whenever you have a drink of tea or coffee, squeeze and relax them.'
JASMIN: 'I think my vagina is very tight, like a clam.'
THERAPIST: 'Maybe the entrance to it is. You must have realised when you have a sexual massage that you lubricate when you get aroused.'
JASMIN: 'I would only get wet when I know Ali is not going to try to put his finger inside me and I can enjoy him touching my clitoris. I do trust him.'
THERAPIST: 'That is good. I am pleased that you can become excited and that Ali can also ejaculate this way.'
JASMIN: 'That is something I was meaning to ask you. Could I get pregnant when he comes outside of me, when he is on top of me?'
THERAPIST: 'Yes, it would be unusual but it has happened to some people.'
JASMIN: 'I do not really want to get pregnant just yet. You see, I am afraid of the pain.'
THERAPIST: 'There are ways of having painless childbirth, you know. Women nowadays do not have to go through natural childbirth if they do not want do.'

It was useful to pick up this reaction from Jasmin at this stage of therapy, although she had mentioned pain and childbirth earlier on. It meant that at the next stage of the couple's therapy a sexual massage was recommended for homework in which Ali would be asked to sit on the bed, with his head resting on the bed head. Jasmin could stimulate his penis and control where the sperm went. This policy actually worked later and she was relaxed about it.

A physical examination is advisable at a fairly early stage or when the woman has learned to relax her PC muscles. When the therapist is medically qualified this can be done easily as trust has built up. If the therapist needs a colleague to carry out the examination it is a good idea for the therapist to be in the room to establish confidence in the procedure. Jasmin's physical examination was given by an understanding female colleague who took a lot of time to relax her. She explained to Jasmin that this was not a full examination and all she would do would be to put one finger inside her using KY jelly. During the first half hour only two-thirds of a finger could be inserted, then Jasmin relaxed more and allowed the doctor to insert the full length of her finger. Ali was requested to do the same thing under supervision and Jasmin accepted this. They were both thrilled. They were asked to practise this daily at home and given some KY jelly.

The KY jelly was an important factor in the success of finger penetration. They had not used KY jelly previously and Jasmin was able to use it when she inserted her own fingers and later even explored her vagina.

The main problem during their therapy turned out to be Ali's poor erections. When they reached the seventh session it was necessary to cross-examine Jasmin tactfully and individually to make sure she was not sabotaging the therapy as she was afraid of penile penetration.

THERAPIST: 'You do not seem to enjoy touching Ali's penis these days.'
JASMIN: 'It's all right.'
THERAPIST: 'Do you think about penetration and Ali putting his penis inside you?'
JASMIN: 'Sometimes.'
THERAPIST: 'Are you worried it will hurt?
JASMIN: 'Yes, it can get quite large.'
THERAPIST: 'Is that why you don't want to stimulate him?'
JASMIN: 'Yes.'
THERAPIST: 'I know you said you did not like the idea of glass dilators, but we do have a special plastic dilator in the clinic which is not so bad. Perhaps you could try inserting that when you are on your own and relax deeply, keeping it inside you for one hour.'
JASMIN: 'Yes. Can I have a look at it first?'
THERAPIST: 'Of course.'

This arrangement worked well as preparation for penile insertion. Jasmin was more willing to stimulate Ali. Eventually sexual intercourse did take place in the woman above position under her control. She revealed the fact that she hated the idea of being pinned down by him in the missionary position. She had requested that Ali should wear a sheath and he found this difficult but accepted her terms. Occasionally Ali lost erections but was generally potent.

Although the last part of therapy consisted of reassuring Jasmin about childbirth she remained apprehensive about the whole idea and the pain she associated with it. Therapy was terminated after eleven sessions and they were both pleased with results.

Two years later they telephoned from Pakistan to announce the birth of their son delivered by a caesarean. Everyone was delighted and this included their families who had pressurised them to reproduce. Often Eastern and African families impose much more pressure on childless couples than European families do. It is useful to be fully aware of some of the cultural influences in relationships and marriages, especially religious attitudes.

On analysis, Jasmin's vaginismus problem was complicated by her interaction with Ali. She was all right working on PC muscle control and relaxation on her own, but she was afraid of losing control over the situation when Ali became potent. This can often happen in cases of vaginismus. It seems that such women almost deliberately select passive and compliant partners. If things change too much the woman becomes threatened.

References

1. Masters, W.H. and Johnson, V.E. (1970) *Human Sexual Inadequacy.* Churchill.
2. Kinsey, A.C. *et al.* (1953) *Sexual Behaviour in the Human Male.* Saunders.
3. Kaplan, H.S. *The New Sex Therapy.* (1974) Brunner-Mazel, New York.
4. Littlewood, R. and Lipsedge, M. (1982) *Aliens and Alienists.* Penguin.
5. D'Ardenne, Patricia. (1986) 'Sexual dysfunction in a transcultural setting'. *Sexual and Marital Therapy.* Vol. 1. 23–34.

Chapter 6

Difficult Cases to Treat

Problems associated with erectile dysfunction can be difficult to treat. Sometimes seemingly easy cases of premature ejaculation start out as being simple when referred. However, by the time the client has been on a clinic waiting list for several months, complications like erectile failure during penetration may develop. Ali is a good example of how complications can occur with premature ejaculation when there is some impotence as well. At the opposite end of the ejaculation continuum is delayed ejaculation and this is difficult to treat, although the man may remain erect for hours on end.

Curiously, women who complain about pain are usually relatively easy to treat, once they have learned to relax and forget bad associations. Women's orgasmic problems can be difficult to treat in association with a partner. It is easy enough for most women to climax with masturbation; it is when they want to transfer their knowledge and confidence to sharing an orgasm with a partner that some difficult can occur.

Often a partner can complicate the issue if the non-sexual relationship is unstable. This can happen with either the male or female partner. Marital difficulties can make people very aggressive during therapy, especially if one partner blames the other for the problem and does not want to attend therapy to help or be supportive. In this type of case the relationship needs to be examined and this can increase the time that therapy takes.

Some people argue that it is easier not to treat each individual partner rather than the couple. Sex is usually a joint activity if there is a partner so it is preferable to give conjoint therapy. Single people can be more difficult to treat.

Situational orgasmic dysfunction

In the early days of sex therapy most of the women with orgasmic problems were divided into those women who had never experienced orgasms and those who could climax by masturbation but not with their partner. Nowadays referrals mainly consist of these latter, situationally anorgasmic, women. The other group of women who had never experienced an orgasm probably have been helped by their general practitioners or women's groups. Women's magazines provide a lot of information about arousal and several books are available. Sometimes women who have read *Becoming Orgasmic* by Julia Heiman and the LoPiccolos[1] have been able to succeed in carrying out stimulation tasks on their own, but when they get to the last part of the book where sharing with partner tasks are recommended they are confronted with difficulties.

Another group of women in this category are those who can masturbate with their partner present, indeed with penile containment, but they want a 'no hands orgasm'. They desperately want the type of orgasm they read about that other women obtain through their partner's penile thrusting, without simultaneous manual stimulation. In the early days of sex therapy these women would be encouraged to try to achieve this, but nowadays most therapists would inform such a client that she should learn to accept the situation but she could try some additional techniques to achieve an orgasm from intercourse alone. The ideal most women would probably like to achieve is an orgasm by intercourse alone, at least part of the time. According to a *Forum* magazine questionnaire for readers, only one-fifth of women in the survey found they could obtain an orgasm without clitoral stimulation, while three-fifths needed vaginal plus manual stimulation.

Few epidemiological surveys have been carried out to show the incidence of anorgasmia. The Hite Report[2] did reveal that only 30 per cent of American women are ever orgasmic during intercourse.

Situational orgasmic dysfunction does not imply low sexual interest or poor response. The woman normally responds sexually with normal responses as far as the plateau phase. Her difficulty may be solely the inability to succeed with orgasm, despite every effort, during which she is both excited and lubricated. After much effort she may become sore, embarrassed or fed-up and desist. Maybe her partner has climaxed and he cannot continue for another half hour. This leaves her to face a lengthy 'resolution phase' in a state of unrelieved sexual tension. Of course, she would be advised by a sex therapist to masturbate at this stage but some women would say that this would defeat the purpose and they prefer to tolerate the painful effect of building up unrelieved sexual tension.

Sometimes the cause of this difficulty to let go is related to an inhibited personality with a lot of self-control. Such a woman might think she would look silly or make a fool of herself by urinating or fainting whilst climaxing in front of a partner. Often there are relationship difficulties. Sex can become a power game for some couples and this can be related to the provision of adequate stimulation. Most therapists believe the cause to be frequently psychological. These psychological causes can result from a strict upbringing and poor sex education.

Occasionally the dysfunction may be related to serious illness or the action of drugs – particularly those used for depression or anxiety. Some women ascribe their difficulty to the contraceptive pill which may well alter sexual responses. There is a current belief that after childbirth slack PC muscles may make orgasm more difficult.

A case of situational anorgasmia

Leila, a 42-year-old Egyptian television researcher, came to the clinic on her own. She explained:

LEILA: 'I did not want my husband to attend. I see my problem of not achieving an orgasm with him as one I would like to solve on my own. In any case, he considers me dominant and over-emotional.'
THERAPIST: 'Do you consider that is the case?'
LEILA: 'I suppose I am dominant, because I was a feminist early on in Egypt. That was before I met him. The strange thing is that he wanted a liberated university woman. He is an archaeologist and quite academic.'
THERAPIST: 'Did your family approve of the marriage?'
LEILA: 'Yes. Of course, it was not arranged. Neither of us would have tolerated that sort of situation but, oddly enough, Ahmed is just the sort of man my mother would have chosen for me. I don't think his family would have chosen me though.'
THERAPIST: 'How did you meet?'
LEILA: 'It was very romantic, at a place called Abu Simbel where some magnificent statues were being raised to avoid the flooding of the Nile. I was involved in a TV programme and had to research some of his work.'
THERAPIST: 'Was it love at first sight?'
LEILA: 'I liked the way he talked and his personality. Physically he did

not look the strong outdoor type who would be good at a 'dig'; he looked more like an academic. You know, glasses and all. I don't rate my appearance as fantastic but that's going back twenty years and I had youth on my side then.'

The above account shows that Leila expressed herself well considering it was the first assessment interview. She did not appear to be inhibited.

Further conversation with Leila revealed that her two children had grown up and now that she had more time to herself she wanted to achieve an orgasm with Ahmed. Sometimes establishing how much stimulation a partner provides is hard to discuss or describe, but this was not so with Leila:

THERAPIST: 'Do you consider that Ahmed makes love in the way you want him to?'
LEILA: 'Yes. He is quite sensual. He knows how I like to be massaged and masturbated. Initially he had trouble finding my clitoral glans, but he soon got used to pulling the hood back and touching me in the right place. He read some sex books and after that he varied the pressure and aroused me.'
THERAPIST: 'Do you ever have a climax during foreplay with Ahmed touching you?'
LEILA: 'I don't think I could get quite excited enough. I can only really climax when I masturbate. I used to feel quite guilty about that once but I got used to it. The main trouble started when I started affairs at 18 at university in Paris. I used to try sex with different boys, hoping to get a climax, but I never did. I got a bad reputation for a quick turnover of boyfriends. I was labelled a flirt, and that worried me until I joined women's lib and realised that I had freedom of choice. It is my body and I have the choice to do what I like with it.'

The above interview, when analysed, shows that Leila enjoyed talking about sex and appeared to be quite mature over discussing her high turnover of boyfriends and admitting some initial guilt. She seemed confident about asking Ahmed for stimulation.

Leila talked a lot during sessions and was quite clever over preventing Ahmed from attending therapy. Homework which included Ahmed had to be done by remote control and he was given the instructions by Leila who appeared to enjoy stage-managing the situation. Homework tasks were given where she was asked to fantasise, to see whether her difficulty lay in fantasising. Her fantasies were always most interesting and she had no difficulty over this task. She could have written excellent scripts for erotic movies.

One of the characteristics of women with situational anorgasmia is that they cannot let themselves go sufficiently during intercourse to tip over into orgasm. One method of helping a woman to do this is to ask her to practise exaggerating her movements before and during orgasm when alone and later to transfer the activity to a partner situation. Leila could effectively let herself go either alone or with Ahmed. When asked to exaggerate some of the sounds and movements she made just before orgasm whilst masturbating she had no difficulty, nor did she find this inhibiting to do in Ahmed's presence. They had to play a cassette tape in the background to prevent the people in the next door flat from hearing.

Other American techniques were used in which Ahmed provided intense clitoral stimulation before he started more vigorous penile thrusting. The surprising thing about Ahmed is that he was given all these instructions and was remarkably compliant and potent throughout. He had excellent control, according to Leila. She had reached a stage in therapy where some discussion with Ahmed was essential. The need to get Ahmed to attend was handled as delicately as possible:

THERAPIST: 'We have now gone through seven sessions and I feel progress is slow. It would help me a lot to discuss things with you and Ahmed.'
LEILA: 'No. I don't like that idea. I told you that the first and fourth time I saw you.'
THERAPIST: 'What a pity that you will be unable to make further progress.'
LEILA: 'I do not want Ahmed to interfere with my therapy.'
THERAPIST: 'The thing is that I cannot recommend any more homework without discussing some points with the two of you.'
LEILA: 'That is unacceptable to me.'

The above dialogue was rapidly becoming almost like a battle between patient and therapist which is a bad policy. At this point some therapists would terminate the therapy but there are some alternatives:

THERAPIST: 'I would be sorry to terminate therapy when I think things can still change. Would it be possible for me to write to Ahmed or phone him?'
LEILA: 'Why?'

THERAPIST: 'Perhaps he has certain hang-ups himself and maybe he is unaware of them but they are turning you off.'
LEILA: 'That could be possible, but I don't think that is the case. He would like me to shave off my pubic hair and I have tried that but I find it unpleasant.'
THERAPIST: 'What about bringing him along next week?'
LEILA: 'Would you be seeing him on his own?'
THERAPIST: 'I have not yet decided. No, I shall see you both together.'
LEILA: 'All right. I shall ask him, but I'm not sure he will agree to come here.'

Leila did not seem keen that Ahmed should spend time on his own with the therapist. This could have been because she disliked being discussed behind her back or possibly because she was jealous.

Ahmed accompanied Leila to the next session and the tension between them was obvious. Each was equally dominant and they were competing in a power game. At 45 Ahmed looked much older than Leila as he was overweight. He talked a lot and competed with Leila, but the same applied to her. Ahmed did appear to be sincere and keen to help Leila. The bombshell was dropped by Ahmed early on in the session when he announced:

AHMED: 'Of course, Leila is quite a jealous woman. She is suspicious of me most of the time. Did she tell you of my affair? She has never forgiven me for that, have you darling?'
LEILA: 'No, we have not spent too much time discussing you and your affair. It's not very interesting or relevant.'
THERAPIST: 'I thought it would be useful if we talked about some of the things you could do together.'

In a few minutes Ahmed had provided some extremely useful information which provided the key to Leila's reluctance to include him in therapy. She had never mentioned his affair; indeed, when her case history was taken she had remarked that neither of them had affairs. Although Ahmed's announcement of the affair was of great interest the therapist deliberately appeared to attach little importance to it, so as not to embarrass Leila and draw attention to the fact that Leila had not even disclosed this affair.

Seeing the couple together made the therapist realise that better communication and harmony between them needed to take place before they could enjoy sex. After half an hour's discussion a strategy of trying to get them to please each other non-sexually and do something positive was put into action. It was clear that they needed some marital therapy and contract therapy was the answer.

Often clients find it difficult to think of a positive task they would like to request of one another, but this was not the case with Leila and Ahmed:

LEILA: 'When I return home from the office Ahmed is surly. I feel he is not pleased to see me.'
AHMED: 'No, because I have usually waited so long. I would like her to come home earlier.'
LEILA: 'I do try to.'
AHMED: 'It does not seem so to me. It's usually after 8 pm almost every night, apart from Friday and the weekend. That's one of the reasons I had an affair; I was lonely.'
LEILA: 'Oh come on, Ahmed, it's the meal that you really want.'
THERAPIST: 'I suppose you must get hungry and angry.'
LEILA: 'He should cook something himself.'
AHMED: 'I do not know how to. I have tried and the pie got burned.'
THERAPIST: 'If you could cook something quickly and easily, like in a microwave oven, Ahmed, would that be easier?'
AHMED: 'What a good idea!'
THERAPIST: 'Would you be more pleased to see Leila then? Would it reduce your anger?'
AHMED: 'Yes, but I would still like her to return one hour earlier.'
THERAPIST: 'Could you manage that two nights only, Leila?'
LEILA: 'Yes, if I worked longer the other two nights. At least we could have two pleasant dinners together during the week. I could use the microwave oven myself when I am late. Would you be pleased to see me under those conditions, Ahmed?'
AHMED: 'Yes, darling. Do you recommend a particular microwave oven that does not burn things, Doctor?'

The above dialogue illustrates how tasks can be arranged amicably. The therapist suggested a compromise, with Leila returning home earlier half the time, and she was mature enough to agree to this. She went along with the microwave idea and was even willing to adapt it to her requirements. It was now Ahmed's turn to make his request.

THERAPIST: 'We must not forget that Ahmed has agreed to cooking two meals a week for himself. If you also are more welcoming towards Leila when she returns home is there anything you would request of her?'
AHMED: 'You mean when she returns home?'

THERAPIST: 'Either then or at any time.'
AHMED: 'Yes, it's her smoking that I dislike, especially when we make love. I would like her to stop smoking.'
THERAPIST: 'That is really like a negative request for stopping something. Could you try to rephrase it in a positive way?'
AHMED: 'When we make love, darling, could you use a mouth wash?'
LEILA: 'That really makes me laugh. You've never made out it was that bad before.'
AHMED: 'Maybe you did not listen.'

The tasks were agreed to and no sexual homework was given for the week. When they returned the next week they were more composed and pleased with themselves, but there was still some tension. They had tried to carry out the tasks but Leila had only managed to return home early one evening, although at least she had telephoned to say that she could not make it. If a set task is only half successful it is still advisable for the therapist to be rewarding and praise the client. This also applies to the slightest effort made by the client. Ahmed had bought the microwave and succeeded with it.

Further contract therapy was arranged during the second session that Ahmed attended. Leila wanted Ahmed to welcome some of her feminist friends to the flat when it was her turn to hold the meeting. Reading between the lines, it seemed that he did not like her friends visiting and this was her way of getting him to agree to her holding the meeting in the flat in the first place. Ahmed agreed and in return wanted Leila to meet him occasionally for lunch. They carried out these tasks.

The third therapy session that Ahmed attended was like a 'fireworks session'. Their love-making was discussed and various complaints were aired:

AHMED: 'Leila is so directive.'
LEILA: 'Your stomach is not very attractive, Ahmed.'
AHMED: 'At least I don't smoke and I climax when I want to.'

This type of discussion can be helpful for a while, to get the couple to release their tension, but they can then be channelled into a more positive direction by the therapist:

THERAPIST: 'You have spent 15 minutes discussing negative aspects. Leila, is there anything you like about Ahmed's love-making?'
LEILA: 'Yes. He does touch me nicely.'
THERAPIST: 'Could you tell him that now?'

LEILA: 'Yes, I like the way you touch, Ahmed.'
AHMED: 'Thank you. I like your body, Leila, and the way you use it. You give good oral sex too.'
LEILA: 'I wish I could let go totally when you give me oral sex, as you do it well.'

It is preferable to get the couple to address each other when discussing positive aspects of their sexuality.

Some helpful material came up in the above third session and some sexual tasks were suggested to Ahmed and Leila. She was asked to masturbate herself and almost reach the point of no return, stop and then get Ahmed to stimulate her. They were requested to do this in a dark room and to listen to music of their choice on a cassette tape. This was recommended so there would be some distraction and Leila would not have too much attention focussed on herself.

When they returned for their fourth session together Leila had not been able to get an orgasm with Ahmed touching her and she was disappointed:

LEILA: 'It does not work. It almost does, but each time Ahmed touches me I immediately lose the sensation I have when I do it. This happened on three separate occasions and in the end I did something I regret. I actually masturbated myself as I felt so frustrated.'
THERAPIST: 'There is nothing wrong with that. It's quite normal. Do you think Ahmed objects?'
LEILA: 'It's not what I want. It's not perfect. I must be an idealist.'
AHMED: 'Your standards are too high, darling. I don't mind.'
LEILA: 'I do.'
THERAPIST: 'Let's try an experiment for your homework. Half the time I would like you to continue the previous homework but if you do not get a climax with Ahmed, continue masturbating yourself and climax that way. The rest of the time I would like you to try to use a vibrator. I suggest that you hold the vibrator, Ahmed, and when Leila stops stimulating herself you use the vibrator on her clitoris.'
AHMED: 'I am prepared to try anything, but we haven't got a vibrator.'
LEILA: 'That's no problem. I have seen them at the drug store.'

The therapist was surprised at how willing they both were to try something like a vibrator, as many couples resist this idea. However, both Leila and Ahmed were quite scientific in their approach to therapy. The more surprising thing is that although she was not achieving her ideal orgasm she did manage to climax with him present. We later discussed that and they mentioned the fact that they thought their relationship had improved. They spent more time massaging than quarrelling. Ahmed had even made Leila a surprise microwave dinner.

When they returned a week later the vibrator plan had succeeded. This was a big step in therapy as Ahmed had applied the vibrator and she had climaxed. They were both pleased, but Leila still wanted to climax naturally with him inside her. They were instructed to try intercourse and for Ahmed to use the vibrator simultaneously. This worked, but Leila felt she was becoming dependent on the vibrator.

They had a break in therapy when they visited their relatives in Alexandria. During that month they experimented further and Leila found she could get a powerful climax if she stimulated herself at the same time as Ahmed thrusted. She declared this was not ideal but somehow it did not matter so much any more. Therapy was terminated. After a six months' follow-up, the situation was found to have remained the same, and Leila still had not achieved a no-hands orgasm.

Leila and Ahmed had been a difficult couple to treat. Although her goal was not achieved, they ended up having a more satisfactory and realistic sex life. Obviously the marital contract therapy was an essential ingredient in teaching them to enjoy one another's company more and to be less dominant. Leila's attitude towards sex changed and sex was no longer a power struggle between them.

Erectile dysfunction

The word impotence, meaning a lack of power, has now been changed to erectile dysfunction. The term really means the persistent inability to obtain and/or maintain an erection sufficient for penetration and conclude sexual intercourse to the satisfaction of the male. Masters and Johnson considered that a failure of erection in 25 per cent of attempts at sexual intercourse constituted a 'persistent inability'.

Secondary erectile dysfunction in which the man has been potent for some time then for some reason becomes impotent is the most common male disorder. Some cases are relatively easy to treat if therapy is provided early on or if the problem is mild and only happens occasionally. It is also easier to treat a man who can penetrate but loses his erection shortly after that stage.

If a man suffers from primary erectile dysfunction and has never had an erection strong enough for penetration this is a rare problem which is difficult to treat and the cause is usually physical. Most men would opt for a penile implant to solve the problem if there was no indication of any erections in an investigation which included spending several nights in a sleep laboratory. Masters and Johnson found only 32 such men over an eleven- year period. If such a man can obtain an erection during masturbation but not with a partner, he is suffering from 'primary situational erectile dysfunction' and the cause is psychological.

Secondary situational erectile dysfunction is common and associated with partner problems. Maybe such a man can get a good erection with his lover but not with his wife. Therapy might be complicated and most therapists would recommend that such a man first finished his relationship with his lover.

It is difficult to assess how common erection problems are in the general population. When *Forum* advertised for impotent volunteers amongst its readers to test a new serum for impotence they received over 3000 replies, although only 100 men were needed for the trial. It is twenty years since Kinsey found it affected one male per 1000 at the age of 20, rising to 26 per 1000 at the age of 45. Most younger men do not require as much penile stimulation as older men in order to become erect.

Most erection problems have a psychological cause. The psychological causes are a complex of personal and socio-cultural effects. Anxiety is probably the most common cause, resulting in negative conditioning. Sexual behaviour or the sexual act becomes associated with some unpleasant anxiety-producing event or events and this association has been learned and incorporated into the mind of the man concerned. Thus, when the need for erection arises, instead of feeling the pleasure of sexual arousal the man feels worried or anxious. Unpleasant emotions inhibit the erection. Anxieties of this kind may be related to multiple unpleasant events which have taken place or are anticipated: a sexually repressive childhood, hostility towards the partner, fear of pregnancy, a fear of disease (especially AIDS), fear of discovery, fear of rejection, fear that erection problems will recur, stress, overwork, a fear of past physical illness recurring like a heart attack, and also a fear of premature ejaculation. One of the strongest fears such a man can have is that his sexual performance may be insufficient to satisfy either internal ideals or the imagined demands of a partner. In erection problems there is a high frequency of 'performance anxiety'.

Negative conditioning provided by a repressive upbringing is probably one of the commonest, most pervasive causes, resulting in the idea that sex is sinful and dirty.

The possibility of organic disease should always, however, be considered before the condition is diagnosed as psychological. An important question will help to make the distinction. Can the man obtain a good erection during masturbation, during dreams, when awakening, or with another partner? If the answer is positive then physical and organic causes can be excluded. When the answer is negative a physical examination is necessary to exclude local causes such as phimosis or deformities of the penis. Various drugs can cause erection problems, like anti-depressants, alcohol or anti-hypertensive drugs.

If the erection problem is due to anxiety it is easy enough to treat by relaxation and desensitisation techniques. A recommended book, *Men and Sex* by B. Zilbergeld[3], makes helpful reading, especially the section on sexual myths. Each sexual myth described by Zilbergeld, like 'a man always wants and is always ready to have sex', can be discussed with the client.

Poor erections due to a lack of sex education, disgust or guilt are relatively easy to treat. Books and videos can be suggested. It is necessary for the therapist to ask questions later about the books recommended, to make sure that the client is actually reading them and is not phobic over such matters. Information and reassurance can be given in a relaxed setting. It is also advisable to make the sessions quite light-hearted and occasional jokes go down well.

Many men report erection problems because they do not get sufficiently aroused, but they are not anxious or guilty. This type of problem is easy enough to treat. More difficult clients are those with partners who are no longer attractive or are in a bad relationship. It is also more difficult to treat a man who wants to be heterosexual but it is only attracted to men.

The case of a man with an erection problem

A single American man with situational erection problems came for therapy. Mark presented problems from the beginning of therapy. As a successful 37-year-old banker, he never had time to attend therapy and used to cancel his appointments. Usually before therapy starts a contract is drawn up so that the client gets an idea of the number of sessions involved and a conception of the types of homework tasks required. Mark was seen for private therapy and happily put his money down for the first half of therapy, but having only attended two out of five sessions he needed a confrontation:

THERAPIST: 'Mark, I am concerned about your attendance rate. It's awful.'
MARK: 'Don't worry. I know I have cancelled visits I've already paid for.'

THERAPIST: 'It's not the money I am worried about – it's the time. When you cancel I can't arrange another appointment and there is a long waiting list.'
MARK: 'Look, I'm sorry, it won't happen again. I really want help.'
THERAPIST: 'Are you sure you really want therapy? You started off all right doing the tactile tasks on your own like massage and masturbation. I notice when it came to suggesting you should share this with a partner you were reluctant last time I saw you. Have you shared the massage?'
MARK: 'No. There was no time. I had to work late and then business contacts came over from New York and I had to entertain them. It would be much easier if I were married and had settled down; at least there would be someone to take their share of the load.'
THERAPIST: 'You have had bad luck over so many broken engagements.'
MARK: 'Yes. If I got my problem sorted out I'd be fine. Once a woman realises I can't get a hard on she rejects me.'

Previously, while his case history was being taken he had rationalised his failure with women as being due to his Jewish background. He had said he was in a 'Catch 22' situation where he only got turned on by gentile girls but his family wanted him to marry a Jewish girl. This new explanation that he was a failure due to his erection appeared to be a new excuse.

The therapist had noticed that when homosexuality was discussed Mark had been quite defensive about this topic and strongly denied any such behaviour. Attraction to other men seemed like a possible explanation of his homework and attendance failure. The subject was delicate, however, and needed to be carefully assessed.

One way of investigating what really arouses a client is to show slides of different sexual situations and people and measure how erect the client is whilst viewing the material. Mark was quite willing to undergo penile plethysmography tests to examine his erection in association with anxiety tests. In the laboratory he only responded to slides of men and became fully erect. After this type of test it was easy to discuss his possible attraction to men:

THERAPIST: 'You had no difficulty over getting erections when you viewed slides of men, but the women left you cold.'
MARK: 'I was aware of that. The fact is that I withheld information from you when you first talked to me,'
THERAPIST: 'That's not unusual. Tell me about things.'
MARK: 'I've never had a male partner. It's too late now with the AIDS

scare. I don't even want to try. I sure feel better now I'm telling you this. I've never been attracted to a woman but I do want to marry and have kids.'
THERAPIST: 'Don't worry. Let's talk about some of the ways of achieving your goals.'
MARK: 'Wait a minute. How normal is my response?'
THERAPIST: 'Many men respond to slides of men but the majority respond to slides of women as well.'

The above revelations were not very surprising to the client or the therapist. The therapist was reassuring and matter-of-fact about the situation and willing to try to help Mark achieve his goals:

THERAPIST: 'Let's be plain about things in your own interest. When you masturbate are your fantasies about men?'
MARK: 'Yes. I told you I did not have many fantasies but I actually do. I imagine seducing bronzed young men on tropical beaches. That makes me really erect.'
THERAPIST: 'Your current woman friend at present is someone you told me you had been dating for several months now.'
MARK: 'Yes. Surprisingly, she is an Orthodox Jewish girl. She does not want sex before marriage so she has not put me to the test.'
THERAPIST: 'Have you got a photo of her?'
MARK: 'No, but I could get one. Why?'
THERAPIST: 'I would like to describe a method of 'orgasmic reconditioning' for you to change your attitude towards her. You masturbate using your regular fantasies and at the point of orgasm switch to looking at her picture.'
MARK: 'That's very cool.'
THERAPIST: 'Yes. The idea is to associate her with an orgasm and pleasure. Then you imagine her earlier on each time you masturbate so you become conditioned to feel sexually aroused by her.'
MARK: 'I'll try anything.'

Remarkably, the above case turned out to be a success. He married his woman friend, whom he never wanted to attend therapy sessions or to know about his real responses.

How to overcome resistance to therapy

Mark's failure to carry out homework and attend therapy sessions was dealt with in a tactful manner, by the therapist trying to find out the cause of this. Resistance often occurs in therapy and difficulties may happen at any stage.

Initial case history forms

The first sign of resistance to therapy may be suspected if a couple fail to return the initial clinic forms that are sent out for them to fill in before they attend. This can result in a reminder letter, but it is a bad sign.

The assessment interview

(1) Attendance failure
Sometimes a client fails to attend the assessment interview or postpones it at the last minute. If a couple have an appointment to attend together one partner might fail to attend. These are bad signs. Some therapists might be tough-minded and say 'too bad', but most therapists would give the couple another chance – maybe telephoning or writing to the mising pair.

(2) Commitment to therapy
Assessment can usually be a good indicator of whether each partner is committed to therapy. Is one partner having an affair that he or she will not suspend for the sake of therapy? Most therapists would not agree to treat the couple if this is the case. Are both partners inconsistently reporting facts, i.e. how frequently they have sexual intercourse or who usually initiates lovemaking? The therapist should discuss this inconsistency of reporting facts. Is one partner complaining that the problem is due to the other partner and he or she should be responsible for therapy? The therapist can explain that sex takes part in a relationship and is the responsibility of both partners.

Resistance early in therapy

(1) Failure to do the homework
Excuses of being too tired or indisposed or too busy to do the homework are common. The therapist should be patient and try to find out why this is happening. If the homework is for the couple to do a massage together and they have failed to do this perhaps the room is too cold, in which case they could have a bath first whilst they heat the room. Maybe the thought of being nude embarrasses them and they could be allowed to wear some clothes initially for their next homework.

(2) Negative experience
Mutual massage can be an excellent indicator of direct sabotage, from 'It's no go – I have not done *that!*' to one partner pouring the massage oil over the other's head. At this stage it is useful for the therapist to have some idea of how tense the couple is and how the partners behave when touching and how anti-massage they are in the clinic setting. The couple should relax and then be asked to hold hands, touch and gently stroke each other's arms. If they fail or refuse to do this at all, this is a therapy 'danger signal' and care needs to be taken to get them to do their massage very gradually at home. Perhaps their next homework task could be for them to sit opposite each other with only their feet touching, drinking a cup of tea.

Other complaints are associated with touch; some clients complain that they feel nothing, others say they are too ticklish. The therapist should get the couple to be more communicative at the time of touching and to tell each other what they like. Feeling ticklish is often a sign of too light pressure during massage.

(3) Aggression
Direct resistance can take place where one partner refuses to do the massage or picks a quarrel just before, and this is easy for the therapist to assess and deal with by making a direct request to carry out the massage during the next week. Indirect resistance is more difficult to deal with: one partner might say the massage was hopeless, and he or she did not like one area to be touched and disliked touching his or her partner, or it was a waste of time as he or she felt nothing. Such a person should be asked which area of the body they do enjoy being touched. Another way of resisting massage is for the unwilling partner to fall asleep, this being an act of passive aggression.

It is essential to assess whether resistance to massage is due to fear or hatred of the partner, and to counteract these fears by systematic desensitisation tasks of partners touching in the presence of the therapist. The therapist should provide time for the couple to air their aggression and ill-feelings about their sex lives. This is a good opportunity to set marital contract therapy tasks for the couple to carry out. Some individual tasks like bathing or massaging the body when alone should be given. This is an excellent way to see if hostility is directed towards the partner or comes from within.

(4) Breaking rules
This is quite common as often couples get so carried away by the non-sexual massage that they indulge in mutual masturbation or have sexual intercourse. The therapist should not be too disciplinarian

about this if it only happens once, but should tell them not to do it again as it can spoil future therapy. If it happens again the therapist should spend more time finding out why one or both partners want to break the rules.

Resistance in the middle of therapy

(1) Resistance to masturbation

Sometimes individuals or couples start off well with the non-sexual homework but once individual masturbation or other tasks are suggested they encounter difficulties. Excuses might be made that it was impossible to find the stimulating parts and no feelings of pleasure were experienced. The therapist should explore further their attitudes towards masturbation and discuss fear, anxiety or disgust over this task and be reassuring and encouraging. The therapist could get the client to look at his or her genitalia in a mirror and check the parts.

(2) Resistance to shared masturbation or genital sensate focussing

This stage can present several difficulties. The male can touch the female's genitals in an unsympathetic way, by being rough or failing to use the correct amount of jelly that she prefers. She can spoil a session by touching his penis uncaringly – after he has shown her exactly how to do it. The therapist should check that the couple have actually understood the instructions and maybe provide a second physical examination for the couple in which they examine each other. A series of explanations should also be offered to the couple to explain their difficulties. If the same problem occurs again the couple could go back a step to non-sexual massage.

(3) Complaints that the homework sessions lack spontaneity

Often one or both clients will say that the homework is too set or formal. This is a common complaint and can be dealt with by the therapist explaining that it is better to know exactly what is going to take place as this can be reassuring. The therapist can also add that in any case when the couple were left to their own devices to be spontaneous they had a problem.

(4) Oral sex difficulties

By the time the oral sex stage has been reached difficulties in therapy should have been smoothed out. Oral sex is usually a good way of bridging mutual manual masturbation and sexual intercourse, but it can lead to anxiety or fear. Many women are apprehensive about fellatio and genuinely worried over gagging, but if some women wanted to sabotage therapy at this stage, this would be an easy time to do it. One way of coping with this objection is for the man to lie on the bed with his hands tied down, so that he is in her power and she can be in full control of oral kissing: he cannot hold her head down and thrust his penis into her mouth. Similarly, the male might need to be desensitised to cunnilingus. The therapist could recommend the spreading of jam or honey over the genitals to make oral sex more palatable. The therapist should show enthusiasm and encouragement.

Difficulties encountered at the later stages of therapy

(1) Heterosexual intercourse

The last therapy stage of sexual intercourse could involve resistance, especially as the first recommended position, the female superior position, is one that some partners find unmasculine. The therapist can discuss the advantages of this position for both partners, emphasising that it reduces the man's anxiety as he does not have to check that he is erect and his partner can guide his penis. The woman can be reassured that she is free to move in this position and not trapped.

Other positions like the 'feel free' position can be recommended as good for manual stimulation of the clitoris if the woman finds this difficult in the 'woman above' position. Some couples like the 'rear entry' position and need reassurance that it is not too animal-like.

(2) Fear of failure

Sometimes clients do very well but towards the end of therapy they might have a relapse and worry that this will happen more often. The therapist should reassure them that this is perfectly normal and they have done well in therapy and now know how to cope with an occasional relapse. They should be told that the more they worry about this the more frequent the relapses will be. It is also relevant to discuss the relationship between stress and relapses.

(3) Terminating therapy

Some clients become too dependent on the therapist and worry about finishing therapy. The therapist should encourage such clients to discuss their fears. Halfway through therapy it is a good idea to assess progress and how much longer therapy might take, and then to repeat this assessment after every third or fourth session. A follow-up of three months should be arranged for all clients, if possible.

Useful therapy techniques

(1) The therapist's attitude

The therapist should be as relaxed and comfortable as possible with sexual terms. A friendly atmosphere should be established, maybe by asking the clients about social or work activities they might have mentioned or by discussing children's progress. Occasional jokes are acceptable as laughter breaks down sexual barriers and anxiety. The therapist should give the clients *permission*; this is usually contrary to their upbringing and other authority figures who have been condemning over sexual matters.

(2) Self-disclosure

This is rather a controversial topic in therapy. Some professionals do not agree to the therapist making any personal comments about his or her attitudes or behaviour. Most therapists, however, would agree that sometimes a quick personal comment can be very effective at the right time.

When a client is anxious about masturbation and asks the therapist if he or she approves of it, it would be perfectly acceptable, for the therapist to admit to having masturbated. It would probably not be acceptable, on the other hand, for a therapist to reveal his or her masturbation techniques. Similarly, sexual intercourse positions can be discussed and a therapist could reassure a client about a position which is causing concern by saying: 'Yes, I enjoy the rear position. It's quite acceptable'. Sometimes a therapist might disclose having personally overcome a sexual problem like situational anorgasmia.

(3) Reassuring clients that their experiences are not abnormal

Sometimes partners who are seen for couple therapy see their experiences as isolated and abnormal and label themselves as freaks. It is often better to see people in a group therapy situation to avoid this stigma. Often gay couples say they feel abnormal attending a sex clinic where the majority of couples are heterosexual. They should be reassured by the therapist that other homosexual couples attend therapy although there are actually fewer such couples in the general population.

Clients often see oral sex as dirty or abnormal and they need to be reassured that it is all right; perhaps some self-disclosure coming from the therapist is advisable. Sometimes a video of sexual activity can be helpful when a client continues feeling anxious about some particular aspect of his sexual experience or behaviour. Seeing someone else talking about such matters or doing them can have a powerful 'modelling effect.'

(4) Role playing

Sometimes telling a client how he or she should cope with certain situations is not enough and it is good for them to rehearse the appropriate dialogue. The therapist could act out a situation in which the client says no to a request from an over-demanding partner, but suggests a massage instead. The client can then role play the situation. Other role playing situations can be helpful when one client is dominant. The therapist can ask the couple to reverse roles so the partners get some feed-back about their behaviour.

(5) Paradoxical intention

Occasionally a suggestion made by the therapist which is the direct opposite of what a client would expect can help to overcome difficulties. A man with an erection problem might be told not to try to get an erection during sexual message, but to aim for enjoyment of the actual massage. A woman with situational anorgasmia might be asked to avoid having an orgasm with her partner. The aim here is to make the woman less goal-oriented and to appreciate foreplay more.

(6) Confrontation

When therapy is unsuccessful for no apparent reason and the couple are doing their homework but reporting failure a confrontation can be useful. The therapist could ask them why they think they are failing. Perhaps additional work is needed on their negative thoughts and attitudes.

Sometimes it is helpful for the therapist to suggest possible explanations. Maybe they need to relabel their responses. A male client might be saying that he feels therapy is failing because he is not getting erect during mutual sexual massage, and the therapist could ask him if he is enjoying the massage and feeling aroused. Also, the partner should be asked about her enjoyment – probably he is manually satisfying her and this is a positive aspect to the therapy. Often clients tend to focus too much on their own responses. Trying to please a partner can be positive and rewarding.

Really difficult clients are easy to spot early on if they do not respond to the above suggestions. Sometimes they are waiting for permission to end their relationship.

References

1. Heiman, Julia, LoPiccolo, Leslie and LoPiccolo, Joseph. (1986) *Becoming Orgasmic: A Sexual Growth Program for Women*. Prentice-Hall International.
2. Hite, Shere. (1976) *The Hite Report*. Dell, New York.
3. Zilbergeld, Bernie. (1980) *Men and Sex*. Souvenir Press.

Chapter 7

Low Sexual Interest

Low sexual interest is recognised by sex therapists as a common problem nowadays. It has taken therapists a long time to agree on the meaning of this term. Academics have argued over the terminology of libido or low sexual interest for many years. Freud referred to the libido and this was later renamed sexual drive or appetite by psychologists. Kaplan called it sexual desire and wrote a book[1] about it. Nowadays all these terms are often used interchangeably.

Whatever the label given to it, the client with low sex interest is the most common referral problem in my surgery. It took a long time for sex therapists to recognise the problem and devise effective techniques to help people who wanted to increase their sexual interest. Masters and Johnson did not even include low sexual interest as a classification of a disorder when they published their new therapy methods book, *Human Sexual Inadequacy*[2] in 1970.

Low sexual interest is not a problem if both partners have the same level of interest and do not want to make love that often. It only becomes a problem if they want children and have sexual intercourse so infrequently that the possibility of pregnancy is low.

Discrepancy in the sexual interest of couples

The most common cases involve one partner having a normal or perhaps high level of sexual interest which does not correspond with the other partner's low sexual interest. This can result in unhappiness and misunderstanding. Usually the goal of therapy is to change the sexual interest of the couple, attempting to increase the low sexual interest of one partner and maybe decrease the sexual interest of the other. This type of compromise is a much fairer deal than focussing attention on changing only one partner.

There are various underlying causes of low sexual interest. A frequently presenting cause is sexual boredom. The couple might have been together for several years and practise the same script every time they make love so that every move becomes predictable. Perhaps one or both partners are seeking sex outside the relationship. Often if one partner is much more highly sexed than the other an affair can result.

Sex outside the relationship can be exciting for many people. There is an element of sexual novelty in an affair. Some people might have regular affairs with a high turnover of new sexual partners, although recently the growing problem of AIDS is having an effect on fidelity. Sex outside a relationship can be high risk sex, not only because of the risk of AIDS. Japanese findings[3] have shown that heart attacks for men are more common in the lover's bed than the domestic bed.

Often, if one partner has a low sexual interest, he or she feels inadequate and imagines the partner having sexual adventures with other people. This can lead to suspicion and paranoia. Suspicion can work the other way around and the partner with the high sexual interest sometimes imagines that the partner has a low sex interest because he or she is too tired to make love at home due to carrying on affairs outside.

An additional cause of the discrepancy of sexual interest between heterosexual partners is biological. Kinsey observed that men reach their sexual peak during late adolescence, whereas women attain their sexual peak in their early forties. Usually older men and younger women become sexual partners and society supports this system, whereas an older woman can be accused of baby-snatching if she partners a young man in his early twenties.

Tact is a much needed quality when interviewing anyone about an affair. Traditional sex therapy for couples used to be conducted with both partners present, but it is preferable to allow for confidentiality when discussing delicate issues that one partner might want to conceal from the other. Some therapists think it is advantageous to bring up the subject of affairs in therapy and let the couple discuss this. I consider it is preferable to allow couples some individual privacy but if one or both admit to an affair and want to discuss it during therapy then this is reasonable.

Most people think that women are always the ones with low sexual interest and that men have a higher sexual interest. This attitude is misleading and is a result of man being labelled the 'hunter and great lover'. Most of the sexual record-holders are men, like Don Juan or Casanova. In reality, just as many men present with low sexual interest as women. This would be expected according to Kinsey's findings, as men reach their sexual peak during late adolescence. However, social attitudes preval that when women become menopausal they quickly lose their sexual interest.

Often couples coming for therapy want to know how abnormal they are and whether other couples exist with similar problems. It is quite in order to talk about the frequency of low sexual interest and couples often want to know whether middle age or old age will affect their sexuality. Again, Kinsey's findings can be discussed and couples can be reassured that it is normal to have sexual intercourse less frequently as age advances.

A discrepancy of sexual interest in couples can be caused by marital problems and it is wise for the therapist to explore this area thoroughly, even though the couple might appear to be happily married.

Profile of a male with low sexual interest

Paul, a 42-year-old stockbroker, was referred for sex therapy as he had a nine-year history of low sexual interest. This affected his 38-year-old wife, Martha, who ran a successful antiques business but felt rejected by her husband.

When Paul first arrived at the clinic he presented a rather unattractive picture. His expensively cut dark grey suit did not hide his paunch. He was obviously overweight but so was Martha, although she disguised this better with her smart tent dresses and eye-catching Victorian jewellery.

Although Paul had been sent away to a school which did not provide any sex education he had been interested in sex and his sisters' female friends in the holidays. His parents had discouraged this healthy attitude and during swimming parties had been very strict over changing arrangements. As he was the only male adolescent present he had become quite self-conscious about his developing genitalia. His father did tell him that sex with girls was immoral and if he got any girl pregnant he would be in big trouble. Paul read up the subject of sexual development and became quite knowledgeable although he associated the subject with anxiety and the fear of getting a girl pregnant.

At university, where he studied economics, there were not enough women to go round but Paul managed to date his sister's friend who was studying fine art at an art school in the same town. His sexual interest was high and they had a good sexual relationship during the term, but sex was not possible at holiday time. During the summer term things were good as they enjoyed sex outdoors when it was warm enough. This happy relationship came to an abrupt end when his girlfriend went to Italy for a year and met and married an Italian.

Paul took quite a long time to get over his first love. He worked hard for his degree and did well. During this time he masturbated once a day to relieve his sexual tension. He had no guilt over this activity and obviously his sexual interest was high. Eventually he got quite a good job on the Stock Exchange, due to his excellent family connections. At this stage of his life he presented an attractive front, as he played tennis well and was a junior partner in an important firm. He did not find it at all difficult to have several affairs with extremely desirable women. He went the usual night club rounds and as a good dancer was popular with the women in his circle.

At the age of 28 he met Martha at a weekend houseparty. It was love at first sight for him. Martha was the niece of one of the partners in the firm and the couple were socially extremely well suited to one another. A good sexual relationship developed and Martha was pleased to relate to Paul. Her only misgiving was that she had met Paul on the rebound. She had previously been engaged to someone who had broken it off and she still liked this man physically more than she was attracted to Paul.

Their wedding was the social event of the year and their honeymoon in Mustique was successful. Sex was good and frequent. Both of them had orgasms and enjoyed each other physically. The relationship was good and Martha enjoyed entertaining. They were keen to have children but this did not happen. For three years they did not worry and then they went to a fertility clinic for advice. They were lucky as Martha became pregnant that same year and gave birth to a much wanted son and heir.

Paul's low sexual interest occurred after the birth of his son. He had tolerated the pressure put upon him to make love during Martha's fertile times but had felt that he was being forced to have sex or used as a stud. He did not want to go through the same procedure again when Martha enthused about having another child. He started to avoid sex and worked longer hours. This coincided with extra work and prestige in any case, as he was made a partner in the firm. Martha felt neglected and took to drinking too much sherry whilst she waited for Paul to come home. Gradually, dining alone during the week became her custom and she would drink over half a bottle of wine, followed by brandy. Eventually food and drink became her main interest and over a period of six years her weight increased.

Paul's low sexual interest was not helped by Martha's appearance. Nor was he a model of male attractiveness. Lunch-time drinking and heavy eating were his pattern and an early evening snack and drink with his colleagues led to further weight problems. He no longer had time to play tennis or dance. Their garden was managed by two gardeners so he did not even have to mow the lawn. He only realised the extent of Martha's drinking when he noticed one night that she had finished a whole bottle of wine. They discussed the drinking problem and Martha dried out at a health farm.

During Martha's convalescence her therapist suggested that she should take up some occupation to interest her and she chose the antiques business as something she already knew well. This proved to be a big success and she flourished financially, but her therapist had failed to curb the eating habits which diminished her sexual attraction and decreased Paul's sexual interest in her even further.

Both Paul and Matha attended for therapy. They were highly motivated as they wanted to live together and have some sort of sex life. They had avoided sexual intercourse for two years. Martha masturbated on her own, but Paul did not have the need to masturbate. When interviewing Paul, several things came to light:

THERAPIST: 'How have you managed to do without sex for so long?'
PAUL: 'I suppose two years is a long time. I have not really missed it as I feel so tired after work.'
THERAPIST: 'What about weekends, you must have more time then?'
PAUL: 'Not really; we socialise a lot, you know.'
THERAPIST: 'Is that your choice?'
PAUL: 'Half and half. Martha likes entertaining and we both combine this with business quite a lot.'
THERAPIST: 'Are there any other reasons why you don't make time for sex?'
PAUL: 'If you want to know, I find Martha gross. She is well groomed and all that but I like a woman with a good figure and when she takes her clothes off she looks a mess.'
THERAPIST: 'Have you told her that?'
PAUL: 'No. It was bad enough when I confronted her about her drinking. She had therapy for that and is moderate in her habits now but she eats more than she ever did.'
THERAPIST: 'Have you ever suggested dieting?'
PAUL: 'Sometimes, but she does nothing about it.'
THERAPIST: 'Are you happy with your weight?'
PAUL: 'No. I've been drinking less at home, but I guess it's the alcohol at work.'
THERAPIST: 'What about dieting?'

PAUL: 'That would be difficult with business lunches and that sort of thing.'
THERAPIST: 'Maybe you could suggest a diet to Martha and you could both eat less at home. Is there any other reason why you don't fancy sex?'
PAUL: 'No.'

The strategies the therapist chose here were quite straightforward. Paul's sexual interest was low but he first rationalised this by making excuses about his work. Admittedly his working hours were too long but he was avoiding the issue of Martha as a sexual stimulus. He was probably being loyal to her and not wanting to blame her, so he needed to be prompted over discussing her sexual appeal. Some therapists would not have persisted in exploring the reasons for Paul's low sexual interest but it is always useful to sound people out about how they appeal to one another physically, especially as some of the initially shared exercises, like massage, involve being in the nude.

Obviously some sort of dieting or the wearing of certain articles of clothing would be helpful before massage therapy was advised. The therapist needs to be tactful in drawing attention to weight problems, and Martha had already commented that Paul was overweight and paunchy but sensitive to criticism. When the therapist brought up the subject Paul was asked if he was satisfied with his weight. This was an approach in which the therapist does not appear to be critical. When it was suggested to Paul that he should go on a diet with Martha, Paul was being put in the 'supportive role' over dieting in order to help *her*.

Later during therapy they both lost weight. Paul took a long time to change his overwork routine and take exercise. He initially objected to spending time on stimulation therapy exercises devised to increase his sexual interest. He said he did not have time to read.

Life style

Many clients do not appreciate that spending time on therapy exercises can enhance their life style. They are willing to attend for therapy but are often not keen to do the exercises which do not interest them.

Paul had a particularly stressful life style. He increased his work load by being physically available during evening hours. He commuted to work by train. This was not particularly stressful as he travelled first class. One of the gardeners doubled up as a chauffeur to transport him to the station which was quite near home. He had never considered walking to the station or taking any exercise. He lived a very unhealthy life and was under pressure at work. The therapist tried to change the situation but it was uphill work.

THERAPIST: 'Could you take a daily break from work and do something physical?'
PAUL: 'Like what?' (He laughed at this point and the therapist smiled.)
THERAPIST: 'Is there a gymnasium in the City?'
PAUL: 'Yes, but it's not exactly near my office.'
THERAPIST: 'How long would it take you to walk there?'
PAUL: 'It's quarter of an hour away. I suppose you are going to suggest I walk it?' (Laughter again.)
THERAPIST: 'Well, it's better to be moving than sitting frustrated in a taxi in a traffic jam. We've talked about stress and you have said that moving about reduces your stress – you don't feel cooped up then.'

Paul's laughter was associated with embarrassment. He did not like the idea of exercise. The therapist was firm and already knew about a gymnasium for businessmen in the City.

Often clients are unaware of their reactions to the stress they are subjected to. Usually they are pleased to learn to relax and put what they have learned about stress management into practice. It is much easier to convince clients that time spent on their health is important. It makes sense to confront them with the idea that better health means better sex. It is more difficult, on the other hand, to try and get clients to spend time to become more sensuous, or even to appreciate their senses.

The following conversation shows what heavy going it can be to persuade someone like Paul to make time for homework.

THERAPIST: 'When you came here initially we talked about your senses and you said you quite enjoyed looking at women.'
PAUL: 'Yes. I remember you asking me if I bought sex magazines. I certainly don't have time for that sort of thing.'
THERAPIST: 'But you did tell me that when you were trying to get Martha pregnant you used to look at pictures in magazines and get quite aroused by them. Do you now associate this type of picture with stress as you had to get an erection and be sexually active for four nights in a row?'
PAUL: 'No, it's not that. It's just that I have no reason for looking at pictures like that nowadays.'
THERAPIST: 'We have been talking about your trying to fantasise as part of the programme related to increasing your sexual interest. Perhaps you could try reading some erotic literature like *Fanny Hill*?'

PAUL: 'I read that at school but it did not do much for me.'
THERAPIST: 'What about a more up-to-date book about women's sexual fantasies? Would you be interested in reading about them?'
PAUL: 'Yes. I might be.'

Paul needed to be more motivated to look at erotic literature or pictures as a homework task. Sometimes clients do not like going into a shop and purchasing magazines. An easy way out is to suggest videos for them to view, but often these are in bad taste. There are not many suitable videos on the market. The ones available are more suitable for showing at stag parties, but some videos like *The Devil in Miss Jones* are artistically presented. Another way of overcoming resistance to homework is to ask the partner with the high sexual interest to purchase the magazines or books and leave them around.

Some therapists tend to be too authoritarian about homework and this can mean that the client stops attending. Allowing a partner to gang up with the therapist to use forceful tactics can be fatal. It is better to be persuasive and use a back-up of research results and science for what the client is being asked to do.

PAUL: 'I don't really know about reading that book, *My Secret Garden*[4]. It sounds a bit unlikely.'
THERAPIST: 'A lot of people have said that they find these fantasies sexually arousing.'
PAUL: 'Yes, but that's like hearing about personal recommendations for some really useless tonic.'
THERAPIST: 'Yes, I also prefer objective experimentation and there are research studies available with plethysmography measuring penile tumescence when reading such stories.'

Another approach the therapist can try is that there are many attractive women in the City and it is not difficult to fantasise about them. That is not going to take much time whilst walking along the street!

It took many more therapy sessions than originally predicted for Paul to change his life style and put time aside for homework that was not directly related to his health.

Trying to help a couple to change their life style is like recommending suitable activities in marital therapy. Often one partner is more perceptive than the other and thinks of all the solutions. It is useful to find out how they both spend their time and what they would both ideally like to do together, apart from trying to engage in sexual activities. Many couples have conflicting interests and it is helpful in therapy to try and find an activity of mutual interest which will bind them together and provide positive reinforcement. Taking up a new sport can be a good thing, as they are both beginners and can progress together.

One activity which many couples enjoy sharing and which enriches their sensuousness is cooking a meal together. The preparation of some curries is an interesting activity with delicious aromas, although the disadvantage for some clients is that it is time-consuming. It could be argued that if something is absorbing then it is good for one's health not to feel that it is necessary to hurry. Chinese and Japanese cookery are also recommended; these are quicker to prepare for people who argue that they have little time. Clients can progress at a later stage to Indian cookery.

Going for a walk can be an enriching experience if it is done in a leisurely manner. Visits to art galleries or museums can be enjoyable. It is worthwhile mentioning to clients that it is nice to revert to courting days when they might have held hands whilst sharing this type of activity.

The last stage of changing the life style is to inform the client how to find time for massage and lovemaking – perhaps to put aside time in the afternoon to have a massage, if they complain of fatigue in the evenings.

The senses: stimulation therapy

Many people are not fully aware of the effect of the senses on sexual interest. Indeed, people like Veronica (see later in this chapter) are quite unaware of the wide range of sexual stimuli which their senses can provide.

Many people are conditioned to respond sexually to certain types of stimuli. The process starts early on and continues through a person's life. It is probably at its most powerful when the individual is sexually developing and makes the initial association between sexual excitement and whatever event or stimulus happened to be around at the crucial moment. This may explain why people respond sexually to a wide range of stimuli, ranging from tribal sex for Veronica to rubber aprons for a male client. These stimuli may vary in their power to evoke a sexual feeling; they may be very slight or have all the power of a fetish.

One method of *stimulation therapy* involves teaching clients how to appreciate their senses. Men are usually slower than women to appreciate touch. It is useful to suggest to clients the sensory qualities they should seek out, like rough/smooth, warm/cold, and hard/soft dimensions. Some clients dislike the feel of vaginal lubricant or sperm. These clients need to be desensitised and a good step on the way to providing the real thing is to get them to break an egg in a bowl, dip their hands in it and rub in the substance.

Human skin is probably the most satisfying object to touch, especially when it is warm and soft. Of course, touching oneself is often not as satisfying as being touched by someone else, but clients report that rubbing themselves with bath or massage oil can be very rewarding.

Some people need to be educated to appreciate the connection between sound and sex. Many clients have not explored the range of music that could arouse them sexually. Some strong rhythms can have a sexually arousing effect. The beat of a primitive drum can lead to frenzied sexual activity among tribes who practise such rituals. Some clients have reported being carried away by making love to Ravel's *Bolero*, others have preferred Indian evening ragas or reggae music[5]. It is a good idea to recommend listening to different types of music if this has not been tried.

Other people find the spoken word very exciting and can get aroused by listening to excerpts from erotic literature. Some cassette tapes available on the market are quite arousing. *Leaves From My Diary*[6] is a tape about a woman who has sexual adventures. Many people are stimulated by stories in which there are detailed descriptions of sexual behaviour.

Some people prefer to listen to erotic tapes of other people making love. *The Sounds of Sex*[7] is a Japanese tape in which a man and woman make love and have few inhibitions. Often sounds made by a partner during lovemaking can be stimulating but the previously passive partner needs to learn to breathe more heavily, sigh, giggle, groan or scream. This can be done by 'modelling' techniques in which the client sees another person doing this on a video and joins in during therapy. The client is then asked to practise this at home. If this is embarrassing and there is concern that neighbours might hear, it is advisable to recommend that the radio could be turned on as well to conceal some of the sounds.

The sense of smell can be one of the neglected senses which can be developed. People vary considerably in this respect, and conditioning has often had a powerful influence. A man might, for example, associate a certain scent with a particular woman who rejected him, and this might make him dislike another woman wearing the same perfume. Similarly, a woman might dislike the smell of Harris Tweed, associated with the jacket of a previous partner.

Recommending a massage oil with a perfume is such a personal thing that it is better for a single client or couple to go to a shop and select their own perfume by the use of perfume testers. Some people like light flowery perfumes, but others prefer heavy, sophisticated perfume. If partners choose a perfume for their massage oil it is essential that they both appreciate it, otherwise it is better to choose a more neutral aroma.

During sexual excitement, sweat glands produce considerable odours which both sexes might find arousing and it would be a pity to disguise these natural odours with perfume. It is advisable to find out what people like. The smell of sweat in a sexual setting can excite some people. The specifically sexual smells of the genitalia can be the most arousing smells and their effect is enhanced by oral sex. On the other hand, some sexual smells can disgust partners and if this is pathological and due to anxiety some desensitisation should be provided.

It is generally agreed that few people find the odour of cigarette smoke attractive. Smoking in the bedroom can be a disagreeable activity, unless both partners are smokers. On the other hand, burning incense can have a delightful effect and can also conceal the smell of stale smoke or cooking smells.

Visual stimulation is often the most obvious of the senses when it comes to sexual arousal. It is not necessary to explain the connection between sex and sight to most people. Some people are more aroused by certain parts of the body. In an English newspaper study it was revealed that women on the whole were turned on by men with slim hips. Men were more or less divided into 'breasts' and 'legs' enthusiasts. Clients should be asked if they find particular parts of the body exciting, and whether they like a partner to be clothed or unclothed, or in transition from one state to the other? Some people like clothes themselves and might enjoy materials like leather or satin. Black materials with a sheen are popular.

Some people need to be more aware of just looking around themselves and appreciating scenery and people. It seems strange to have to tell a client to take a walk in the park on a summer's day and look around and aesthetically and sexually appreciate some of the sunbathers.

Pictures of the opposite or same sex can be sexually arousing. Photographs are usually more powerful than drawings and paintings in terms of sexual arousal. Some people would prefer their sexual stimuli to be alive or at least moving in films. Some people can get sexually stimulated by looking at cricketers or tennis.

Both men and women occasionally reveal anxiety that they might become aroused by the sight of a person of the same sex: for example, a man seeing another man in a film with a rising erection becomes aroused himself and fears he is a homosexual. In fact it is normal to have a degree of homosexual interest and a client should be reassured.

Erotica and pornography

Arguments over the difference between erotica and pornography still prevail. Pornography is easier to define as it originally meant 'licentious writings' which Ancient Greek prostitutes used to read to their clients. Erotica is a poem or art associated with love, with artistic merit. Aesthetic merit is notoriously difficult to judge, but so is pornography. Legally in the UK it is defined as 'that which depraves and corrupts'. One man's meat is another man's poison and some might find a picture disgusting which others would find pleasing and arousing.

As people vary so much the therapist should give some guidance in the form of recommended books, magazines and films. Many people think that women do not respond to erotica. Kinsey, four decades ago, produced evidence that women were turned on only by romantic material, and that arousal by explicitly sexual stimuli was more common among men than women.

In the sixties and seventies, however, a female sexual revolution took place, probably associated with reliable contraception. Women demanded their own erotica and magazines like *Playgirl* and *Viva* were produced. In the eighties such magazines have become unfashionable, partly due to feminist propagandists such as Susan Griffin[8]. The feminists point out that women are used as sex objects and certain parts of their torsos are used in a fragmented form in sex magazines. This is probably true, but there is no reason why men should not complain in the same way when their bodies are used as pin-ups. Men, however, seem to take such things in their stride. Exploitation is another argument used by people like Andrea Dworkin[9]. It is easy to understand that it is wrong to exploit children and animals, but adults do have a choice. (Stimulation therapy does not, therefore, recommend 'kiddy' or 'animal' porn.)

Nowadays a wealth of scientific evidence is available that women do respond to erotica. Initially physiological measurements of sexual arousal were limited to men. Their erections can easily be measured by wearing a small cuff around the penis; this cuff is sensitive to stretching and provides a reliable measure of erections. Women's sexual responses are less obvious and accurate measurement of their sexual responses occurred late in the history of sexology. Vaginal blood flow is the best measure and this is achieved by the insertion of a probe into the vagina which provides a feedback of blood flow through light or heat methods. The therapist is interested in what type of erotic material produces an increase in blood flow for individual clients. Do clients fantasise effectively?

Of course, the whole purpose of providing erotica in therapy is to teach clients how to fantasise effectively and thereby increase their sexual interest. There has been much debate over the type of material used to achieve this. Some European studies show that women get more turned on than men in response to erotic stories. The explanation given is that women have more vivid imaginations. Julie Heiman's studies on Long Island[10] show that if women hear stories in which they initiate sex they are more aroused. In her study she reported that men were also more aroused when women initiated sexual activity.

Gillan and Frith[11], however, reported little difference between English male and female students in response to viewing erotic videos. Neither sex responded as well to stories on cassette tapes. Their research supported other European studies in which the content or type of lovemaking played a significant part. Sexual intercourse in the missionary position was arousing for both sexes but men were more aroused than women by less conventional positions and oral sex.

Stimulation therapy studies carried out by Gillan[12] in London and Rochford showed that clients increase their sexual interest after such therapy. This therapy even worked effectively when women suffering from low sexual interest attended group stimulation therapy with their partners. One finding of interest is that the mode of stimulation was not significant. In the London study, clients were either given auditory or visual stimuli during their therapy. There was no difference in effectiveness between these stimuli and no sex differences either. The clients in the control therapy did not increase their sexual interest. The control therapy consisted of deep relaxation and minimal stimulation. Patients were asked to talk about their sex problems and then an effort was made to steer them away from sex topics and to discuss other non-sexual matters.

The use of erotica in stimulation therapy is well established. This method does help clients increase their sexual fantasies. Some sex clinics have books, slides and videos available for viewing. A recommended list is provided in the Appendix.

Therapy for a woman with low sexual interest

On the whole, women are more aware of their senses, especially touch. In present day society, women have more opportunity to dress in a more colourful and individual manner. This did not apply to Veronica who came for therapy wearing a most drab grey dress with a brown jacket. She would not have looked out of place as governor of a women's prison. She obviously did not need to look elegant at work and it was hardly surprising to learn that she was an entymologist and already distinguished in her field at the age of 36.

When we took her case history and discussed her senses it turned out that nothing aroused her sexually. She seemed to have come from another planet when we brought up the subject of touch; she had never stroked cats or dogs or picked up little children. She had spent most of her teenage years peering through a microscope in her father's laboratory in Africa. Her father was professor of botany in a prestigious African university and he had provided a rigorous research programme for her instead of encouraging her to go to parties and meet youngsters of her own age. Her mother was dead, so she had no-one to guide her in her choice of clothes. In fact, most of her clothes were almost randomly ordered from a catalogue, so she never felt and appreciated the texture of materials in shops. Her younger brother was mainly interested in golf, much to the annoyance of her father who disapproved of such an activity.

Her brother's womanising was even more disturbing to her father. As far as her father was concerned, Veronica was sensible and well-behaved in having no boyfriends.

At the age of 18 Veronica won a scholarship to Cambridge University to the delight of her father who encouraged her to go to Girton. Before she left home he brought up the subject of sex and warned her not to let anyone touch her. She had spent all her adolescence without one kiss on the lips and hardly thought about sex. She remarked that she knew all about masturbation and had tried it but she did not find it particularly wonderful and preferred to study.

Her study record at Cambridge was immaculate. She once brought some pictures from the family album to the clinic and she was evidently pretty in those days. Her double first was expected as was her excellent research for her PhD on the tsetse fly. In a way, she could be described as emotionally cold and calculating over sex. She had put all her energy into her studies so as to achieve her doctorate, but she had decided to try having sex as soon as her thesis was complete. It was not difficult for her to find a partner as clever and attractive women were in very short supply in her world and she had turned down many offers of dates for seven years.

The lucky man who initiated sex with her was a fellow African field worker who had faithfully followed and admired her during their three years of field work on similar subjects. He was very good looking and bright, and had come from a background very different from Veronica's colonial upbringing. His tribe had encouraged him to attend the missionary school and he had progressed rapidly to getting a research post at the local university. His lovemaking had been gentle and considerate and he had not mentioned the strange fact that she was a virgin.

Veronica did not enjoy her first experience and thought that perhaps she felt socially guilt-ridden as her lover was black. She dismissed this idea, but her second partner was white and still unsatisfactory. She analysed the situation and decided to sleep with a woman next when she returned to Cambridge to present her thesis. She considered the possibility that she could be a lesbian, although she was not attracted to women. She did not enjoy sex with a woman either, although she formed her first close relationship with her and decided to remain in the country to be near her woman friend.

Curiously, that was the sum total of her sexual partners. She remarked that she felt like a freak and that she had first thought there could be something hormonally wrong with her, though hormonally everything was satisfactory. She had finally tried taking testosterone and her sexual interest had been a little higher but she was worried about the side effects and was appalled by the growth of some hairs on her chin. It was good to hear her confessing a small degree of vanity.

Stimulation therapy was highly appropriate for Veronica but it took her time to appreciate her senses. The first breakthrough in therapy occurred when she returned to the clinic having been asked to try touching her skin with various materials.

VERONICA: 'Silk certainly has a nice texture compared with cotton. I suppose I like the smooth, warm textures. I tried Vaseline and did not like the cold slimy feeling it produced. I'm surprised I have not experimented before – the nearest thing I ever got to was making mud pies at home.'

THERAPIST: 'You have done well. How did you get on with your body homework?'

VERONICA: 'Initially I felt rather stupid sitting in the bath and massaging myself with bath oil, but after a while I found it quite pleasant. I can see how you are educating me over touch and I appreciate what you are doing. I had no trouble at all when it came to

looking at my genitals in the mirror and naming them. I bought that book by Betty Dodson[13] about masturbation. You said I could read the books later but I should try and get them now. I looked at some of the drawings of other women's genitalia and some of them looked like mine. I find the range of genitalia interesting.'
THERAPIST: 'Did you read what Betty said about masturbation?'
VERONICA: 'Yes. I still don't think it is very effective for me. I wish it was, as I feel I am missing out. I suppose you are going to ask me to spend time on masturbation as a homework task? What if I don't feel like it?'
THERAPIST: 'I am not putting pressure on you to feel like it, all I would be asking you to do is to experiment with touching your genitals and experimenting a bit to see what feels best. Maybe you like soft and slow stroking or perhaps you like stronger pressure.'
VERONICA: 'I can try.'

The above dialogue shows that Veronica was motivated and would continue to educate herself as far as touch was concerned. She needed some encouragement with the masturbation homework.

Several weeks later Veronica was getting some pleasurable feelings during masturbation, but her sexual interest was low and she did not look forward to the homework although she did it automatically. She was having difficulty with fantasising. She had read the recommended book, *My Secret Garden*, and had found it amusing but not erotic.

The following conversation is taken from her most difficult therapy session where she needed help to come to terms with fantasies which made her feel guilty.

THERAPIST: 'Surely you have fantasised at some point of your sexual development, Veronica?'
VERONICA: 'No.'
THERAPIST: 'Everyone has fantasised at some time or other but lots of people prefer to forget their fantasies as they are socially unacceptable. If that's how you feel it's quite normal.'
VERONICA: 'Really?'
THERAPIST: 'Yes. No-one is asking you to act out your fantasies.'
VERONICA: 'It would be hard to do that as they are associated with tribal lovemaking. See, I've told you, so you know now.'
THERAPIST: 'Thanks for sharing that with me. I'm not saying how terrible it is, am I?'
VERONICA: 'No, because you are permissive and you understand me.'
THERAPIST: 'I'd really like you to think about this tribal fantasy and when you masturbate deliberately think of the scenario and enjoy it.

Don't worry what anyone else might think about it, as your thoughts are private.'

Veronica returned to the clinic a week later and reported that she had enjoyed an orgasm on three occasions and was already accepting her fantasy and thinking about sex when she walked along 'The Backs' at Cambridge. From then on she made good progress and chose her woman friend as a partner to experience massage with. This proved to be beneficial and led to mutual masturbation. Summing up therapy, probably two factors were essential ingredients in stimulation therapy for Veronica: tactile stimulation was encouraged and put into practice; her fantasies were approved of and encouraged.

At 'follow-up' six months later Veronica reported that she was pleased with her relationship with her woman friend and that they masturbated one another to orgasm regularly.

She was quite objective about her therapy and considered she had done well in only ten sessions. She had found it upsetting that her tactile sense was undeveloped as she correlated this sense with femininity, but remarked that she had overcome this by spending a lot of time experimenting until she felt confident that she fully appreciated her sense of touch. She confessed that touching her woman friend had provided the greatest amount of pleasure for her. She also derived much satisfaction from being touched and cuddled.

Fantasising had not been easy for Veronica and she revealed that she had bought Susan Griffin's book during therapy but had not admitted reading this as she thought she might annoy the therapist. She also remarked that she had bought a recent book by Anne Dickson called *The Mirror Within* and found the advice, humour and women's fantasies useful.

Veronica's final remark was that she had found stimulation therapy useful and this had given her an opportunity to catch up on what she had missed out on.

References

1. Kaplan, Helen. (1979) *Disorder of Sexual Desire and Other New Concepts and Techniques in Sex Therapy*. Brunner-Mazel, New York.
2. Masters, W.H. and Johnson, V.E. (1970) *Human Sexual Inadequacy*. Churchill.
3. Ueno, M. (1963) 'The so-called coition death'. *Japanese Journal of Legal Medicine*. 17. 333–40.
4. Friday, Nancy.(1975) *My Secret Garden*. Virago/Quartet.
5. Gillan, P. 'Stimulation therapy for sexual dysfunction'. *Brit.Jrnl. Sexual Medicine*. (June 1978)
6. *Leaves from my Diary*.(1975) Distributed by Stag Tapes. Findraus Ltd.
7. *The Sound of Sex*.(1970) CF 315 Ultra Stereo. Satellite.
8. Griffin, Susan.(1984) *Woman and Nature – The Roaring Inside Her*. Women's Press.
9. Dworkin, Andrea.(1981) *Pornography – Men Posessing Women*. Women's Press.
10. Heiman, Julia.(1975) 'Lady's Relish'. *Pyschology Today*. Vol. 1. No.4. June.
11. Gillan, Patricia and Frith, Christopher.(1979) 'Male-female differences in response to erotica'. *Love and Attraction*. Edited by Cooke, Mark, and Wilson, Glenn. Pergamon Press.
12. Gillan, P. 'Group therapy for increasing the sexual interest of female patients and their partners'. (See above in *Love and Attraction*.)
13. Dodson, Betty. (1975) *Liberating Masturbation*. Box 1933, New York 100011.

Chapter 8

Individual Therapy

Originally only conjoint sex therapy was provided in clinics. This policy has gradually changed and most clinics now have devised programmes of therapy for single people without partners. Often people with partners also seek individual therapy if the other partner blames them for the problem and refuses to attend. Sometimes couples are unable to attend together in any case. Occasionally therapists prefer to single out one partner for more intensive individual treatment during sex therapy.

Usually a single person with a sex problem finds it difficult to relate to the opposite sex. Such a person feels anxious about sex and very worried about potential performance involving someone else. The therapy policy for sexually insecure individuals is to encourage them to gain confidence by giving them tasks to carry out when alone. When this goal has been achieved they are ready for the next stage of finding a partner.

It is preferable for most individuals with sex difficulties to have group therapy as they lose their sense of isolation when meeting people with similar problems in groups. For many individuals, asking them to join a group is like a vicious circle as they are afraid of other people knowing that they have a problem or are sexually inexperienced. They decide against the group and reinforce their sexual isolation. Many single people have deep-seated fears that if they do not have a partner of the opposite sex they will be labelled gay as people will think they indulge in covert homosexual activities.

One of the ways a sexually inexperienced person can gain sexual confidence is by learning how to succeed with a partner and going through 'surrogate therapy'. The therapist provides a temporary sexual partner for the client. This latter therapy is highly controversial and is provided in few sex centres. Encounter groups and massage parlours can provide stepping stones for increasing sexual confidence.

Social skills

Many inexperienced men with sexual problems do not have a regular partner, and probably have only tried to make love with a couple of partners. They fail to succeed sexually, brand themselves as failures and avoid sexual encounters after this.

They tend to see sex as quite a mechanical process and this can be the cause of the trouble as they fail to develop relationships. Trying to get them to change their attitude towards sex and looking for relationships is hard work in therapy. Many of them lack social skills and are afraid of meeting and mixing with people.

At this stage it is useful to describe persuading a man called Philip how to change his attitudes. Philip, a 29-year-old man, was persuaded by his well-to-do family to come for some sex therapy. He has been socially quite isolated for five years as he went to an art school but only stayed on the course for a couple of years. He has painted unsuccessfully since then and his family refused to let him register as unemployed. He was afraid of women and sex and had erectile failure:

PHILIP: 'I tried to have sex on several occasions when I was at art school. I had two girlfriends. But every time I kissed them I lost my erection in minutes.'
THERAPIST: 'How long did your first relationship last?'
PHILIP: 'About three weeks, but I can't really remember.'
THERAPIST: 'How often did you go out?'
PHILIP: 'About twice a week. But I gave Janet up when I could not get an erection with her.'
THERAPIST: 'What about your second relationship?'
PHILIP: 'That lasted less than a month. I met her on Christmas Eve and we finished a week after the New Year. I could not even get an erection with her after Christmas. By the way, I am ashamed to tell you I was drunk when I met her on Christmas Eve.'
THERAPIST: 'Have you tried to have a non-sexual relationship with a woman?'
PHILIP: 'No. There would not be much point, would there?'
THERAPIST: 'There would from the point of relieving your anxiety. I think you are so keen to have sex that you have a performance anxiety, whereas if you tried to make friends initially there would not be so much emphasis on the sexual side of things.'

PHILIP: 'I am not much good at making friends.'
THERAPIST: 'We can rehearse some situations and I can help you.'

This sort of situation can be exasperating for the therapist as obviously Philip is using women as sex objects. It would be foolish at this stage to confront him over his attitudes; it is better to guide him tactfully away from the idea of meeting women just for sex and then abandoning them when he has erectile failure. Philip needed to learn social skills when he met anyone, not just women.

THERAPIST: 'I would like you to pretend you are going to an evening class and meeting some of the people there who are quite friendly. I shall pretend to be one of your fellow students, and you could ask me my name and smile at me.'
PHILIP: 'Hello. What is your name?'
THERAPIST: 'That was fine; you sounded friendly, but you looked down most of the time. Could we repeat the introduction and can you look at me when we talk this time?'
PHILIP: 'All right. But I don't like looking at women to start with. I feel shy.'
THERAPIST: 'You are a painter, so try to look at their faces and imagine you are painting a portrait.'
PHILIP: 'All right. Hello. What's your name? Mine is Philip.'
THERAPIST: 'That was really good, you looked straight at me. You did that well.'
PHILIP: 'Did I?'

Philip smiled and was more at ease because he had been praised.

Several sessions were spent teaching Philip how to talk with and respond to people he met. He then registered for a local history evening class. He was in the conspicuous position of registering late, but he had rehearsed how to deal with this and managed adequately.

The next step was to get him to rehearse inviting one of the men students out to the local bar after the class. Things worked out unexpectedly well as one of the men invited Philip for a pint. When they were at the pub, Dick, the fellow student, confided in Philip that he would like to pick up some girls on Saturday night at a local dance. Philip had agreed to join him but afterwards said he had cold feet and was dreading it.

PHILIP: 'After two pints I think I overdid it agreeing with Dick to go to this do on Saturday.'
THERAPIST: 'What are you afraid of, Philip?'

PHILIP: 'That a girl will find out that I can't get an erection and will tell Dick.'
THERAPIST: 'That is hardly likely to happen, as we have already discussed your policy over meeting a woman. You agreed that it was preferable to start a friendship initially and see what that led to. If that is the case, there will be no kissing or making love when you meet, not for some time, in fact. Your erection is not going to be judged by anyone.'
PHILIP: 'All right. But I don't like going to dances in any case.'
THERAPIST: 'That does not matter – it's trying something out that is important. Are you worried that when you ask a woman for a dance she will refuse?'
THERAPIST: 'Yes. I don't like being left out.'
THERAPIST: 'Let's be realistic. A lot of women do refuse but let's think how many would accept – would you say a third of the women you asked?'
PHILIP: 'Probably half.'
THERAPIST: 'Then you are a lucky man. Have you watched how often other men get turned down?'
PHILIP: 'No. I don't notice things like that.'
THERAPIST: 'What do you do when you get rejected? Do you move on to ask the next lady?'
PHILIP: 'No. I leave.'
THERAPIST: 'But that's a shame as the next lady might accept you and dance.'
PHILIP: 'I feel bad and I want to get out immediately. You don't know what it's like.'
THERAPIST: 'Yes, I know what it is like to be rejected by someone, but I am not going to let one person put me off. I would say to myself I expect I only appeal to half the people I would like to and be philosophical about it. You can't win everything.'
PHILIP: 'You're all right because you are a therapist.'
THERAPIST: 'That does not open the door to me for everything. Look, I've had to learn to relax over certain things. I am going to ask you to listen to your tape and take stimulus 1 and imagine that you have been rejected by a woman you ask for a dance. You stand there and relax when this happens and go on to invite the next lady.'
PHILIP: 'Just like that?'
THERAPIST: 'For stimulus 2 I would like you to imagine that you have been rejected by four women in a row and you are asking a fifth.'
PHILIP: 'You must be joking!'
THERAPIST: 'You say to yourself that you are not going to be put off, even if you go round the whole dance hall. Don't feel humiliated –

someone will dance with you. Now let us practise; I'll take the part of the woman you invite to dance and refuse to dance with you. Try and keep calm and relax as much as you can. See how you feel.'
PHILIP: 'All right.'

Persuading Philip not to feel rejected was hard work and took a long time in role playing. Eventually he seemed well rehearsed and ready to try out the task *in vivo*. Obviously it would have been helpful to have practised the situation in a group therapy setting, but much of the shaping of the desired behaviour can be done in individual therapy social skills training.

A week later Philip returned looking pleased with himself. Philip and his friend had enjoyed the dance and met two women. At first the task did not work and when the first woman rejected Philip he left the dance and stormed off outside feeling angry that his friend had been successful and he had not. He relaxed enough under the circumstances to return and dance with the next woman he invited.

Philip had made arrangements to go out in a foursome the following Saturday to the local pub for a drink, but felt nervous about it.

THERAPIST: 'It should be all right. You did very well inviting Sheila out.'
PHILIP: 'I did not ask her. Graham made the arrangements as a foursome. I said nothing.'
THERAPIST: 'She must have liked you to accept. Did you give her a lift home?'
PHILIP: 'No. I didn't ask her. She went in her girlfriend's car.'
THERAPIST: 'Oh. Was that the other woman in the foursome?'
PHILIP: 'No, someone else, I did not meet her.'
THERAPIST: 'Can we talk about your date now? In what way do you feel nervous?'
PHILIP: 'I really like the look of Sheila but I don't feel up to making love and not getting an erection.'
THERAPIST: 'But, Philip, we discussed all that last time, the idea is just to be friends at first.'
PHILIP: 'If I don't do anything perhaps she won't want to see me again.'
THERAPIST: 'The whole idea is for you to enjoy her company.'
PHILIP: 'What if she asks me for a lift home?'
THERAPIST: 'That's fine. You can give her a lift without making love, can't you?'
PHILIP: 'What if she wants me to kiss her goodnight?'
THERAPIST: 'You can give her a friendly kiss.'
PHILIP: 'She might think I'm queer if I just do that.'

THERAPIST: 'That's a ridiculous conclusion. Just try a friendly kiss and hug if you feel such a gesture is essential.'
PHILIP: 'All right. It's also talking I am nervous about. I dry up in conversations.'
THERAPIST: 'What do you feel confident about discussing?'
PHILIP: 'Art, but she might not be interested in that.'
THERAPIST: 'You could try talking about that as most people have some interest in art. What does Sheila do for a living?'
PHILIP: 'She is a dental receptionist.'
THERAPIST: 'What are her hobbies?'
PHILIP: 'I don't know.'
THERAPIST: 'You could ask her.'

The therapy session continued with trying to find suitable topics of discussion like holidays, sport, music, television programmes. Philip rehearsed some of these topics and became more confident.

After three more sessions Philip had got to a stage in therapy where he had progressed considerably. He and Sheila were becoming good friends and he relaxed with her. The amusing thing is that Graham lost out on his date by being too fast with her, but he had no difficulty finding another woman friend. At this stage it is advisable for the therapist to question the client about sexual arousal and find out how anxious he is about his sexual performance.

THERAPIST: 'It's quite a long time since we talked about sex. I know you told me you kiss Sheila goodnight. Do you still feel tense about this?'
PHILIP: 'No. I get erect when I kiss her but she doesn't know that.'
THERAPIST: 'Has she asked you in for coffee?'
PHILIP: 'No. She shares her flat with another girl.'
THERAPIST: 'So you kiss her goodnight outside the front door?'
PHILIP: 'No, in the car actually.'
THERAPIST: 'So you get aroused sitting in the car when you kiss Sheila?'
PHILIP: 'Yes, I get an erection then. It's not very comfortable as the steering wheel gets in the way.'
THERAPIST: 'Have you tried sitting in the back with Sheila?'
PHILIP: 'No. That's too obvious. You know I really do like her. I think I could try having sex with her soon.'
THERAPIST: 'You know the rule you agreed with. You said you would not make love yet. Having a massage together would be a good plan for the next stage. You could take it in turns to massage one another. I am going to give you these massage instruction sheets to read and imagine.'
PHILIP: 'Thanks. You talked about that last time.'

THERAPIST: 'This book, *The Massage Book* by Downing[1], is quite useful. You could show it to Sheila and say you bought it recently and would like to try out some of the recommendations. I would like you to use your therapy tape and imagine massaging Sheila's back initially with some massage oil. Then you could imagine that she is massaging your back. It would be rather difficult doing the massage in the car. What about asking her to your place?
PHILIP: 'It's too public. My parents hang around.'

Planning a campaign to arrange massage for a couple with accommodation problems is difficult. Sometimes a weekend away can be the answer, but this can lead to nervousness and an expected sexual performance. Philip's problem was solved by Sheila who invited him for Sunday lunch only four days after his last therapy session. They landed up in Sheila's bedroom.

PHILIP: 'Sheila liked the sound of the massage. I described it to her as I did not have the book with me.'
THERAPIST: 'Did you enjoy massaging Sheila?'
PHILIP: 'I felt a bit nervous to start with. She said she liked it but I was pressing too hard.'
THERAPIST: 'Yes, people vary a lot according to what sort of pressure they prefer. Did you like the way Sheila massaged you?'
PHILIP: 'Yes, it was nice but it was a bit too gentle, I think.'
THERAPIST: 'Did you tell Sheila you would like more pressure?'
PHILIP: 'No.'
THERAPIST: 'You could tell her next time.'
PHILIP: 'I don't think I could. It would sound too much like complaining.'
THERAPIST: 'Not if you say it nicely. Let's role play it. I'll pretend to be you and you be Sheila. Here we go: 'That's really nice Sheila. I would like it if you could press a bit more on my shoulders.' Now you try saying that, Philip.'

Trying some role play over individual requests can be helpful and a client's behaviour can be shaped. It is advisable to start with giving a partner some praise before asking for specific acts. Philip had done quite well over the massage in Sheila's bedroom, he had even got an erection which they both ignored.

Sometimes it can be difficult for a partner to turn down the request the other one makes as anxiety increases. Teaching a client to say no to a partner can be a useful procedure in therapy and Philip needed to be prepared for this.

THERAPIST: 'If Sheila asked you to have sexual intercourse with her, how would you feel?'
PHILIP: 'Scared.'
THERAPIST: 'Would you say no?'
PHILIP: 'No. I suppose I would try it.'
THERAPIST: 'Not only would that be breaking therapy rules but it would do yourself harm. You are doing yourself down.'
PHILIP: 'But that's easier than making a fuss.'
THERAPIST: 'You don't need to make a fuss about saying no. You can simply say that you don't feel like making love yet. You feel more comfortable at present massaging her and having fun that way.'
PHILIP: 'She won't think much of me as a man. I am being like a woman making an excuse because of a period or a headache.'
THERAPIST: 'Do you think all women think that all men should be ready, willing and able?'
PHILIP: 'Yes, and I think I would lose my erection.'
THERAPIST: 'You have not been asked to get an erection yet.'
PHILIP: 'Maybe not, but I think about it.'

At this stage quite a lengthy discussion followed about Zilbergeld's male myths and how men are conditioned into thinking they must be willing to have an erection and sex at the drop of a hat. Philip was asked to read *Men and Sex* by Zilbergeld[2] for the next therapy session in order to discuss some of the myths. The last part of the therapy session was spent teaching him how to say no to a partner. He needed a lot of role playing to change his atttitude. He left the session not looking totally convinced, but promising to stick to mutual massage for another week, avoiding genital touching and sex.

When Philip returned a week later he looked pleased and had enjoyed the massage, asking Sheila to increase her pressure. Sheila had not requested sex and he had gone shopping with her on the Saturday. They had bought Zilbergeld's book and discussed it.

PHILIP: 'I was very surprised when Sheila said she agreed with some of the myths you and Zilbergeld talked about. She said also that she was glad I was not fast, as most men demanded sex before they had even got to know her and she never wanted to see that type of man again.'
THERAPIST: 'I am so glad that Sheila appreciates you.'
PHILIP: 'I am also surprised that you are right and you are nice about it. My mother would be crowing and saying "I told you so".'
THERAPIST: 'How did the massage go?'
PHILIP: 'Well, I felt more relaxed. Sheila was very frank about things. She said she finds it difficult to get an orgasm during sex and that she

prefers it with her finger. I was shocked by her telling me that. What do you think?'
THERAPIST: 'She sounds very natural and honest. I like the way she seems. Did you tell her you have problems too?'
PHILIP: 'No, of course not, that would be demeaning wouldn't it? I mean it's different for a man.'
THERAPIST: 'I think you could lower your level of anxiety if you revealed that you sometimes find it difficult to get fully erect.'
PHILIP: 'Really?'
THERAPIST: 'Yes, because you would not be worrying about what she would think if you did not get a full erection, as you would be preparing her for the worst.'

The therapy session continued and some role playing was used to help Philip tell Sheila that he had a problem. In the end he was quite natural over his revelation and it did not even sound rehearsed:

PHILIP: 'I think I can say it right to Sheila now. How does this sound: "Last Saturday you were very frank telling me about your problem with getting a climax. Sometimes I find it difficult to get erect. So, I have a problem too."'
THERAPIST: 'That sounds fine. I am sure that after you have told Sheila this you will relax well. You might even try stroking one another's genitals if you feel like it.'
PHILIP: 'But I would start to worry about my erection'.
THERAPIST: 'Your goal would be to enjoy the activity; you do not have to achieve an erection at this stage.'

It can be difficult to convince a client that an erection is not required when he is so performance-orientated. Under these circumstances it can be useful to get the man occupied with trying to please his partner and once his mind is taken off getting an erection the fact that his partner is excited can arouse him. The therapy session continued and Philip discussed how to arouse a woman. Previously he had not fully understood how this was done.

Philip progressed well in therapy and gained confidence about making love with Sheila. At one stage he lost his erection whilst having oral sex as he felt nervous the first time he did this. It was suggested at this stage that he should ask Sheila to come for a couple of therapy sessions with him, but he turned down this idea. In fact, he never told her that his problem had been solved by therapy. It was interesting that although he had experienced difficulty with oral sex, when he made love for the first time with Sheila, in the woman above position, he had no trouble in maintaining his erection. Most men have bad associations with lovemaking in the man above or missionary position as this is the position that they connect with failure. Once they are advised to try a new position they lose the bad associations with failure and rapidly gain confidence. Also, they can be told to lie back and enjoy sex!

Gaining sexual confidence

Of course it is easier to treat someone who has had some sexual experience, although limited, like Philip. It can be difficult describing sex to a person who has never masturbated or kissed. Men who fall into this category are statistically unusual but quite a lot of women do not know what masturbation is or are too embarrassed to try it.

Social skills training is often helpful for a lack of confidence and experience. Obviously a virgin male needs to succeed in his first lovemaking session, but if he is anxious he will encounter problems from the start. It is interesting to see how animal breeders solve this problem; they usually mate the inexperienced male with an experienced female and this leads to success. It makes sense for an inexperienced man to find an experienced woman, but this is not always easy as he has no confidence. Few single men like a woman to know that he is inexperienced so ways have to be found for such a man to cope and therapy sessions can produce coping methods.

Jim came for therapy as he lacked confidence and experience. He had masturbated, obtaining good erections and a strong ejaculation. He revealed that he was not very interested in women but liked the look of some men and had sexual fantasies associated with men when he masturbated. He was keen to develop a relationship with a woman, and hoped this would lead to marriage. The idea of a homosexual relationship had been considered by him but he was terrified of catching AIDS, a subject he knew plenty about as he was a doctor. He had been approached by quite an attractive male registrar colleague in the hospital where he worked but had turned down the offer. He had taken out a nurse several times and liked being friendly with her but felt no sexual attraction towards her.

After three therapy sessions Jim revealed the fact that he felt almost phobic about women.

JIM: 'Although I have never made love with a woman I feel rather put off when I think of their genitals.'
THERAPIST: 'What puts you off?'

JIM: 'It's the combination of odour and stickiness. There is a fishy smell down there. I could never give a woman cunnilingus – the thought of that would make me vomit.'
THERAPIST: 'I suppose you have clinically examined a lot of women and you have had no emotional involvement and do not associate this area with pleasure. How do you feel when you examine a man's penis?'
JIM: 'Fine, it's not sticky and clammy. I must say I do not like examining uncircumcised males – they tend to smell more.'
THERAPIST: 'I suppose you are circumcised yourself?'
JIM: 'Yes.'
THERAPIST: 'How do you feel about your own genital odours?'
JIM: 'My hygiene is immaculate.'
THERAPIST: 'I did not mean that. What I meant is how do you react to your own semen when you masturbate?'
JIM: 'I suppose it does have a slight odour, but it is my own smell, so I do not think about it. I don't think I would mind the smell of another man's semen, but I don't think I would like to get it on my hands.'
THERAPIST: 'Is that why you are afraid of homosexual activity?'
JIM: 'Of course not. I would dislike the idea of anal intercourse, as it is unnatural and associated with AIDS.'
THERAPIST: 'A lot of gay men these days indulge only in mutual masturbation.'
JIM: 'Right. I would like to know why we are discussing men. I only talked about women with you in the last session and I want to succeed with a woman.'
THERAPIST: 'It's only because I am interested in your attitudes towards genital odours and secretions.'
JIM: 'Do you think I am abnormal?'
THERAPIST: 'No. Many men are anxious or phobic about women's genitals.'

At this stage in therapy Jim has revealed his dislike of female genitalia. He appears to be more neutral towards male genitalia, but guarded about his sexual attitude towards men. A decision needs to be taken by the therapist on what to advise. If it is suggested that he should try to find a female partner his disgust towards her genitalia will put him off, but he could be desensitised over his attitude. If the therapist suggests that Jim should experiment with a homosexual relationship he will probably be very angry. The therapist risks antagonising Jim but it is worthwhile at this stage tactfully to outline a possible treatment plan.

THERAPIST: 'It's quite difficult to suggest a therapy programme without offending you.'

JIM: 'Go ahead. I am not worried about your offending me, I am interested in your ideas about me.'
THERAPIST: 'I would like to suggest a parallel programme for you in association with either male or female partners.'
JIM: 'Are you suggesting I am bisexual?'
THERAPIST: 'You only have to read Kinsey to realise that most people are basically bisexual but are orientated more towards one sex than the other. Were you interested in psychiatry when you were a medical student?'
JIM: 'Not much, but I'd quite like to know more about your reference to Kinsey; someone else mentioned his work somewhere along the line.'
THERAPIST: 'What I would suggest is that you have desensitisation therapy to make love with a woman, so you can get confident over touching her body, particularly her genitals.'
JIM: 'Does that mean I would have to relax daily by playing the tape and imagining stimuli related to genital odours and secretions?'
THERAPIST: 'That's right. I would give you items to imagine associated with making love to a woman. It would be good if you could find a girlfriend as well, rather than sitting there imagining what it would be like.'
JIM: 'That's not easy. It's like committing myself. I don't like the idea of misleading a woman so as to use her body.'
THERAPIST: 'Would you prefer to meet a surrogate partner?'
JIM: 'Yes, I have heard all about that in the newspapers. I would be prepared to try that. Can you arrange it?'
THERAPIST: 'Not directly, but there are places you can be referred to where you can have some counselling and surrogate therapy.'

This plan worked quite well. Jim knew about the surrogate therapy scheme and appeared to be quite matter-of-fact about it. Some clients are much more shocked by the idea of a surrogate. It is interesting to note that Masters and Johnson[3] did provide surrogate therapy for male patients but abandoned this scheme because of legal problems.

Jim seemed very reasonable until it came to bisexual discussion.

JIM: 'That sounds fine. What about the parallel plan you mentioned?'
THERAPIST: 'Yes, that would involve your experimenting with finding out whether you were happier with a male partner.'
THERAPIST: 'I hate the idea of being branded queer. Are you suggesting I approach a man?'
THERAPIST: 'I am suggesting that you could consider this idea.'
JIM: 'Are male surrogate partners provided?'

THERAPIST: 'In the States there is such a service, but here you could read one of the gay magazines with advertisements.'
JIM: 'To be frank I would like to see what it is like with a man, but my fear would be catching AIDS.'
THERAPIST: 'I can understand your fear; this is a highly emotive issue. I am not suggesting anal intercourse, although this is legal between consenting adult males in this country. What I am recommending is that you could try mutual masturbation with another man. How do you feel about that?'
JIM: 'That would stop me worrying about AIDS. Talking about it with you helps. It's not so terrible when we discuss it dispassionately. I could never talk about homosexuality with my colleagues as they would condemn me. I would like to try it, but I have reservations about it; my feelings are mixed.'
THERAPIST: 'We could devise a desensitisation programme for you to try, if you want.'
JIM: 'All right, but I would also like to try the surrogate partner.'
THERAPIST: 'Yes, that sounds sensible, that's why I suggested a parallel therapy programme. You could prepare both at the same time, and then choose which plan you are most comfortable with when you experiment in reality. You should have built up confidence through your desensitisation programme to try making love with a man or woman.'

The above session had reached a satisfactory conclusion and Jim had confessed that he would like to experiment with a male partner, but he had been extremely cautious over admitting this. The therapist had left open the idea of his experimenting with either a male or female partner, according to what he felt comfortable with. It is always preferable for the client to make the final decision over sexual orientation.

Gaining sexual experience

Surrogate therapy is one of the ways in which a sexually inexperienced client can obtain sexual experience but this is a highly controversial issue and not recommended by all therapists.

Many therapists consider that obtaining sex with a surrogate is a short-cut to sex, as it eliminates the social side of a relationship. Other more liberal therapists argue that this helps the client as he or she has failed in a social setting and become phobic of sex, therefore it is preferable for such a client to find a suitable and cooperative sexual partner who will be sympathetic.

Some therapists refuse to acknowledge the positive conditioning effect of such therapy. If a man has failed to have intercourse with his partner and seeks the help of a surrogate and is successful with her he will associate sex with pleasure and will have a better chance of succeeding when he returns to his partner. Other therapists say, however, that this is a way of avoiding coming to terms with the regular partner as he is seeking sex elsewhere.

Martin Cole[4] recommends surrogate therapy for male and female clients. There is more activity in this field in the USA and Canada, although Masters and Johnson no longer include surrogates in their therapy due to some legal problems. When they did use this method[3] various surrogates were attached to their practice and they were able to interview both the client and the surrogate after their massage or sexual foreplay. The advantage of surrogate therapy is that a client knows that the surrogate is aware of his problem, their relationship is not dependent on sexual success and so the client's performance anxiety is considerably reduced. The surrogate knows how to relax the client and how to be reassuring throughout.

Jim's progress is interesting to follow. He went through the parallel programmes and listened to his tape and desensitised himself to touching a woman's clitoris and to vaginal containment. He tried to picture himself with a surrogate and imagined massage tasks and genital touching. He knew that sexual intercourse would be banned on the first occasion of surrogate therapy, but he was asked to imagine eventually having intercourse with the surrogate in the woman above position. The other parallel programme involved approaching a male partner and maybe later enjoying a massage. Jim did not want to get involved in mutual masturbation with another man, because of his worry over AIDS as this would place him in the 'high risk' group. Although he felt happy over approaching a man for a massage he decided that the surrogate therapy would be the better choice as he would have the opportunity to make love with an experienced woman and although he might be treating her as a sex object there would be a contract between them and no ties over forming a lasting relationship.

During the eighth therapy session the methods of surrogate therapy were outlined:

THERAPIST: 'You will initially meet Dr X who will explain a bit more about your first session.'

JIM: 'What if I don't like the look of the woman?'

THERAPIST: 'Dr X will introduce her to you and obviously you are not expected to go through with the therapy if you dislike her. One of the disadvantages of surrogate therapy is that there is a shortage of women who want to help in this way and Dr X has already told me that the choice for you is limited to only two surrogates who are available.'
JIM: 'What will happen when I have chosen my surrogate?'
THERAPIST: 'Dr X will explain to you both about massage and then you will go with your surrogate to a comfortable room where you can massage one another.'
JIM: 'That will be a strange experience for me, as I have never done that before. It's mutual massage, isn't it? Shall I massage her first or will she massage me?'
THERAPIST: 'She will massage you and help you to relax. Of course you both take off your clothes and use some sort of body oil. Sometimes it's a good idea to have a shower first together and I am sure that can be arranged.'
JIM: 'What happens next?'
THERAPIST: 'The first time you only massage one another and after you have done that you discuss things with Dr X who will let you know when you are ready for the next step which is mutual masturbation or what Masters and Johnson call 'genital sensate focussing'.
JIM: 'I have to touch her clitoris and arouse her.'
THERAPIST: 'Yes, like you imagined on your tape when you did your desensitisation exercises. Of course, you can take your tape with you and if you feel tense about the situation you can play your tape beforehand.'
JIM: 'That sounds fine. But what about sexual intercourse? Am I expected to go ahead with that?'
THERAPIST: 'Eventually but not yet. I will let you know when to aim for such a thing. Then it is up to you. You judge how you feel when the situation arises.'
JIM: 'I am not concerned with how I feel or my confidence. What I am worried about is her hygiene; how can that be guaranteed?'
THERAPIST: 'You can't totally guarantee any woman's hygiene.'
JIM: 'Maybe not but the risks with a surrogate are higher.'
THERAPIST: 'Yes, I agree with you. There are ways of getting round this, of course. You do not have to go the whole way, you could wear a sheath. Here I am giving you advice when you know the answers yourself as a medical man.'
JIM: 'You told me early on in therapy that I had conditioned too well to the idea that sex was dirty and women were whores. I suppose an element of that has remained with me.'

At this stage the surrogate therapy was in question and it was hard for the therapist to judge whether Jim's queries were associated with an emotional block towards sex with a woman or based on realistic worries about disease. He raised no objection to mutual masturbation so the desensitisation therapy associated with female genitalia had worked. His objection to sexual intercourse seemed fairly well founded. Of course, clients do not all have to have the same goal of sexual intercourse in surrogate therapy and mutual masturbation can be the goal. It is up to the client to decide upon appropriate goals.

After two weeks Jim returned for therapy. He had got on well with the surrogate, but had found Dr X too authoritarian. Dr X had simultaneously reported that Jim was extremely awkward over decision-making and had rather poor social skills. When questioned about sexual progress with the surrogate Jim had done fairly well with the massage:

JIM: 'She did help me to relax and we had a shower together. She has a warm personality. Her body is all right, she is quite nice and slim. When we got to the genital stage I must admit I started to get anxious but it was all right, in fact I got an erection when she touched me.'
THERAPIST: 'Did you feel excited when you touched her?'
JIM: 'No. I did not feel anything. I felt neutral. Touching her did nothing for me.'
THERAPIST: 'Did you touch her before or after she had touched you?'
JIM: 'Afterwards. I had quite a good erection to start with but rapidly lost it after I touched her. This happened on three separate occasions.'
THERAPIST: 'What were you thinking of when you touched her? Were you able to fantasise?'
JIM: 'No. I was thinking of what it would be like to be inside her.'
THERAPIST: 'Were you thinking about hygiene?'
JIM: 'Not really.'
THERAPIST: 'Were you thinking about men in the way you fantasise when you masturbate on your own?'
JIM: 'On and off I did have that type of fantasy, but that faded rapidly when I saw her. I have concluded that I would not want sexual intercourse with her.'
THERAPIST: 'I think you have done very well in surrogate therapy. You do not need to go any further at present, as you have now had some contact with a woman. You were under no obligation to conclude with intercourse. What would you like to do next?'
JIM: 'The alternative of seeing what it is like with a man is open to me. I have bought some magazines which I find stimulating. I am thinking

of applying to a box number rather than joining a club, as that would be too public. I must admit that I feel nervous about the approach.'
THERAPIST: 'We can take some stimuli connected with your anxiety for desensitisation.'

Jim finally met a man he was attracted to quite early on, after only a couple of replies. He was lucky. His partner was looking for a clean and reliable man, so Jim's obsession with hygiene was a positive factor in the relationship. They both enjoyed mutual masturbation and Jim's erection was good when he pleasured his partner.

Jim did benefit from surrogate therapy as he gained quite a lot of useful experience although this did not lead to a relationship with a woman. He did sort himself out and looked on a relationship with a man in a more positive light because of the surrogate therapy.

Several other male clients, especially male virgins, have benefitted from surrogate therapy in order to gain sexual experience.

Clients who benefit from individual therapy

Sometimes couples present for therapy and one or both partners might be taken out of conjoint therapy to be given individual therapy.

Certain types of clients are particularly likely to benefit from individual therapy and the following list is a guide to choosing such suitable individuals:

(1) Clients who need sex education, as they are misinformed, ignorant or need reassurance. This can happen with couples, when one partner is well informed but the other needs guidance.
(2) Clients with a genital phobia need some individual therapy, mainly consisting of desensitisation.
(3) The fear of masturbation needs separate densensitisation therapy and reassurance and permission from the therapist.
(4) Clients with poor fantasies need extra individual therapy, especially if this is connected with increasing the libido.
(5) If a client has been assaulted or raped, especially as a minor, individual therapy needs to be provided.
(6) Abortion therapy is advisable, both before and after the operation.
(7) When a client is advised to terminate an affair some individual therapy is useful.
(8) Role playing can be given to individuals, especially if an individual

is involved in a dominant relationship and they are both in conjoint therapy.

(9) Women with vaginismus often need some initial densensitisation *in vivo* with the therapist present, in order to gain confidence over inserting fingers into the vagina.

(10) Men with premature ejaculation should have some individual therapy when their homework 'stop start' tasks are explained.

Therapy should be as flexible as possible and it is up to the therapist to intervene and suggest separate therapy sessions for individual partners if there is some sort of crisis or unexpected problem in therapy.

References

1. Downing, George. (1972) *The Massage Book*. Random House.
2. Zilbergeld, Bernie. (1980) *Men and Sex*. Souvenir Press.
3. Masters, W.H. and Johnson, V.E. (1970) *Human Sexual Inadequacy*. Churchill Livingstone.
4. Cole, Martin. (1985) 'Surrogate sex therapy'. In W. Dryden (Ed.): *Marital Therapy in Britain*, Vol. II. Harper and Row.

Chapter 9

Women's Sex Therapy Groups

The Americans led the way with group sex therapy for women. Group therapy started with programmes for women who had primary anorgasmia and later groups were formed to include women with situational and secondary anorgasmia. Lonnie Barbach is considered the pioneer of such groups. Although her book, *For Yourself – The Fulfilment of Female Sexuality*[1], was written in 1974 it still is very up-to-date. There are some lively sections on opportunities for women to experiment with and enjoy masturbation and pornography. She utilised LoPiccolo and Lobitz's[2] masturbation training programme. Her main research has been on anorgasmic women, but instead of talking about anorgasmic women she refers to 'pre-orgasmic' women. This implies orgasms for all women and avoids the pejorative implications of the term 'non-orgasmic'.

The West Coast of America, where Lonnie Barbach comes from, is regarded as a sexually progressive and permissive area. New York is probably the only East Coast competitor, where Betty Dodson's book, *Liberating Masturbation*[3], caused such a stir in 1974 that it was driven underground. Some of the drawings in the book are very fine, especially drawings of the female genitalia resembling orchids. Betty is well known as an artist and some of her drawings of women masturbating encouraged women with masturbation problems to ask her about much matters. Eventually, so many women were interested in these techniques that Betty ran groups for them, based on body relaxation and appreciation with a focus on bio-energetic techniques. The women were quickly desensitised to anxieties concerning their body imagery as Betty insisted that all the women were nude for all the groups. The women showed one another their individual masturbation techniques and Betty discussed any blocking or hang-ups that they had.

The groups were based on carefully programmed activities which started with sex education, body appreciation and masturbation confidence.

The programme

Most women's sex therapy group programmes, however, are based on tasks which are discussed in the group and carried out at home. The number of sessions varies from about six to ten or more sessions. Usually therapy is carried out on a weekly basis. The following programme is fairly general and based on American and European group sessions[4,5,6]:

Session 1

Initially the women sit in a circle with the therapists and each woman introduces herself, revealing her sexual problem as well as telling the group something about herself. It can be quite a good idea to break the ice by going round the circle discussing hobbies as a start. The women are usually quite anxious at this stage and a group relaxation session can be helpful. A brief period of relaxation can be set aside for each subsequent session. Slides or pictures of female genitalia are shown and sex education is provided. Then homework is outlined and each woman is requested to take a bath at home and relax and experiment with touching areas of the body. A bath oil is recommended. Of course, in certain areas of the world where there is a shortage of water this task has to be modified and the women are asked to sit comfortably and experiment with touch. After doing this task they are asked to examine their genitalia in a mirror and identify the different parts shown on an accompanying diagram.

Session 2

A discussion of homework for each woman is a regular procedure throughout all of the subsequent sessions. During the group session the structure and functions of the female genitalia and PC (pubococcygeal) muscles are discussed and illustrated by slides. PC muscles instructions are given throughout therapy with increases in the number of practice contraction times and type and response. Homework also consists of feeling the genitals but not trying to become sexually aroused.

Session 3

Initially, this session consists of talking about individual thoughts and feelings associated with self-stimulation. The therapists suggest that each woman should try experimenting with different methods of rhythm and touch when masturbating.

Session 4

Sexual fantasies are discussed and various erotic books, magazines and films are recommended. In addition, the physiology of the four phases of sexual arousal as described by Masters and Johnson are explained. The women are also asked to carry out homework, exaggerating any stage or movements associated with masturbation that embarrass them. This latter method is paradoxical as they are deliberately having to do something they feel awkward with.

Some therapists recommend the use of a vibrator at this stage. If the clinic does not provide vibrators the women are asked to purchase them.

Session 5

Role playing of orgasm is a task that many women find difficult if they have never had an orgasm. The women are asked to exaggerate their movements and sounds and asked to breathe loudly, grimace, and so forth. It is useful to practise moaning, groaning and screaming in a group situation. A tape can be useful in breaking down inhibitions and desensitising the women to this task. This task is given as homework in combination with many of the activities already described, such as fantasising and practising PC muscle exercises whilst masturbating.

Session 6

The focus during this session is on sharing some of the previous activities and tasks with a partner. If no partner is available the women are requested to imagine sharing the experiences with a future partner. The sharing is carefully graded to desensitise anyone who feels awkward over massage or masturbation with a partner. At this stage a modified Masters and Johnson programme is outlined together with instructions for the woman above position and the 'feel free' position.

Session 7

This is a review session in which the women are given an opportunity to discuss at length any doubts or difficulties they had.

Research in the UK has included various assessments before and after group therapy. Questionnaires like 'the orgasmic response scale' which are related to the group members' sexual behaviour and other ratings related to their psychological state are useful. Another measure which has been of interest in the UK has been psychophysiological measurement related to the blood flow. Before and after therapy most women attend a laboratory session in which a probe is inserted into the vagina to measure changes in the blood flow in response to various stimuli. The stimuli include erotic pictures and sounds, fantasising, and vibration of the glans clitoridis at a frequency of 80 cycles a second. The object of this exercise is to compare the women's responses before and after therapy to see if any change has taken place.

Advantages of women's groups

It is most advantageous that the women in the group can identify with one another and support each other in their therapy. The women can often feel comforted that their problems are so similar. Many of the women would have felt abnormal and isolated before coming to a group.

Sometimes in therapy the therapist comes over as authoritarian and disapproving if an individual client does not do her homework, but in a group situation the women often take responsibility themselves for disciplining members who fail to do their homework. The women in the group as well as the therapist or therapists can offer advice and suggestions. Many of the women in the group will have had different experiences and can thus provide a lot of valuable information.

Another advantage of a group is that films shown to individuals can cause anxiety; it is much better viewing slides or videos in a group situation and sharing the experience. A modelling effect is useful in a group; if one woman strongly objects to masturbation and all the other women are enthusiastic about it the isolated woman's attitude is probably going to change. In a group where all the women are anorgasmic it is very encouraging when the first woman in the group becomes orgasmic and this influences the other women. Practising orgasm role playing can be less inhibiting in a group.

Probably the greatest advantage of a women's group is that women are more comfortable discussing their sexual problems together, without the presence of men. Many women would be put off by the knowledge that men find their problems stimulating and get erotic pleasure from listening to them describe how they masturbate or use a vibrator.

Disadvantages of women's groups

Often women, especially those from Europe, do not like joining a group initially. Group dynamics can cause problems like competition. Sometimes the more verbal groups members can dominate the group. Therapists have to be careful to allot each woman in the group a fair amount of time to report their homework experiences.

Another disadvantage can be that some women do not like discussing sex with other women and perhaps fear lesbian involvement. This is rarely expressed as a fear but is occasionally mentioned. The loss of confidentiality is another fear women have in a group. Some group organisers do not accept women from the same town in the same group.

The major disadvantage of the women's group is that partners do not attend. A partner might feel excluded and angry about this. Some therapists arrange for partners to attend halfway through. Other therapists see the partners before and after the group to explain and advise how to cope with situations.

How to run a group

It is easier, although obviously less economical, to run a group with two therapists rather than one. Often non-verbal communication can be a useful way of assessing group dynamics and as one therapist talks and interacts with a group member the other therapist can observe the other members and study their reactions. One therapist can take on 'the tough role' if members do not carry out their homework and the other therapist may choose to be more permissive.

At the start of a group the therapists should agree how they are going to structure the programme. Sometimes groups are run by a therapist who is teaching a trainee therapist how to run groups and obviously the experienced therapist will be the main authority, but arrangements should be made to give the trainee therapist plenty of say and responsibility.

At the beginning of a new group session it is a good idea for the women to discuss their sexual problems when introductions take place. It is helpful for the therapist or therapists to use some self-disclosure at this stage but this type of self-disclosure should be brief:

THERAPIST A: 'I once had a sex problem myself and that's how I got involved in therapy. I found I could get an orgasm if I masturbated but I could not share this with my partner. I found I could not climax with him but thought it unnatural to ask him to use his finger to stimulate me. I never asked him to help but secretly blamed him for not doing this. Then I realised that I should ask him and benefited from this.'
THERAPIST B: 'I grew up in quite a repressive and inhibiting family. I was terrified that they might find out that I masturbated so I used to do it furtively in case they could hear. It was difficult to get a climax as I had to control my movement and breathing.'

The first thing the women benefit from is learning how to relax. This is their first joint activity and is usually positive. The therapists, if there are two of them, can take it in turn to relax the group as this activity should take place on a weekly basis, each time the group meets. Another shared activity is viewing the slides of genitalia and often there is no need for the therapist to intervene and reassure a woman who shows disgust as one of the other group members usually points out the acceptability of such a picture.

At the beginning of each session it is advisable to discuss homework. Each therapist can take it in turn to discuss homework activities with each woman in turn – allowing intervention by the other therapist or the other women, of course, when appropriate. If everyone gangs up and is very unpleasant to one group member, one of the therapists should take her side and be supportive.

Therapists vary in their policies for trying to motivate the group members. Of course, it is bound to be a competitive situation, and this is advantageous for most people. However, in the case of the woman who makes little or no progress it is good to reassure her that the therapy is greatly pressurised and the pace is fast, but later on there will be a rest pause and she can make up for lost time then.

Research carried out by Gillan and McMullen[7] showed that intensive two-day 'marathon' therapy can be effective but most therapists prefer to run groups on a weekly basis.

The last question is whether it is better to run homogeneous groups where all the women have anorgasmia or whether to include those with situational anorgasmia. Such heterogenous groups work well as clients who are situationally anorgasmic can tell the primary anorgasmics about orgasms.

Progress of a woman with anorgasmia

Camilla was extremely reluctant to attend a group in the first place and she needed a lot of persuasion finally to take the plunge. Camilla, aged 28, came from Trinidad, and had never experienced an orgasm. She thought she was missing out and decided to have therapy when the opportunity came for her to discuss some of her problems with a behaviour therapist.

It was only because she suffered from migraine that she was referred to the clinic in the first place for biofeedback therapy to help her with her headaches. When discussing some of her symptoms the subject of sex was brought up, but she did not like the idea of having help in a group:

CAMILLA: 'Yes, of course I would like to have an orgasm. The women in the cutting room where I work are always discussing it and I feel I miss out. However, I prefer to have help from you on my own, like I am doing now. I do not like the idea of a group.'
THERAPIST: 'Why not, Camilla?'
CAMILLA: 'Well, I am quite shy and not at all extraverted. I could not talk to people in a group like that.'
THERAPIST: 'But you do talk with the other women at work about sex.'
CAMILLA: 'No I don't. I hear them discussing it, but I say nothing.'
THERAPIST: 'Don't forget that all the women in the group would have a sex problem and would be like you.'
CAMILLA: 'What, from the Caribbean?'
THERAPIST: 'No, I did not mean that. I meant that a lot of them would never have had an orgasm.'
CAMILLA: 'I see. Actually being in a group with people from back home would make matters worse for me. You already know the culture.'
THERAPIST: 'That you are Indian and do not participate in carnival?'
CAMILLA: 'The other women are probably more confident than I am.'
THERAPIST: 'Not necessarily. Why don't you give it a try?'

Camilla finally decided to join the group after the various methods and activities had been explained to her. When she heard that it was necessary to discuss her hobbies she panicked and said she had no time for hobbies because after working as a tailoress she was worn out. It was suggested that she could talk about cookery. It so turned out that there was another Caribbean member called Doreen, a hairdresser who came from Jamaica and also had no time for hobbies. She had decided to talk about reggae. Camilla first made friends with her and then with all the other women. The positive feature of women's groups is that there is plenty of warmth and support from members.

At the first session Camilla described her problem:

CAMILLA: 'I have never had an orgasm and would like to experience this.'
THERAPIST B: 'Have you ever masturbated?'
CAMILLA: 'No. I told Patricia (Therapist A) that when I had therapy for my headaches.'
THERAPIST B: 'It's good to share your experiences with all of us here. I myself had problems over getting orgasms so I can understand how you feel. Did your headaches get better?'
CAMILLA: 'Yes, I learned to relax and that helped. Also I was stressed under certain circumstances and I had some cognitive therapy to learn to cope with these situations.'
THERAPIST B: 'That's good. You might be able to help other people relax.'

Therapist B had done well with Camilla as she had identified with her and drawn her out in a discussion of her therapy for her migraine. She had also pointed out that Camilla might be able to help over relaxation. Of course, Therapist B had been prepared in advance concerning Camilla's problems.

During the slide presentation, Camilla said nothing, but when she received her homework sheet to fill in after taking her bath and sitting and observing her genitals she spoke:

CAMILLA: 'What if the clitoris is difficult to find as the labia are large and cover it like one of the slides you showed?'
THERAPIST A: 'You can pull your labia minora to each side with two hands then hold this area open with one hand and look in the mirror with the other. It should not be too difficult.'

At this stage one of the women in the group called Daphne tried to help:

DAPHNE: 'Perhaps it's a matter of pulling back the clitoral hood to find the glans. It took me a long time to do this as I did not understand when I looked in the mirror last year what I was supposed to be looking for.'
CAMILLA: 'Thanks, I could also try that.'

All the women agreed to try the task but after the session Camilla wanted more reassurance:

CAMILLA: 'Could you tell me again what to do over the homework?'
THERAPIST A: 'Look, Camilla, it's not really fair if you are having extra time like this. You should ask your questions in the group.'
CAMILLA: 'I never really wanted to join a group in the first place.'
THERAPIST: 'Yes, I appreciate that, but if all of you in the group come and want further explanations after sessions it's difficult to arrange because of the extra time. Also it's helpful for the other members to share your problems. You are part of the group now, you know.'
CAMILLA: 'Okay.'
THERAPIST: 'In any case, you do have written instructions over your homework and I suggest that you go home and try the tasks. You should actually have a relaxation session first and listen to your tape which we have provided and imagine identifying your genital areas.'

The therapist had to be hard on Camilla, as obviously if all the group members wanted individual sessions after the group the group would disintegrate. It is best immediately to discourage individual help and to allow questions only in a group setting.

When the group met the next time an announcement was made to allow any of the women present to ask anonymously those questions that they particularly felt shy about.

THERAPIST B: 'At the end of the last session we forgot to mention that although we cannot allow individual questions after the group we do allow unsigned written questions which can be put in the box outside the door before sessions.'

The women quite liked this idea.

Camilla had found the homework difficult but had actually succeeded in finding the required genital parts. She was pleased and Daphne spontaneously praised her:

DAPHNE: 'Gosh, Camilla, that's really good. Last week I did not think you would be able to find your glans.'
THERAPIST B: 'Yes, you have done very well. How did you feel about touching this area when you were looking for the right parts?'
CAMILLA: 'Not too good. I felt it was a bit like masturbating.'
DAPHNE: 'I felt quite aroused; you don't have to be ashamed, you know.'

Sometimes spontaneous remarks like this can be a tremendous help to a participant who feels shy and embarrassed. The therapists knew that further embarrassment could be caused by the next homework task of touching the genitals and they predicted that several members of the group might raise objections. Doreen, the Jamaican hairdresser, was quite verbal during the sessions. Like Camilla, she was anorgasmic and had never masturbated. She was married and expected her partner to take responsibility for her orgasm. Doreen's partner was only interested in sexual intercourse and needed little foreplay. Camilla had a visiting man friend who came to her flat about once a month, on a Sunday. He had tried to give some clitoral stimulation but she had become tense. When the task of touching the genitals was described Camilla said nothing, but Doreen raised objections.

DOREEN: 'This task is really masturbation, isn't it? Why don't you call it that?'
THERAPIST B: 'We have not labelled it that as we are not asking you to masturbate. We want you to become confident over finding the stimulating parts of your genitals with your finger. You said, Doreen, that your husband never stimulated you properly. If you could learn to show him the right areas this would help him.'
DOREEN: 'I could not do that as I don't know.'
DAPHNE: 'That's why you are being asked to find out for yourself now. In any case, what's wrong with masturbation? A lot of you in this group have hang-ups.'
DOREEN: 'You are not the therapist to make remarks like that.'
THERAPIST A: 'Everyone is allowed to say what they want, so, Doreen and Daphne, you can both make comments. We don't expect everyone to agree.'
DOREEN: 'If you are so clever and know so much about masturbation, Daphne, how come that you don't get an orgasm?'
DAPHNE: 'That's why I am here. I get close to it so I'm in the second league.'

The therapists were concerned as they could see that Doreen and Daphne would be at loggerheads during therapy because they were both equally articulate. During this clash Camilla looked worried.

THERAPIST B: 'Camilla, you look worried. Are you happy about trying to touch your genitals?'
CAMILLA: 'I feel a bit like Doreen and Sandra. Sandra said in the first session that she did not like touching herself down below as it felt cold and wet.'
THERAPIST B: 'Does it feel like that for you?'
CAMILLA: 'Probably more warm and wet.'
THERAPIST A: 'Being moist in this area is good as lubrication is a positive thing. It's easier to get aroused if you lubricate well.'

DAPHNE: 'Sometimes I find that if I am too well lubricated I cease to have feelings in my clitoris.'
THERAPIST A: 'That can happen sometimes, but it's better to be too well lubricated than to be very dry.'

When the women returned a week later and discussed their homework, Camilla was pleased with her progress:

CAMILLA: 'I found that I was quite relaxed and that I could touch my genitals easily. Each day I did it it was easier.'
DOREEN: 'Well, that makes two of us. I did not feel happy about it but it was okay. I felt rather dry and wondered why.'
THERAPIST A: 'You have both done very well. But let's take one at a time and continue with you, Camilla. Did you find anything difficult?'
CAMILLA: 'Not really. I suppose the most difficult thing is to find my clitoral glans but it gets easier as time goes by.'

The therapist did not allow Doreen to take over at this point of questioning when each woman had her turn to discuss progress.

When the next stage of touching the genitals was outlined, Camilla did not look at all comfortable but as usual said nothing. Doreen spoke up:

DOREEN: 'What you have outlined is masturbation, although you will probably deny that.'
THERAPIST A: 'No, I am not denying it. There is nothing wrong with masturbation if it helps you to gain confidence in your own sexuality.'
DOREEN: 'Well, I am a Christian and I think it's wrong.'
DAPHNE: 'I am a Christian, too, and there is nothing in the Bible to say that masturbation is a sin.'
DOREEN: 'Yes, there is. What about Onan spilling his seed?'
DAPHNE: 'You have it wrong. He deliberately did not ejaculate inside his brother's widow as he did not want to impregnate her.'
DOREEN: 'I think you are being disrespectful.'
THERAPIST B: 'Look here, let's try and keep the atmosphere warm as we want to help one another.'
THERAPIST A: 'Daphne's point is valid. Masturbation is not forbidden in the Bible. The point I want to raise about masturbation is that it is a means to an end. We are not asking you to spend your sex lives masturbating if you prefer to transfer your activities to sex with a partner. Some of you, on the other hand, might prefer to masturbate on your own. It's your choice.'

The therapists complemented each other in putting an end to Doreen's objections. Therapist B was the peacemaker but Therapist A was firm and directive. Sometimes a plan of having one therapist as a policy-maker and 'an authority' is useful.

At this stage Camilla made a comment:

CAMILLA: 'I agree with Patricia about Onan, but I do not feel right about masturbating.'
DAPHNE: 'Why not? Your clitoris is there for a purpose.'
CAMILLA: 'I think it's for a man to touch.'
DAPHNE: 'That's really sexist. That's what men say; it's their propaganda. I say it's your own clitoris and you can do what you want with it. It's your choice. Right?'
CAMILLA: 'Yes.'
JENNIFER: 'My worry about masturbation is that it is an end in itself and could stop a person, male or female, from progressing to a partner situation.'
CAMILLA: 'That's really what I mean, Daphne.'
DAPHNE: 'Why do we always need to think about partners and pleasing them? What's wrong with pleasing ourselves?'
JENNIFER: 'Well, I would like to have good sex with a partner. That's why I came to this group.'
THERAPIST B: 'You are all here for different reasons and that's good. We do not expect you to have the same desires and motives. Some of you have partners and obviously want to build up your sexual confidence to share your pleasure with your partner. Others who do not have partners want to find out what an orgasm is like and to take it from there.'

Masturbation is always a controversial topic in women's groups. It is obviously helpful to include in the group some women who approve of masturbation. In the group selection procedure it is always possible for therapists to balance a group if all the women already registered hate the idea of masturbation. The therapists could wait for some women who are positive in their attitude to register although this situation would be unusual as the majority of the women who apply to join groups do not disapprove of masturbation. They usually are not confident or have problems associated with achieving an orgasm when they masturbate. Of course, statistically, there will always be some women who have never masturbated. It is also difficult to assess whether some women are telling the truth; if they object so strongly to masturbation they might not admit to having tried it.

A negative attitude towards masturbation is often expressed by women who come from different cultures. Caribbean women often disapprove of masturbation because of their religious upbringing, especially Roman Catholics.

Muslim women also have reservations about masturbation, although they are willing to try it. Muslim women, on the whole, are unwilling to join groups, as their husbands or families do not like the idea. Some men are worried that more liberated westernised women will influence their wives. Some African women are very unfortunate if they come from a tribe where clitoridectomy is performed and the clitoris is cut off. This barbaric act certainly almost prevents any response from the surrounding nerves.

Therapists need to be firm about getting the women at least to try masturbation and usually some other group members support them. Both Camilla and Doreen objected to masturbation. When they returned to the group both had sabotaged their homework.

CAMILLA: 'I did not have as much time this week as I had to work overtime.'
THERAPIST B: 'What? At weekends as well?'
CAMILLA: 'Not on Sunday, but I go to church on that day.'
DAPHNE: 'You don't go to church all day, do you?'
CAMILLA: 'No, but I help with Sunday school. After that I had a migraine.'
JENNIFER: 'You sound as though you did not want to do your homework. How is that you made time the weeks before; were you on holiday?'
CAMILLA: 'No.'
JENNIFER: 'You and Doreen are the ones who do not like the idea of masturbation, aren't you?'
DOREEN: 'Well, I tried but my husband wanted to know what I was doing. He put me off, as he wanted sex. I know you did mention we should tell our partners that we are having therapy and do not want sex but it's difficult.'
JENNIFER: 'So you found a good excuse for one night?'
THERAPIST A: 'How many times did you actually try the masturbation programme, Doreen?'
DOREEN: 'Once, actually. I did have the bath and try to relax about twice, but my husband keeps on coming into the bathroom.'
JENNIFER: 'Can't you lock the door?'
DOREEN: 'No, he would break it down.'
THERAPIST A: 'Do you really not want to do the masturbation task, Doreen?'
DOREEN: 'No. You see the truth is that my husband objects.'

THERAPIST A: 'I think we should do some role play at this stage in which you explain the situation to your husband so that you could get more privacy to do your own thing. Then you will get more confident about carrying out your homework.'

Doreen and some of the other women did the role play and Doreen ended up speaking quite firmly:

DOREEN: 'No dear, I really do not want to share my homework with you. I prefer to do the tasks on my own, like the other women in the group. When I am ready to involve you later I will be pleased to let you know.'
THERAPIST A: 'That sounded good, Doreen.'
THERAPIST B: 'Yes, it was convincing. Let's go back to you, Camilla. Could you make some time to do your homework this week?'
DAPHNE: 'You can make excuses but you don't make any progress.'
CAMILLA: 'I can try.'
THERAPIST B: 'You don't look convinced, Camilla.'
CAMILLA: 'No, I feel it's wrong to masturbate. It could affect my eyes and give me migraine.'
THERAPIST A: 'Where did you learn that, Camilla?'
CAMILLA: 'I don't remember. Someone back home must have said it.'
DAPHNE: 'What a stupid thing, you must be really crazy to believe it.'
THERAPIST A: 'It's not that illogical for people to become anxious about masturbating and to worry so much that they get tension headaches. The mind can affect the body. What I suggest you could do is to take a lavender oil bath and really relax in it and burn some incense and then take the incense into your bedroom and try the homework.'

It was good that Daphne had spontaneously criticised Camilla. Therapist A did give Camilla some support when she was under attack but remained firm with her. The policy paid off as when Camilla attended the group the following week she had made some progress:

CAMILLA: 'It was much easier than I thought. I burned some sandalwood incense and this took me back to my roots. I remembered some of the thoughts I had about sex, but it did not put me off. I touched myself and found it was quite nice. My clitoris got bigger, like you said.'

Camilla succeeded in obtaining an orgasm by the fifth session. The other women were all very warm and thrilled; only Daphne was cool and envious. Doreen was particularly pleased and supportive.

Although Camilla was the shy one of the two Caribbean women she actually succeeded earlier than the extraverted Doreen. It can be a delicate situation in a group if there is an ethnic minority which forms a support system and a member of the majority group appears hostile. On the other hand, it can be very good for women of all cultures to discuss attitudes and learn about one another in a permissive atmosphere.

A case of control

Daphne was happy talking about masturbation and criticising the others, but her biggest hang-up was her inability to let herself go. Not only did she like controlling others but she liked to be in full control of herself. She was unable to have an orgasm. She had attended a women's group which had been psychoanalytically orientated and had come away from the group realising that she disliked her father who represented a threat of disorderly behaviour with his drinking habits. Daphne had never been drunk. She had eventually turned against men, although she had tried marriage, and had landed up in a happy lesbian situation.

When Daphne was asked to exaggerate any stage of masturbation that worried or embarrassed her she was willing enough to try that out.

DAPHNE: 'Well, that's a new approach. They did not include that at the Centre. It makes sense.'
DOREEN: 'It might be all right for you, but I dread to think what my husband will think.'
DAPHNE: 'That's the trouble with men, they are always suspicious.
DOREEN: 'I would rather live with a man than a woman. It's not natural how you are.'
DAPHNE: 'Why don't you mind your own business.'
DOREEN: 'It is our business in the group. You might stand a better chance of having an orgasm with a man than a woman.'
DAPHNE: 'I have already tried it with a man and it was no good. You aren't doing so well yourself, are you?'
DOREEN: 'Yes, I am. Bert agreed to let me do my exercises in peace.'
CAMILLA: 'You did all right, Doreen.'
DOREEN: 'No one has done as well as you, Camilla. Some people are jealous.'
THERAPIST A: 'There is bound to be some envy when one woman succeeds so early on – all of you are at different levels in any case.'

JENNIFER: 'It's like we are handicapped.'
THERAPIST B: 'That's a good way of putting it.'

The therapists did not interrupt when the discussion on lesbianism took place between Daphne and Doreen. If things had got more heated it would have been reasonable for the therapist to intervene. Jennifer was the rescuer as she broke up the tension by generalising. Homosexuality is an extremely emotive issue in Caribbean culture. Homosexuality has always attracted disapproval and tension has mounted since the publicity on AIDS. Originally paedophiliacs were condemned but recently prejudice towards gay men has increased and this has generalised to gay women.

Daphne had been in a women's group previously and knew the answers to prejudiced attitudes towards lesbianism. She occasionally was over-defensive towards Doreen. Sometimes women from Indian and African cultures can be intimidated by women like Daphne, but Doreen took the situation in her stride.

THERAPIST A: 'Let's continue the discussion of exaggerating things associated with masturbation that cause anxiety, Daphne.'
DAPHNE: 'I think I would exaggerate my breathing and movement.'
CAMILLA: 'I suppose we have to make sure that the neighbours do not hear us.'
THERAPIST B: 'You can always play a cassette tape in your bedroom.'
DAPHNE: 'I am prepared to do anything to make things work.'
THERAPIST B: 'You should not strive too much for a climax; try to concentrate on the task of exaggerating. Also don't forget the element of enjoyment in your homework. Some of you make heavy weather of it.'

Women like Daphne try too hard and are so performance-orientated that this finally inhibits their goal. It was hardly surprising the next week, when the group met again, that Daphne had not achieved an orgasm. The therapists had discussed a policy in advance to pay special attention to Daphne's responses when the practice task of role playing an orgasm was required of the women. The policy, if Daphne did not do this properly, was for one therapist to be very critical of her and the other to be somewhat supportive and act as Daphne's friend, but to be firm nevertheless.

THERAPIST: 'We want you to pretend to have an orgasm and role play what would happen. You can listen to this tape and join in the

screaming, moaning and heavy breathing. Does anyone feel awkward over this?'
DAPHNE: 'I don't particularly like this type of task but as I failed with the last lot of homework and did not get an orgasm I am prepared to try.'

When the women and the therapists practised the task Daphne hardly responded at all.

THERAPIST A: 'I did not see you joining in, Daphne. You said you were going to scream, grimace and breathe heavily like everyone else.'
THERAPIST B: 'Perhaps you feel too embarrassed.'
DAPHNE: 'I do feel awkward.'
JENNIFER: 'So do I, but we are all doing it together.'
THERAPIST B: 'That's right. When you are alone no one will be watching.'
THERAPIST A: 'I think you are too afraid to lose control, Daphne, so you might as well forget about having an orgasm.'
THERAPIST B: 'What do you think will happen to you if you do lose control, Daphne?'
DAPHNE: 'I think I might faint or urinate on the bed.'
THERAPIST A: 'There is nothing wrong with that, get a towel and put it under you and let it all hang out.'
THERAPIST B: 'You could try that, Daphne. It would not be so bad if you fainted, would it? No one is going to criticise you.'
DAPHNE: 'I have never fainted.'
DOREEN: 'If you really want to see people let themselves go you should join the Baptists.'
DAPHNE: 'Is that a joke?'
DOREEN: 'No, I'll take you there this Sunday if you like.'

This was one of the most surprising invitations of the group. Usually the women had met for a drink after the group session. Friendships had formed like Jennifer and Daphne who had gone together to buy magazines to help them fantasise. The meeting did actually take place and Daphne and Doreen became friends. Two weeks later Daphne did become orgasmic but by that time she had also bought a vibrator. Daphne did not know whether to thank the Baptists or the vibrator for her orgasm.

Jennifer: problems with sexual fantasies

Sometimes women have problems over fantasising. They feel it is wrong to think about things they find stimulating but which could be classified as kinky. Jennifer had secondary anorgasmia, she had been able to enjoy orgasms when she was younger but by the age of twenty she no longer had orgasms although she was happy about masturbating.

Jennifer's main problem was that she totally stopped herself from fantasising when she masturbated. She had reached the fifth session in therapy and she was still making little progress. Various books had been recommended but Jennifer was not enthusiastic about them:

JENNIFER: 'I thought *My Secret Garden*[8] was shocking. I can't imagine women having those sort of fantasies.
CAMILLA: 'I agree with Jennifer. I particularly disliked the fantasy of the dog licking cake mix off a woman's pussy, I mean her genitals. But I quite liked the woman having to do it at knife point fantasy.'
JENNIFER: 'But that's rape.'
CAMILLA: 'I know, it makes me feel bad liking the fantasy.'
THERAPIST B: 'That's quite a normal response, Camilla. You can feel aroused by something you know would be horrific if it happened in reality, because it is only a fantasy.'
THERAPIST A: 'That's right. We said before that you must give yourselves permission to think about what you like. Try to think back to when you were developing sexually and remember what you thought about sex then and what you thought it would be like to make love.'
JENNIFER: 'It's hard to remember. I can think of a French film I once saw that was sexy, but that's about all.'
THERAPIST A: 'That's fine, try to remember that. Do any of you have access to erotic videos at home?'

The usual answer to this question is that the men in the house have crude pornographic videos, but nothing really suitable. Some clinics show films or videos designed for therapy. Some of the tapes can be quite erotic and may be used as an aid to fantasy. It can be quite erotic for women to see videos of other women or men masturbating, or of couples enjoying foreplay.

Jennifer's story has a happy ending, thanks to a trip to Amsterdam. Although she had not become orgasmic by the time the group ended she decided to go on a trip to Amsterdam. She was confident enough to go with her two friends to various 'Live Sex Shows' which included sex between women, sex between a man and a woman and a mini-orgy. She described the experience as unbelievable and returned to London with enough fantasies to last her a lifetime.

She returned to London with a mini-library of sex books and arrived at the Women's Group follow-up reporting that she had become orgasmic.

Women are very supportive towards one another and appear to do well in groups. It is good to give the ones that have not succeeded another chance by getting them to do some homework and explaining that the course was very demanding, that they could consolidate what they had learned, and come for another follow-up in three months' time.

References

1. Barbach, Lonnie Garfield. (1975) *For Yourself – The Fulfilment of Female Sexuality*. Doubleday.
2. LoPiccolo, J. and Lobitz, W.C. (1972) 'The role of masturbation in the treatment of orgasmic dysfunction.' *Archives of Sexual Behaviour*. 2, 163–171.
3. Dodson, Betty. (1976) *Liberating Masturbation*. Published and distributed by Betty Dodson, Box 1933, New York, New York 10001.
4. Gillan, P., Golombok, S. and Becker, P. 'NHS sex therapy groups for women.' *Brit.Jrnl.Sexual Medicine*. 7 (64). 44–47.
5. Hooper, Anne. (1980) *The Body Electric*. Virago.
6. Dickson, Anne. (1986) *The Mirror Within*. Quartet Books.
7. Gillan, Patricia and McMullen, Susan. (1978) 'Women's Sex Therapy Groups in London'. Paper presented at Rome, World Congress of Medical Sexology.
8. Friday, Nancy. (1975) *My Secret Garden*. Virago.

Chapter 10

Men's Sex Therapy Groups

Zilbergeld's contribution

Zilbergeld in California reported as early as 1975 a successful programme for sexually dysfunctional men attending group therapy without a partner.

Before Zilbergeld's research most clinics accepted only men referred with a partner, as a couple. If a man did not have a partner the clinic suggested he should go and find one. This latter attitude did not make sense as many men needed help from the clinic in order to find a partner. Such men had lost their sexual confidence, or blame had been put upon them by an existing partner who was unwilling or unable to attend for therapy. Other men were single by choice, not having found a partner to settle down with or perhaps preferring a series of one night stands.

A male and a female therapist conducted several Zilbergeld groups for erectile and ejaculatory problems. This research on men's group sex therapy resulted in a sensible and effective series of techniques resulting in 'The Zilbergeld Programme' which has been successfully applied in the USA and Europe.

Emphasis is placed initially on body image and touch. The men are asked to discuss touch in a group session, then they are given homework to explore their tactile sensations. They are asked to select ten different objects varying in degrees of hot/cold, soft/hard, rough/smooth, sticky/non-sticky, and to touch each object and rate it for pleasant or sensual feelings. Many men have never deliberately touched objects before and are quite intrigued. Usually in the discussion, childhood memories are brought up where touching was forbidden and even punished with the words 'Don't touch', which led to guilt and inhibition over touch. Research on child health and development has shown that touch is essential and tactile deprivation can even lead to the death of infants. It appears, during discussion, that there is a sex difference over this aptitude, as women seem to touch things more readily.

Zilbergeld points out in his book, *Men and Sex*[1], that America is a particularly non-touching society. Several men in the British groups suggested that English men rarely touch one another compared with Continental and Asian men. In American society there is the underlying assumption that touch is sexual; if people hold hands this leads to kissing and sex.

Associated with touch is the fact that boys compared with girls do not have as much physical contact with their parents. Zilbergeld refers to the fact that boys have shorter physical contact with their mother than girls have with their father as the concept of 'being sissy' underlies a mother/son relationship. Girls see their mother kissing and being affectionate with friends, whereas boys do not see their father behaving in this manner. Therefore there is a difference in learning between boys and girls. All these facts are brought up in the group and discussed fully.

The men in the groups usually reinforce the fact that touch is associated with the opposite sex and they only touch the same sex in activities connected with sport and being rough. They discuss the fact that women are nice and soft to touch. When they carry out the homework, selecting the ten items to experiment with touching, they tend to rate silk and soft fabrics high on the pleasant scale, whereas cold objects like keys or glass are low, especially if cold and slimy.

The next stage of taking a bath and massaging the body is much more strange to men in a group. Most women in group therapy have no qualms over such a task but men are not used to pampering themselves with massage oil. When asked to experiment with massaging their own bodies after the bath various comments like 'How odd!' or 'Why have we got to do this?' are expressed. Usually, most of the men in the groups who carry out this homework task mention that self-touching is very different to touching someone else.

The Zilbergeld programme consists of each man assessing his body image with a homework task of standing in front of the mirror and looking at his body then turning sideways in the mirror and observing his profile. Both these tasks are carried out nude. Questions are asked like 'Which part of your body do you like or dislike?'. This type of homework can be very revealing and as time progresses the men in the group become increasingly frank about their homework.

Approximately ten sessions cover homework connected with

looking at and touching the genitals. Masturbation tasks are the stop and start techniques for premature ejaculators, and the losing an erection task for men who have erectile problems. The latter task gives a client the confidence to lose his erection deliberately and then find he can get it back.

Perhaps a good way of describing the groups and their advantages and pitfalls is to follow the progress of two men who underwent therapy.

A case of erectile failure

Walter was a 27-year-old PhD student from Los Angeles. He had been very successful with women but had never enjoyed a steady relationship. He was attractive to look at, a typical Hispanic American with dark brown skin and very black hair. He looked extremely relaxed, but this was deceptive and only a facade as he was full of anxiety inside. His field of English Literature was a way of unlocking the chastity belts of many intellectual and well-to-do young women studying English but, instead of enjoying this sexual freedom he was inhibited and anxious, mainly about AIDS, and this ruined his sexual appetite and performance.

Initially he seemed very happy about touching the ten objects. He was obviously an extremely sensual man and liked touching things. He brought a rose to the group and the other men did not tease him or call him effeminate. He was a popular group member with his cheerful manner. His body image work went well and he enjoyed his body, letting the group know that his penis was pretty big.

FEMALE THERAPIST: 'You sound as though you had no problem with your homework.'
HARRY: 'If you are so big how come you can't get it in when you have sex?'
WALTER: 'Because it's too soft.'

Harry was a premature ejaculator who always came outside a woman. From the beginning of the group meetings he complained that his penis was too small. He was also a Nigerian journalist who had some very odd ideas about sex for a well-educated male. He remarked that most women thought Africans were well-endowed. He had already become very animated when the group discussed homosexuality and had almost accused Walter of being gay. Harry denied there was such a thing as homosexuality in Nigeria, telling the group that such people did not exist. Although Walter had not yet revealed his phobia of AIDs to the group he had been very liberal towards the concept of homosexuality, having grown up in California which is quite a permissive state.

During the course, Zilbergeld's myths about male sexuality were brought up and discussed. The men were asked to read the chapter on male myths. Obviously Zilbergeld's myth 'Sex requires an erection' was relevant to the discussion between Walter and Harry.

MALE THERAPIST: 'Let's talk about the male sexuality myths you read about for your homework. Do you agree with these myths, Walter?'
WALTER: 'I find it hard to accept that you can enjoy sex without intercourse, which of course requires an erection which I don't get.'
HARRY: 'Of course you need an erection to get inside. If you come outside it's not proper sex.'
FEMALE THERAPIST: 'But surely mutual masturbation can be pleasurable sex?'
HARRY: 'Not for me, oh no.'
FEMALE THERAPIST: 'Well, it's good for me to have mutual masturbation.'
WALTER: 'Is that so? We learn a lot about women in this group. Don't you like to feel a stiff penis inside you?'
FEMALE THERAPIST: 'Sometimes, but I agree with a lot of women who say that a small finger, skillfully applied, can do more than a big erect penis.'
WALTER: 'I like that!'
HARRY: 'You must be joking!'
FEMALE THERAPIST: 'No, I really mean it.'

This type of self-revelation can be quite useful in a group situation, as most women that men meet reinforce the male myths as they, too, are dishonest about themselves. Zilbergeld found it useful to have a woman therapist to lead the group with a male therapist as the men had the opportunity to learn about women in an informal setting. In this setting it seemed much more natural to discuss very personal sexual details, like being asked whether a stiff penis inside is an ideal. Most female therapists agree that it is easier to reply to questions in a group compared with a one to one situation with a male client where things are interpreted as at a much more personal level.

MALE THERAPIST: 'We all seem to be making the assumption that a man needs an erection to enjoy sex without intercourse?'

HARRY: 'I would have thought that it takes a good erection to enjoy sex.'
WALTER: 'I only feel like a real guy when my penis is hard.'
FRANK: 'That's a real macho attitude.'
MALE THERAPIST: 'You can get very pleasurable sensations and enjoy sex when a woman touches your penis. It does not have to be erect.'
FRANK: 'Yes, that happens to me.'
HARRY: 'But you don't come at all so you are different.'
WALTER: 'That's a mean thing to say, Harry.'
FRANK: I can take it, man, but don't forget I have come in my time. I am a situational delayed ejaculator.'
FEMALE THERAPIST: 'We are always coming up against this barrier of people not understanding one another's problems.'

Sometimes it is good for a therapist to intervene if things are getting out of hand. Often men cannot empathise with one another. In this case the intervention was not essential but it was useful to remind the men that they need to understand one another's problems before making hurtful remarks.

FEMALE THERAPIST: 'You might have hurt Frank's feelings, Harry.'
HARRY: 'This thick-skinned Jamaican is tough.'
FRANK: 'Yeah, man, it takes a lot to put me down. But I've noticed you speak out of turn sometimes about things you don't know about.'
WALTER: 'You can say that again.'

Again, during this particular session personal tensions were building up. Sometimes it is difficult to keep the peace between Africans and Caribbean men. Many Africans regard Caribbeans as inferior and descended from slaves. This creates personal tension and had already come up in the group. Frank had told Harry that Africans themselves had enslaved people from other tribes and that Harry could be descended from such ancestors. It's hard to mix men of different cultures in groups, but on the other hand it is a challenge which can lead to attitude change as the men get to know each other and appreciate their different backgrounds.

The male therapist decided to intervene at this stage.

MALE THERAPIST: 'You made an interesting point Harry about Frank being thick-skinned.'
HARRY: 'He is.'
MALE THERAPIST: 'I suppose this is a quality that we males value. I am

thinking about the Zilbergeld myth that men should not have feelings or show emotions.'
FRANK: 'I see that as macho; it's a matter of conditioning, I would have thought.'

Frank came up with quite sophisticated arguments from time to time. He played bass in a local band at night and worked by day on the buses. He was quite shrewd and usually tactful. The others were somewhat wary of Frank. He was not moulded in their image of what a reggae man is all about, and sometimes he was too articulate for them, except for Walter.

HARRY: 'In my culture we express feelings more than Europeans do. Ibo people are the most expressive people in Nigeria.'
WALTER: 'I wish the same could be said about Americans, especially in situations of mourning, for example. We have to keep a stiff upper lip and not cry at funerals in our culture.'
FEMALE THERAPIST: 'Do you think it's effeminate to cry, Walter?'
WALTER: 'No, I don't personally, but we are culture-bound, I think. Sometimes I feel like crying when I can't get an erection but I hate my feelings.'
FEMALE THERAPIST: 'What if you expressed your feelings?'
WALTER: 'I would not do that; I just make an excuse and say I'm tired, or something like that.'
FEMALE THERAPIST: 'Do you think you would lose a girlfriend if you were more honest?'
WALTER: 'Yes I do, I lose them pretty fast as it is.'
FEMALE THERAPIST: 'Maybe that's because you hide your emotions and appear distant.'
WALTER: 'Yes, I have been told that twice by two different women.'
FEMALE THERAPIST: 'Are you having a relationship now?'
WALTER: 'Yes, but it's not much good. I see her once a week, on a Saturday night. She said she can't understand why I feel tired all the time.'
FEMALE THERAPIST: 'Why not be more direct and tell her you have a problem that you feel upset about?'
WALTER: 'I don't think I could do that.'
FEMALE THERAPIST: 'Let's role play the situation.'
WALTER: 'Okay.'
FEMALE THERAPIST: 'I'll play the part of your girlfriend. What's her name?'
WALTER: 'It's Jean and she is a lot more aggressive than you are. She teaches English at a polytechnic and she is quite a powerful lady.'

FEMALE THERAPIST: 'Is that what attracts you to her?'
WALTER: 'Yes, dare I say it, she's like my mother. She knows how to put a man down.'
FEMALE THERAPIST: 'Walter, I know you have had several years of psychoanalysis and you don't want to go into these details. I think role play would definitely be the thing for you. I'll play the part of Jean. "What's wrong with you Walter, do you feel tired again? You never get a hard on with me."'
WALTER: 'I feel upset. I am always making excuses and saying I feel tired but the truth is that I find it difficult to get an erection in the first place.'
FEMALE THERAPIST: '"That's difficult for you but let's touch each other up. That would be fun."'

This role play went down very well and Walter needed no prompting and he was praised for expressing his feelings.

FEMALE THERAPIST: 'That sounded good, Walter. How did you feel?'
WALTER: 'Foolish. I don't think Jean would respond the way you did.'
FEMALE THERAPIST: 'Could you role play what you think she would say?'
WALTER: '"If you are not tired you can't be attracted to me, Walter. I feel offended by that."'
FEMALE THERAPIST: 'I don't think she would say that and if she did she would not be worth pursuing. Why don't you test her out and actually express some feelings? You sound much more human when you do so. Are you seeing her this Saturday?'
WALTER: 'Yes, I am. I suppose I've got nothing to lose. I spent five years in analysis and got nowhere so I'm prepared to try out some new techniques.'
FRANK: 'That looked good the way you did it, Walter.'
HARRY: 'I think if he talks like that he'll lose her.'
FEMALE THERAPIST: 'I don't agree, but let's see.'

A week later the group met and Walter looked quite pleased with himself.

FEMALE THERAPIST: 'How did things go, Walter?'
WALTER: 'Better than I imagined. I am still dating Jean. It's funny when I told her my feelings she did actually say she thought maybe I found her unattractive, but she put it in a nice way.'
FEMALE THERAPIST: 'Did you suggest some massage and mutual masturbation?'
WALTER: 'Yes, that went all right. She said she liked that sort of thing

but had never suggested it previously as I always seemed too tired for anything. The funniest thing of all was that I did get an erection.'
FEMALE THERAPIST: 'That's really good. I guess no demands were being made of you so you were able to enjoy your erection.
WALTER: 'But I lost it after about five minutes.'
FEMALE THERAPIST: 'Why was that?'
WALTER: 'I don't really know. I guess I was thinking about whether it would last.'
MALE THERAPIST: 'It seems that you have done all right, but fallen into the trap of performance anxiety by thinking about your erection.'
WALTER: 'You could say that.'
MALE THERAPIST: 'This is something I want to concentrate on today in the group and to give you homework to illustrate our discussion. I would like each of you to masturbate at home and deliberately lose your erections and then relax and enjoy the sexual feelings when you touch yourself again.'
HARRY: 'I don't get any feelings when I do myself. I gave that up when I was 14 years old. I think masturbation is dirty and wrong and I have not come to this group for that.'
WALTER: 'I must say I did not think I would be asked to masturbate but I feel more positive about it than you do; at least I know I get a good erection if I play with myself. In any case I think it's good if we go along with what the therapists say; I've scored so far.'
HARRY: 'We don't have to do the tasks, do we?'
FEMALE THERAPIST: 'No one is forced to do anything they really feel uncomfortable with, but if you think in terms of graded tasks that are designed to give you confidence in the future that would be more positive thinking.'
WALTER: 'In any case, Kinsey said that 99 per cent of males masturbate.'
HARRY: 'Yeah, that's in the USA.'
FRANK: 'I would say most men do it, but don't like to admit it.'

Both the therapists, together with Walter and Frank, had tried to be positive about masturbation and were supported by other group members, especially those with European backgrounds. Sometimes masturbation becomes an issue which is divided along racial lines with Africans and West Indians against it. This could be due to strict or religious upbringing, especially where Roman Catholics like Harry had conditioned well. Usually it is better to wait until the next session before pushing masturbation too hard. Then the men who have done the masturbation task return and talk positively about it and the ones who have not carried out their homework feel awkward as they are missing out. Those men with religious objections can also be reassured by telling them that masturbation is a temporary measure to help them solve their problems.

At this stage Walter had not been really honest with the group about his real reason for his erectile dysfunction and his phobia of AIDS. The two therapists decided to discuss the issue of AIDS at the next session and see how the others reacted and precicted that Walter would have a chance to express his opinion.

When the men met for the next session Walter looked quite pleased with himself again.

WALTER: 'I did the homework and lost my erection like you said and got it back by relaxing and having a sexual fantasy and then touching myself. It was good.'
MALE THERAPIST: 'That's fine, so you found it useful. What about you, Frank?'
FRANK: 'Yes, I managed it too, but I never have problems over maintaining my erections. The failure to ejaculate with my partner is my problem.'
MALE THERAPIST: 'What about you, Harry?'
HARRY: 'What about it?'
MALE THERAPIST: 'How did you get on with the homework?'
HARRY: 'I told you I don't do things like masturbate; it's unhealthy.'
MALE THERAPIST: 'How do you mean?'
HARRY: 'It weakens you.'
MALE THERAPIST: 'There is no evidence for that. Who told you that?'
HARRY: 'A priest told us at school.'
MALE THERAPIST: 'Well, I am a scientist and believe you me if there was such evidence it would make the news headlines. It's a myth.'
MICHAEL: 'I used to think the same thing as Harry. I also went to an RC school like you, Harry, but it's nonsense.'
MALE THERAPIST: 'How did you get on, Michael?'
MICHAEL: 'Masturbating and deliberately losing my erection taught me some self-control. When I lost my erection I started to think of times I'd been with my wife and had worried that I wouldn't be able to make it.'
HARRY: 'Well, I don't want to masturbate and be a wanker.'
WALTER: 'Hey, steady on, that's heavy.'

At this stage the therapists decided to bring up the issue of AIDS.

MALE THERAPIST: 'There are various emotive issues associated with sex and masturbation is one of them. Probably the latest controversial issue is that of AIDS. Have any of you got views on this issue? I notice we have not talked about it in the group before.'

HARRY: 'Well, I come up against it in this country as everyone thinks Africans have AIDS. I am an Ibo man and we do not have it in my country.'

MICHAEL: 'It is frightening as a lot of gay men are dying from AIDS. As a gay man myself I have to be very careful, I suppose I'm glad I've lost my sex drive as it's kept me out of trouble for a couple of years.'

WALTER: 'It's not just homosexuals; you should see the latest statistics. I get obsessed with it – it puts me off sex. Sometimes I think of AIDS when I am trying to make love and I lose my erection. It's like a vicious circle – I want to find a steady girlfriend but I lose my erection when I make love so I lose my girlfriend.'

FEMALE THERAPIST: 'But you have not lost Jean, have you?'

WALTER: 'No, I saw her again last Saturday and things went well. We still have not made love but we are enjoying some mutual masturbation. I'm actually maintaining my erection too, which is good news.'

FEMALE THERAPIST: 'Is there anything wrong with mutual masturbation?'

WALTER: 'I guess I've been conditioned to think it's second best, not the real thing.'

FEMALE THERAPIST: 'If people are afraid of AIDS then mutual masturbation can be the answer. At least it makes sex safer as there is no penetration.'

HARRY: 'You would think of an answer to justify anything. Therapists are good politicians.'

FEMALE THERAPIST: 'I am only being realistic and honest.'

MICHAEL: 'It's true what she says. It did start in gay circles and we should try to think of alternative sexual methods to stop it from spreading. Mutual masturbation is suggested by most counselling centres.'

HARRY: 'If it's gays that carry it they should be stopped from having sex at all.'

MICHAEL: 'That's very dogmatic. What do you think we are, lepers?'

HARRY: 'Yes, you could put it that way. That's how some people have treated me because I am an African.'

MALE THERAPIST: 'There are a lot of ignorant people about. Better communication methods should be used to provide facts. In any case we don't want to get into a political discussion here.'

WALTER: 'So perhaps I have a solution now. If I go in for mutual masturbation this will avoid the danger of AIDS. The trouble is what woman is going to tolerate no sexual intercourse?

FEMALE THERAPIST: Walter, you are being emotional again. You have already seen that Jean tolerates this, as you put it. I bet she enjoys it. Have you read the Hite Report about what women say about clitoral stimulation and mutual masturbation?'

WALTER: 'Yes, I have and it supports what you say. But it's very different when you talk to someone sensible like you, a doctor, to what women are really like.'

HARRY: 'Yes, I've never spoken frankly to a white woman before. The ones I knew back home were mostly nuns and you could never talk about sex with them.'

FRANK: 'Did you have fantasies about having sex with white women?'

WALTER: 'I had fantasies about having it with a black woman. I saw this SAR film in San Francisco, something about 'Love in the Afternoon' and there was this black chick on top of this white man. Her breasts were beautiful, they bounced up and down as she moved.'

MALE THERAPIST: 'I am glad we have brought up fantasy as this is something I want to go into. Obviously it's good that you already have some fantasies, Walter, as you can make use of them when you lose your erection.'

It turned out that Walter had an extremely rich fantasy life. In fact he increased his income by writing articles for a Norwegian soft porn magazine. He was relatively easy to treat, in spite of his phobia of AIDS. Eventually he adjusted to the idea of mutual masturbation. Jean told him that she was orgasmic with him and this had happened for the first time for her with a partner. They settled down together after two months and he moved into her apartment. They changed their sexual pattern to full sexual intercourse, but safeguarding against AIDS by using a sheath.

Harry's problem of situational premature ejaculation

Most groups include a troublemaker and Harry certainly knew how to stir up trouble. He was well-suited to his job on a certain well-known daily newspaper, but was disliked by most of the group members, especially Frank from Jamaica. On the other hand, it's always useful to have someone like Harry in the group as he united the others who generally supported anything Harry was against.

Harry came from a rich and interesting background. His father was a priest or seer man in Afa Divination but his mother was a Roman Catholic and he had been brought up as a believer in the faith. He had gone away to a Catholic college and masturbated against the advice of the priest. He then suffered from a guilt complex for his 'self relief' from the age of 14 until the group had almost finished, when cognitive therapy suddenly worked for Harry.

Situational premature ejaculation was Harry's problem. The irony was that he could ejaculate satisfactorily with his wife back home in Nigeria, but was no longer sexually attracted to her now that she had borne him five children. He appeared to have a series of women friends abroad who were willing to have sex with him but his premature ejaculation ruined his pleasure as he always came outside, losing control of himself. He had not returned home for two years and was worried that he might also lose control with his wife. When Harry was assessed and his case history was taken he was very adamant about not discussing his background with members of the group. Oddly enough he was very willing to join a group of men, whereas most clients want individual therapy and are opposed to the idea of a group. As Harry was an investigative journalist we did not rule out the possibility that he might write a piece on the group so we cautioned him about this. He said he would not do that but would like the experience of being a group member.

From the beginning of the group Harry objected to the homework tasks. He did not even like the idea of choosing the ten objects to touch, remarking that he was an Oxford graduate and that this new course was the most surrealistic scene he had ever encountered. He did carry out the task, however, meticulously rating each object.

Harry liked his body and certainly dressed to kill, emphasising his sexual organs which he was proud of. Admittedly he was handsome and physically attractive to women with his lively eyes, nice smile and slim hips. It was when he opened his mouth that his aggression tended to turn people off him.

When the 'Zilbergeld myths' session came up he argued about almost every myth, particularly about Myth 4: 'A man always wants and is always ready to have sex'.

HARRY: 'What's wrong with that? I am always ready to have sex. That's normal.'
WALTER: 'You would not like to be treated like a sex machine and expect to serve every woman who asked for it, just like pressing a button, would you?'
HARRY: 'Why not?'
FRANK: 'You might not feel like it at the time.'
HARRY: 'I always feel like it. Women turn me on.'
FRANK: 'Any woman?'
HARRY: 'Why not?'

MICHAEL: 'That's ridiculous, but I wish I could say I get turned on by a woman.'
WALTER: 'Harry is a sexual robot.'
MALE THERAPIST: 'This myth is reinforced by men like Harry. We men think it's just women who make excuses and feel tired or are hypochondriacs when it comes to sex.'
FEMALE THERAPIST: 'I agree and I suppose I reinforce that model, but when you come to think of it it's impossible for a man to fake an erection whereas a woman can at least pretend to feel like it and fake an orgasm.'
HARRY: 'I always feel like it.'
WALTER: 'Maybe that's because you have problems and feel let down and frustrated.'
HARRY: 'That's really personal, Walter.'
FRANK: 'Think about that one, man. Walter may be right.'

It was the topic of masturbation that really disturbed Harry. Obviously he needed to master masturbation to gain ejaculatory control but persuading him to do this was almost impossible. Even the therapists were becoming exasperated with Harry by the fifth session.

MICHAEL: 'Why don't you listen to the therapists, Harry?'
HARRY: 'I did not come to this group to masturbate.'
FEMALE THERAPIST: 'But if it leads to your gaining control, that's your goal.'
HARRY: 'Today I read about some new research associated with an anaesthetic; perhaps you are not up to date in this country.'
MALE THERAPIST: 'The trouble with that method is that it anaesthetises the woman as well.'
HARRY: 'I don't see that it matters if the man is all right.'
FEMALE THERAPIST: 'It does not necessarily work for the man, either. It's much better to be able to control yourself without the use of drugs. Harry.'
HARRY: 'I wish there were an injection for my situational premature ejaculation.'
MALE THERAPIST: 'Well, you've got to face the fact that there is not and to listen to us for a change. We know you feel guilty about masturbation but you could at least try one exercise we recommend. You touch yourself, stopping each time you start to feel excited and letting the excitement die down and touching yourself again. You should aim to last for fifteen minutes.'
HARRY: 'I'll think about it.'
FEMALE THERAPIST: 'That's not good enough. You don't give us a chance.

At least you would make some progress and be less critical of our methods if you carried out some of the exercises we suggest.'

The therapists had decided in advance to unite and be tough with Harry, rather than relying on group members to do their work for them.

When the group met a week later Harry did not show up. It was interesting that he was still the centre of attention for the group, although he was absent. Walter thought that the topic of AIDS had driven Harry away. Frank suggested that he had been too aggressive to Harry. Michael mentioned that Harry had a phobia of homosexuality, but did not blame himself for Harry's absence. The therapists noticed that the session went better without Harry's constant objections.

Harry turned up for the seventh session. He had left a message about having to leave the country for a few days but the secretary had not passed the message on. When we checked this story the secretary apologised. Harry had actually done the homework:

HARRY: 'Well, I did the stop start technique. I did it all right and lasted fifteen minutes on three occasions. Mind you, I did not like doing it.'
FEMALE THERAPIST: 'You have done really well, Harry.'
HARRY: 'I am pleased you think so.'
WALTER: 'That's fantastic, Harry.'
HARRY: 'I bet you talked about me last week and thought I was not going to return. I bet you were glad, Frank.'
FRANK: 'I thought we had driven you away. Maybe my slave talk was too heavy.'
HARRY: 'I can handle that. I am pleased you missed me.'
MALE THERAPIST: 'We would like you to continue with step 2 of the stop start technique and use a body lotion on your hand next, to simulate the feel of the vagina.'
HARRY: 'You mean I still have to masturbate? How long have I got to do that?'
MALE THERAPIST: 'Until you learn full self-control, Harry.'
HARRY: 'How long will that take?'
MALE THERAPIST: 'It's up to you. At least you can catch up now and you have a good chance of changing your habits and achieving your goals.'
HARRY: 'I still do not like the idea of masturbating.'
FEMALE THERAPIST: 'When you do your homework next try to say to yourself that masturbation is not so bad after all, tell yourself that it's quite nice and it's doing you good. We are asking you to masturbate

and giving you permission to do something you previously felt guilty about.'
HARRY: 'Talk like that won't work with me.'
FRANK: 'Christ, man, you are always so fucking negative.'

Harry did change his attitude slightly and cognitive therapy helped. He needed a lot of encouragement and positive thinking when he was asked to try out the stop start technique with his woman friend:

HARRY: 'Look, it's bad enough doing it on my own, but to get her involved is asking a lot. Look, I haven't even told Jill I go to this group.'
FEMALE THERAPIST: 'Let's role play the situation.'
HARRY: 'I hate role playing. Why not let someone else be me?'
FEMALE THERAPIST: 'All right. Walter, why don't you be Harry, initially?'
WALTER: 'Okay. Is that okay by you, Harry?'
HARRY: 'Yeah, go ahead.'
WALTER: '"By the way Jill. I don't think I mentioned before that I am going to a group for men with sexual difficulties."'
FEMALE THERAPIST: "'No, you haven't. So what sort of sexual difficulty do you have, Harry?'"
WALTER: '"I'm a premature ejaculator."'
HARRY: 'No. Tell her I'm a situational premature ejaculator, Walter.'
FEMALE THERAPIST: '"I don't mind what you call it. Is it curable, Harry?"'
WALTER: '"Sure, if I carry out the instructions the therapists give me. I have done all right so far, but now you are involved I really need you to help me."'
FEMALE THERAPIST: '"I'll do everything I can. Tell me what to do."'
WALTER: '"Let's look at the instruction sheet together and I'll explain the steps."'
FEMALE THERAPIST: 'Now it's your turn, Harry. Walter did that really well.'

Harry did a similar role play but did not sound too convincing. Nevertheless he was praised by the therapists.

It is reinforcing to provide praise for each client, no matter how badly he performs, as he will then have some positive reinforcement to work on. For example, if a client produces poor body movements his verbal delivery could be praised with the words: 'You said the words well and sounded convincing, but your body movement needs to be improved. Your shoulders were very hunched up and you looked depressed, although you sounded great.' Sometimes it is very difficult for the therapist to praise a performance in which the client does everything badly, but there is usually something that can be found to praise before constructive criticism is offered. Praiseworthy achievements could be: the client smiled nicely; his eye contact was good; his posture was suitable; he emphasised the right words; or he was not over-aggressive.

It took a long time for Harry to make progress although he did eventually learn some self-control. He became less guilty about masturbation. His relationship with Jill flourished and at follow-up he reported that they had enjoyed sexual intercourse several times and that he had lasted half the time. The Zilbergeld myths had not really got through to him as he really still only valued sexual intercourse and anything else was a poor substitute. Nevertheless he had made progress; he had changed some of his attitudes and was more tolerant towards the other men at the end of the group.

Frank: a delayed ejaculator

Frank was a fascinating client. He led two professional and two domestic lives. As a bus driver he was like any other Caribbean man in town, but as a bass player in a reggae group he was 'mean' and very sexy. He invited the group to see him perform and most of the men have never forgotten the abandoned way in which he moved.

The two domestic relationships Frank had were revealed halfway through the group sessions when he appeared to confuse the name of his woman Gloria with another woman called Jackie. The truth was that he lived with each of them in turn and had children by both of them. Frank had never formally married and could not be referred to as a bigamist. Sadly he did not ejaculate with either of them.

Frank took the group sessions in his stride and always appeared reasonable over the homework. It was not easy to see how he kept his cool with Harry who must have infuriated him at times.

Men with delayed ejaculation are statistically rare and certainly form the minority in men's sex therapy groups. In the present group Frank was the only delayed ejaculator whereas there were several premature ejaculators, some of whom were also impotent, and several other men suffering from erectile failure only.

Frank was able to ejaculate on his own and initially he had ejaculated with both his partners – enough to produce six children whom he was proud of. His only vice was alcohol. He liked his rum and confessed that this went right back to his Jamaican days when rum was cheap. He readily admitted his drinking problem to the group and the men quickly calculated the negative correlation between the bottles of rum consumed and the number of times he ejaculated. At one stage we discussed the connection between the ability to lose control in any situation and having an orgasm or ejaculating, but this was irrelevant as he expressed his emotions well and was happy to lose control readily through alcohol and marijuana when he played at clubs. He had a lot of insight into his problem:

FRANK: 'It's stimulation I need, man. I suppose I only get that with a new partner, but I don't have time or money to pick up more chicks.'
WALTER: 'Do they have groupies in the reggae world?'
FRANK: 'Yeah, but I wouldn't want to go with little girls. I'm a big man of 38; it would be like doing it with my girl of 17. In any case I can come if I masturbate, but I've got to a stage where Jackie is complaining she gets sore.'
FEMALE THERAPIST: 'What about Gloria?'
FRANK: 'She doesn't even want much fucking these days. She says she is getting too old.'
FEMALE THERAPIST: 'How old is she?'
FRANK: 'She is a bit younger than me. She went off sex when our son came and I don't want to press her, you know.'
FEMALE THERAPIST: 'I understand. So you prefer to work with Jackie.'
FRANK: 'Yes, but I don't want to make her sore.'
FEMALE THERAPIST: 'Are you drinking less this week? Drink could be the reason for your problem.'
FRANK: 'Yes, I thought you would get round to that. Jackie complains about that and says I get too rough with her.'
FEMALE THERAPIST: 'Do you mainly make love at night?'
FRANK: 'Yes, I suppose I've got into the habit of that. Its odd, because I do shift work and could do it during the daytime.'
FEMALE THERAPIST: 'Do you drink during the day?'
HARRY: 'Not usually. I can see what you are getting at.'
FEMALE THERAPIST: 'What are your sexual fantasies like?'
HARRY: 'Okay. I think of good things, chicks and all that. I can get high playing bass.'
FEMALE THERAPIST: 'Do you think of exciting things when you masturbate?'
HARRY: 'Yeah.'
FEMALE THERAPIST: 'What about when you and Jackie make love; do you fantasise then?'
FRANK: 'No.'
FEMALE THERAPIST: 'I would suggest that you try to do that and also to masturbate on your own for a while to get excited and when you are about to ejaculate to tell Jackie to come on top of you in the 'woman above position' and really move, so that you ejaculate inside her.'

FRANK: 'That sounds good but I don't think I could masturbate in front of Jackie and get her to do that.'
FEMALE THERAPIST: 'Obviously this takes time, but I would suggest that you explain things to her and masturbate in front of her this week as the first part of your homework and see how you get on before you continue with the second part next week.'

This procedure worked in a week as Jackie was only too ready to help out if she was not made sore. Frank never totally performed in the way he called 'normal'; he always needed a bit of self-stimulation but got there in the end. The suggestion that they made love more often during the day helped him over making love when he was not inebriated. He commented that since he had solved his sex problem he had not needed the alcohol to obliterate the problem from his mind.

If Frank had not succeeded in getting stimulated by masturbation we would have suggested that he used a vibrator to get super-stimulation. He probably would have needed a lot of persuasion to do that, so it was just as well that self-stimulation proved effective.

Michael: a man with low sexual interest

Michael was not as physically attractive as the other men in the group. He was a 46-year-old cockney plumber and ran his own business and appeared to be prosperous. He lived with a very pretty male photographer who wanted to be anonymous for personal reasons so the group called him 'the photographer'.

The relationship had deteriorated somewhat as the photographer was extremely houseproud and was always criticising Michael for his clumsiness and untidy habits. Michael had no real evidence but suspected the photographer of having affairs. He said he could not complain about this as he had lost interest sexually in the photographer, but could not remember whether this had happened before or after he suspected his partner of having affairs.

Michael did not get on too well with the other men in the group and was socially isolated probably because of his homosexuality and also his awkward manner. He was rather gauche and shy for such a successful businessman.

The subject of Michael's genitals came up early in the group sessions. He disliked his genitals, complaining that they were too small.

MICHAEL: 'I really felt very disappointed when I looked at my genitals.

My penis is very small, but so are my testicles. Looking at them in that manner made me think they were smaller.'
MALE THERAPIST: 'Probably when you get erect you are larger.'
MICHAEL: 'Not that much. In any case, I do not often get erect. I don't seem to think much about sex any more. It's probably my age. It depresses me.'
MALE THERAPIST: 'That's a myth about sex and age. If you think negatively like that you only will yourself into thinking there is no sex after forty.'
MICHAEL: 'That's what the photographer says. He is ten years younger than me, he is very attractive and dreads losing his looks and reaching the age of forty. I reckon he is quite promiscuous as he is attractive to other men. He goes out a lot on his own. Once we used to go out together.'
WALTER: 'Why don't you find someone else?'
MICHAEL: 'It's not easy at my age. Sometimes I think I might be better off with a woman, but I don't get on with women. They dislike me.'
FEMALE THERAPIST: 'I don't dislike you.'
MICHAEL: 'You are not involved with me. You would find me boring.'
FEMALE THERAPIST: 'I do think you should be more positive in your thinking and meet more people. Maybe you could join an evening class.'
MICHAEL: 'I am glad to have joined the group. I was thinking it would be nice to have a drink in the local together after the session.'

At this point there was a silence; no-one spoke. Usually, men are not very gregarious in this type of group and obviously none of the men wanted to accept Michael's invitation and appear to be reinforcing the idea of an affair with him.

FEMALE THERAPIST: 'We can talk about social events at a later stage.'

During later sessions Michael came over as depressed about his situation. When the male therapist suggested role playing Michael's relationship with the photographer, Michael lacked assertion and was not effective. When criticised he became more depressed. Although most of the group members disliked him for his homosexuality they had mixed emotions as they obviously felt sorry for him. They were quite kind over helping out with the role play; even Harry was helpful and joined in, offering to show Michael how to be verbally effective in these circumstances.

The next session Michael reported back:

MICHAEL: 'I did as you suggested, Harry, and the photographer was quite surprised when I told him he was being obsessional about cleaning the bath after I had already done quite a good job on it. He didn't speak for an hour.'
HARRY: 'Ha, ha! I like it!'
WALTER: 'What about the washing up?'
MICHAEL: 'Yes, that was good too. When he said I had not washed the glasses properly and I replied that they were fine by me but if he wanted obsessively to rinse them again he was welcome to do so, the photographer looked astounded.'
FEMALE THERAPIST: 'That sounds great, you have done really well, Michael.'
MICHAEL: 'Thank you. I would have felt happier if the photographer had talked to me, but he just went out, slamming the door.'
FEMALE THERAPIST: 'I hope you kept up the good work, Michael.'
MICHAEL: 'Yes I did but I wonder if it did any good.'
FEMALE THERAPIST: 'How did your masturbation homework go?'
MICHAEL: 'Not well at all. I really can't get an erection and I get very little feeling when I touch my penis. If it was bigger I might feel more.'
HARRY: 'That's a fallacy, man.'
FEMALE THERAPIST: 'Did you fantasise at all, Michael?'
MICHAEL: 'No, I do try, but I really find that difficult. What was the name of the book you told us to buy?'
MALE THERAPIST: 'It was *Tropic of Cancer*[2].'
MICHAEL: 'I could not get it, but I got some Health magazines instead. Some of the guys in the magazines were quite attractive but as soon as I started masturbating I lost my erection.'
MALE THERAPIST: 'But you did get erect to the pictures.'
MICHAEL: 'Yes.'
MALE THERAPIST: 'That's fine. Could you try to develop your fantasies? We can give you a list of video tapes.'
HARRY: 'Is he getting a different list from us, like kinky videos?'
FEMALE THERAPIST: 'There are various lists of recommended literature and some of the video lists are tailored to each client, Harry. You are very persistent.'
FRANK: 'He is curious about the material you recommend. He probably thinks everyone else has a juicier list than he has.'
HARRY: 'This fantasy thing is a lot of balls.'
MICHAEL: 'It's supposed to increase our sexual interest, so I'm keen on it.'
FEMALE THERAPIST: 'I am always telling you about research evidence, Harry, and you rarely take any notice.'

Sometimes it was necessary to be quite rude to Harry; he was the thick-skinned one, much more than Frank who had been accused of this. When it came to the subject of AIDS, Michael could have become the scapegoat of the group, but he was quite honest, admitting that it is associated with gay circles and trying to think of alternative sex to avoid spreading it. Only Harry was aggressive towards Michael and it was interesting that Michael had received enough assertion training to retaliate when Harry suggested that homosexuals should be stopped from having sex:

MICHAEL: 'That's very prejudiced. What do you think we are, lepers?'

During later sessions Michael discussed the topic of AIDS with the photographer who refused to go for a blood test and was not interested in Michael's suggestion that they should try some mutual masturbation to protect themselves against AIDS. The group and therapists were unanimous in advising Michael to split up with his partner and this is what Michael did later.

Things were still not going well for Michael and the photographyer at the end of the group. At follow-up he had decided to split up with the photographer and do up a house on his own. He was more positive about finding another male partner and persistent about stimulating literature and the teasing techniques recommended in masturbation. He considered his sexual interest had slightly increased.

Summing up

Some of these men might have done better in groups which were more homogeneous in terms of disorders. Zilbergeld[3] reported that groups for clients suffering from erectile failure did better than groups of men with mixed disorders. Burbank[4] has pointed out that a sense of homogeneity can be particulary beneficial to those with homosexual problems and problems of sexual deviation. Sometimes, however, arranging homogeneous groups is difficult.

From the above dialogues it can be seen that the male and female therapists worked together, supporting one another when necessary. It is encouraging that clients also gave one another some support, although they were unwilling to socialise like the women in the women's groups.

The findings of Gillan and Yaffé[5] in a research project carried out at Guy's Hospital, London, support Zilbergeld's research that men with ejaculatory disorders do better in groups than men with erectile impotence. In the UK, increasing numbers of men suffering from premature ejaculation combined with erectile dysfunction are being referred to sex clinics. In our experience, if premature ejaculation is combined with severe erectile impotence in which the man never experiences an erection during foreplay and ejaculates with a completely flaccid penis his prognosis is poor, compared with a man who has occasional erections during foreplay.

Lobitz and Baker[6] in the USA reported an important finding for group therapy for single males with primary erectile dysfunction. They concluded that such therapy is not cost-effective compared with similar therapy for secondary erectile dysfunction.

Burbank[4] also stresses the limitations to the treatment of sexual problems by group therapy, such as the discouragement one member can feel if everyone else progresses more quickly than he does. Associated with this is the issue of having group members who have minority (sexual) interests which can inhibit therapeutic change and this can detrimentally affect interaction of group members outside the group.

Cross-cultural sexuality is an issue which is highlighted in group therapy. Two papers by Chipman[7] and Kinzie[8] concentrate on how to deal with the such problems, skills which will be needed increasingly in our culturally and ethnically diverse society.

In terms of economics and therapist efficiency groups have been proved to be effective in the USA and Europe although more administrative effort is required. The final results are encouraging.

References

1. Zilbergeld, Bernie. (1980) *Men and Sex*. Souvenir Press.
2. Miller, Henry. *Tropic of Cancer*. Granada.
3. Zilbergeld, B. (1975) 'Group treatment of sexual dysfunction in men without partners.' *Journal of Sex and Marital Therapy*. 1. 204–214.
4. Burbank, F. (1976) 'The treatment of sexual problems by group therapy'. Chapter in *Psychosexual Problems*. (Ed.) Crown, S. Academic Press.
5. Gillan, Patricia and Yaffé, Maurice. (1981) 'Group therapy for men.' *Brit. Jrnl. of Sexual Medicine*. March.
6. Lobitz, W.C. and Baker, E.L. (1979) 'Group treatment of single males with erectile dysfunction.' *Archives of Sexual Behaviour*. Vol.8. No.2.
7. Chipman, A. (1978) 'Psychogenic impotence and the black man's burden'. *Am.J.Psychotherapy*. 32. 603–12.
8. Kinzie, J.D. (1978) 'Lessons from cross-cultural psychotherapy'. *Am.J.Psychotherapy*. 32. 510–20.

Chapter 11

Sex Therapy in Mixed Groups

Background

Although most of the research has focussed on group therapy for people of the same sex occasionally sex therapy groups have been formed for clients of different sexes or couples.

In the late sixties the author was inundated by phobic patients when working at Rochford General Hospital[1]. A group for phobics was formed. It turned out that some of the women presenting with agoraphobia also had orgasmic problems and some of the men with claustrophobia had erectile and/or ejaculatory difficulties. They were willing to relax with people who had no sexual difficulties and to discuss their problems in the group situation. The outcome was good and the clients with sexual difficulties fared better than the clients with non-sexual phobias.

Later on, in the late seventies at the same hospital, when research was carried out on sexual dysfunction[2] the local general practitioners referred mainly women with low sexual interest for therapy. So many women were referred that two groups were formed. The women usually attended with partners, although some of the men found it difficult to attend on a regular basis, due to shift work. Many of the sessions concentrated on marital therapy for these couples and marital contracts were worked out weekly. There was a high rate of improvement when stimulation therapy was included in the therapy programme and all the women who had stimulation therapy significantly increased their sex drive. At the same time in Northern Ireland, Ethna O'Gorman[3] was treating what she refers to as 'frigid women'; they were actually sexually unresponsive and were treated in a group setting. These women were desensitised in a hospital ward, lying on the beds. Their male partners had discussions in another room in the hospital. Results were encouraging.

In the USA, group sex therapy research had been going on for a number of years. Leiblum and Rosen in 1979[4] devised an interesting format of intensive weekend workshops for groups of individuals or couples. American researchers like Leiblum and Ersner-Herschfield[5] have pointed out the advantages of groups for couples as both partners attend. In other group therapy settings, if only one partner attends the effect of group cohesiveness may alienate the woman from her partner. This applies, in particular, to women whose increased self-esteem and effectiveness are reinforced by the group but alienate her partner. In such cases it might be preferable to include the partner in the group and to work out problems as a couple.

The interesting finding with group therapy is that there is more loyalty to the group compared with individual therapy where the drop-out rate is significantly higher both in the USA and Europe. A London study reported by Kayata and Szydlo[6] demonstrated complete group loyalty with no drop-outs at all in their mixed group setting.

Leiblum[5] pointed out that one disadvantage of couple groups is that one disruptive couple will have more power to sabotage a group than a single individual. It is highly important to select couples carefully and severe marital discord may prove to be a contraindication. The author discovered this in the UK, as one couple with severe marital problems did indeed sabotage a group as the other couples got tired of their constant harangues and attention-seeking conduct.

Although only little research has so far been carried out making a direct comparison between sex therapy for couples on their own and in a group setting, some promising findings were reported by Duddle and Ingram[7] in the UK. In their study, women had the major sexual problems, although women with vaginismus were excluded. They found that two-thirds in both treatment formats benefited from therapy and concluded that group therapy for couples is as effective as conjoint therapy. They reported substantial saving in therapeutic time, but most couples were reluctant to enroll for group therapy.

Mixed groups for individuals

Clinics in the UK were confident about starting single sex groups, first for women then for men, but there was a certain reluctance to initiate mixed sex therapy groups for individuals. Some consultant psychiatrists suggested that patients could be attracted to each other and it could turn out to be like a dating service. More broad-minded people would probably regard this as a positive advantage! In the history of group sex therapy, clients in mixed groups appear to be the Cinderellas of the scene.

When Kayata and Szydlo[6] researched two such groups at The Maudsley Hospital in London, they neatly summed up their feelings about a combined sex group and considered 'it would provide a forum for a healthier balance of ideas, an awareness of opposite sex difficulties and a greater motivation for input and attendance'. They were certainly right about high attendance rate.

In a single sex group, like a men's group, the men are lucky if one of the co-therapists is female and can therefore give them an idea of women's responses and ideas. It is obviously better to have some female clients in the group to confirm such ideas. It is also preferable to have the sexes balanced in terms of clientele when it comes to role play. It is quite hard on a female therapist participating in a men's group to be always the one to do the role play. Some women's groups have been run at Guy's Hospital, London, with male and female co-therapists and this type of group went down well. Contrary to the opinion of some feminists, the women in these groups welcomed the male therapist and were reassured that men, too, had problems. Again, the burden of role play was heavy for the only male in the group and it would have been preferable to have had more men present, but the theory is that this could have inhibited the women.

The criteria for accepting clients for the London mixed group run by Kayata and Szydlo[6] were stricter than those laid down for other groups, but as their mixed group was so successful it is well worth examining their criteria for clients who had originally been referred to The Maudsley Psychosexual Clinic:

(1) They are now (or were in the recent past) sexually active but not married, living with a partner or involved in a long-term, committed relationship.
(2) The sexual problem is not the result of injury or biological dysfunction.
(3) There are no additional serious physical or psychological disturbances (psychosis, chronic depression, severe physical handicaps).
(4) The nature of the problem is dysfunctional rather than perverse, phobic, or related to confused sexual identity.
(5) They are between the ages of 18 and 45.

Probably their reason for restricting the age range was in their words: 'We chose to balance the membership as much as possible as an aid to integration'. Their choice of the word perverse is curious. Their exclusion of phobic clients is debatable. In fact, their group was a highly selected number of clients who did not have the problems of an ongoing relationship to affect their progress.

The London mixed group consisted of fifteen 1–2 hour sessions, which is longer than the usual programme for individual therapy or other sex therapy groups. This probably balanced out the advantage of saving therapists' time which justifies some groups.

Various problems anticipated by the London group therapists were the competitive element in such groups, different goals and the process of self-exposure in front of members of the opposite sex. In order to cope with some of these anticipated problems the group was presented with well thought out guidelines for participation during sessions:

(1) Group members should phrase their comments positively to create a theme of support and optimism.
(2) The elements of confidentiality and trust are of absolute importance.
(3) Each individual's commitment to the group is crucial in terms of attendance, participation and completion of homework and exercises.
(4) The ability to listen is as essential as the ability to disclose in order to achieve constructive group communication.
(5) The group organisers are not trying to succeed or trying to avoid failure. Each member of the group will move at his or her own pace in the realisation that the group is not a 'cure', but a foundation for the development of a satisfying sexual relationship.
(6) Group members are asked not to meet each other socially for the duration of the group since this would alter the group's dynamics. If this does happen, however, the individuals are requested to inform the group of the meeting.

The above guidelines seem sensible, but protect the clients from real-life situations. On the other hand, the first guideline would have made the men's groups (described in Chapter 10) more pleasant and positive.

The male clients turned out to have a wide range of problems, with two men with secondary impotence, one man with primary impotence, one man with premature ejaculation and a fifth man who had never achieved penetration during sexual intercourse, due to anxiety. Two of the three women had primary anorgasmia although they admitted this was not their presenting problem which they admitted was the complete absence of sexual response; the third woman had vaginismus. This latter woman would have been excluded from most women's groups which concentrate mainly on orgasmic dysfunction.

The London mixed group had an additional special individual therapy clause which could be useful to include in other groups. Each client was seen individually by the two therapists for three sessions. Critics could say that this increased therapists' time and was not economical, but it appears to have been a good investment. Each individual client was given a kind of initial 'crash course' consisting of self-focussing and relaxation training. Time was taken to smooth out any difficulties individuals had with these tasks which included masturbatory exercises. The therapists got to know and understand the clients before the group commenced. Obviously self-disclosure would then be easier in the group, each individual having become desensitised to this procedure with the help of the therapists.

The second stage of treatment consisted of fifteen group therapy sessions, bringing the number of sessions to eighteen counting the individual sessions. This was a considerable amount of therapy by behavioural group psychotherapy standards. The group was given the usual therapy tasks like education sessions and the discussion of individual problems. There were four social skills training sessions (but this type of therapy would have been given to previous group sex therapy clients before they attended group sessions, although tasks included self-disclosure and admitting a sex problem).

Analysing the variables involved in therapy, there was emphasis on the physiology of sex with the aid of slides and films, and also on assertion training. Results were encouraging and showed that according to the GRISS (Golombok-Rust Inventory of Sexual Satisfaction) 75 per cent of the group members had significantly improved at the 4-month follow-up. Self-ratings are not as reliable or as objective as questionnaires but nevertheless are used in most American studies and the mixed group members rated themselves as having an 88 per cent improvement rate at follow-up. They showed a similar improvement rate in terms of their therapy goals. There was no significant change in the overall degree of fantasising.

What was extremely rewarding was the fact that group members had changed their life styles. Some had started live-in relationships and others had ended long-standing uncommitted relationships.

Sex therapy for mixed groups is encouraging and successful. It is a good method for getting members of both sexes to understand heterosexual communication and sexuality itself.

Couples sex therapy in groups

For a long time the idea of treating couples in groups was opposed by the senior staff of clinics in several London teaching hospitals. It was suggested that maybe a woman attending the group with an impotent partner might be attracted to and run off with the partner of a woman who was anorgasmic. Some quite emotional discussions took place on this delicate topic.

The work done by Kaplan *et al.*[7] in the USA avoided this problem as all the men suffered from premature ejaculation. Four couples attended therapy and homework included sensate focussing and the stop start technique. After six sessions and at follow-up four out of six men had improved.

A therapy group for men with ejaculatory disorders was formed in London at The Maudsley Hospital by Gillan and Snowden in 1976. The men attended with their partners and the success rate was quite good; two out of three of the premature ejaculators and one of the two men with delayed ejaculation improved. The men remarked that it was interesting and useful to meet other men suffering from sexual disorders, particularly ejaculatory disorders which were different from their own. The success of this group helped establish men's sex therapy groups in the UK.

Although several sex therapy groups had been successfully run for couples in the USA it was not until 1980 that the first mixed couples British group was reported by Duddle and Ingram[8]. This Manchester study faced the usual difficulty of couples refusing treatment if it took place in a group as they did not want to discuss their problems with other people. This obviously was associated with confidentiality which is admittedly a realistic problem that was successfully managed previously in the London mixed group. The possible danger of attraction between the partners of different couples was also emphasised, 'because of the erotic nature of the therapeutic situation'. It would be educational for some of these British medics to take a trip to California and see some of the therapy methods that take place there in jacuzzis or swimming pools! The Manchester groups met for between ten and thirteen sessions. Women had the major sexual difficulties in these groups, although women with vaginismus were excluded as they need a different type of therapy. Duddle and Ingram reported that two-thirds of the group members improved compared with the same success rate for individual therapy.

Rochford General Hospital in the UK has always been progressive and experimentally inclined. When the idea of women with low sexual interest attending a group with their partners was put forward permission was readily given. It was easy to justify a group: if clients objected they were told that so many women in the area wanted a place in the group that there was no chance of individual therapy and if they did not want the place in the group there was someone else on the waiting list. This was not only perfectly true but also effective; only one couple refused group therapy.

One group was disrupted by a couple with an extremely poor marriage in which both partners were articulate and volatile and this probably resulted in uniting the rest of the group. The other groups were more cohesive. Various stimulation therapy tasks were included in two of the four groups. Both men and women in these two groups reported an increased sexual interest when asked to look at sex magazines and listen to sex tapes.

Each group met for six sessions of therapy and results showed an 86 per cent success rate with no drop-outs for couples receiving stimulation therapy together with sensate focussing and other sexual homework tasks.

Couples attending a stimulation therapy group for couples

Session 1

Sally and David presented as a likeable and attractive married couple. Sally was 35 years old and had a job as the personal assistant to a local managing director. At 38, David was a junior partner in a City firm of stockbrokers. They were both given time off from work to attend the General Hospital.

At a first glance they looked like a well-adjusted happy couple, but an analysis of their relationship revealed that Sally did not respond much to David and sent out no sexual messages whatsoever. For an attractive woman of 35, she dressed in a dull manner and wore pastel acrylic suits which added ten years to her age. Her permed hair was always clean and well-groomed, but her hairstyle made her look older than she was. David also looked older than his years in his dark business suit and City hairstyle.

They had married when they were in their early twenties and Sally had never had any sexual experience outside the marriage. David had been out with two women before the marriage and had carried on an affair for a year before Sally found out about it two years ago. She had reacted badly but rationalised David's need to go to another woman as she had lost her sexual interest and did not even want David to kiss her any longer.

Sally had started off with a lower sexual interest than David, but sex had been good from the beginning and she was orgasmic if he stimulated her clitoris. She enjoyed sex until the birth of her second child when she was 31 and then things deteriorated.

The two children – a girl of 9 and a boy of 5 – were very much wanted children. Everything had gone well at both births and Sally could not understand why she had lost her sexual interest after the birth of a son. Sometimes couples groups can lead to individuals reinforcing one another as the following example shows, and the therapist must step in and effectively stop them from generalising.

SALLY: 'I still can't understand why I immediately lost my sex drive when Brian was born.'
TAMARA: 'I can. Exactly the same thing happened to me after Bernard was born and he is my second. I read in a magazine that it's biological. You have your first child and your sex drive is all right so you fall pregnant again, but after that, unless you want another child you lose your libido – I think that's what they call it.'
SALLY: 'Yes, I'm exactly like that. I don't want another child.'
THERAPIST: 'Look, Sally, there is no evidence about this. If there was it would have been an important finding and discussed everywhere. What magazine was it that you read, Tamara?'
TAMARA: 'I can't remember; it must have been a woman's magazine.'
BEN: 'It wasn't *New Scientist* was it, darling?'
TAMARA: 'No, that's a put-down. In any case, I understand how you feel, Sally. It used to make me guilty but it doesn't any more.'
SALLY: 'Yes, I feel guilty, because I feel it's my duty to have sex. I still do it but it does not do anything for me.'
TAMARA: 'I don't do it anymore. Why should one be obliged to?'
BEN: 'I wish you did feel some guilt. At least I would benefit.'
DAVID: 'You're worse than us, Ben.'
THERAPIST: 'That's why you have come for therapy to try and change things. You will find that you are all at different stages. Some of you may have different problems but basically all the women in the group want to increase their sexual interest.'

During this first session the women had quickly become friends and identified with each other. This first session was basically spent on introductions with no surnames being given, another ground rule being that clients should not state their occupation. The author thought the group would be very formal but this was not the case. Each couple had introduced themselves and described their hobbies. The author, who was the only therapist, helped to break the ice:

THERAPIST: 'My hobbies are travelling, cinema-going, eating and drinking.'

This raised a laugh and immediately the whole group became more relaxed. Tamara and Ben were the most confident of the four couples. Ben actually made a joke which must have shocked the others:

BEN: 'I suppose we are all going to have sex here in the clinic.'
THERAPIST: 'Is that your fantasy, Ben? In fact, you are going to be disappointed as I am going to suggest a ban on sexual intercourse.'
BEN: 'I thought something like that was about to happen to me. In any case I've done without for months now so it won't make any difference to me.'
TAMARA: 'That will be a relief for you, Sally.'
SALLY: 'I'm not sure.'
THERAPIST: 'You are all going to be asked to do your first massaging exercises this week at home. I will be giving each of you a massage sheet. When you massage one another avoid touching the breasts and the genitals. How do you feel about this? Sally, let's start with you.'
SALLY: 'I am not too enthusiastic, to be honest with you. I feel it will lead to other things.'
DAVID: 'No it won't, not if you don't want to.'
THERAPIST: 'The idea is that mutual masturbation and sexual intercourse are forbidden, so don't forget that.'
TAMARA: 'I must say I feel negative about the task as I think it's like prick teasing, having the massage and not doing anything else.'
THERAPIST: 'Those are the rules, Tamara.'
BEN: 'Tamara likes to break rules. I am sure I can control myself when I massage her; after all I have already mentioned that I have been impotent on several occasions.'
THERAPIST: 'Well, if any if you feel over-aroused you can always go into another room and masturbate, there is no ban on that, provided it is done in private.'
DIANA: 'I would never do anything like that.'
TAMARA: 'Women do, you know.'
THERAPIST: 'Are you happy about the homework and the massage, Diana?'
DIANA: 'Yes, thank you. It will be strange to touch again as since my libido got low we haven't had much physical contact and I really regret that.'
JOHN: 'I feel it's unfair to touch you, Diana, when you don't want intercourse.'

THERAPIST: 'Do you think all touching should lead to lovemaking and sexual intercourse, John?'
JOHN: 'Yes, I suppose I do. I consider that if I touch Diana she will interpret it as my wanting intercourse and in any case I come quickly and get quite excited when I do touch her. It's not as though she is the only one with a problem.'
DAVID: 'I hope I will be able to control myself. I know I haven't got any problems. I thought to start with that it would be easy to control myself, but when I listen to people like Ben and John I am not too sure.'
THERAPIST: 'Well, why don't we all have a relaxation session now and I shall ask you to imagine some of the tasks when you are relaxed.'

Group relaxation is quite a good exercise for uniting the group in a positive way, especially after a lot of aggression has been expressed. So far the group had been friendly enough, but as there were only three couples the group was quite manageable. The therapist had judged Tamara and Ben as potential troublemakers, Diana and John as rather quiet and Sally and David as a nice couple.

Session 2

When the group met a week later the couples discussed their progress.

TAMARA: 'I must say I enjoyed Ben massaging me, it made quite a change. It was really funny when I massaged him – he got quite erect.'
BEN: 'I found it exciting.'
THERAPIST: 'That's fine. I trust you did not break the rules.'
TAMARA: 'In spite of threatening to do so we did not. If you want to know, I was not turned on like Ben.'
THERAPIST: 'But you were not turned off, Tamara.'
TAMARA: 'Actually, no. It was neutral for me.'
THERAPIST: 'That's fine.'

In fact, the therapist had expected much more hostility and difficulty from this particular couple.

THERAPIST: 'Who else would like to report back on their massage?'
SALLY: 'It was nice. I did not feel threatened and knew we were not going to make love.'
DAVID: 'Yes, I really liked having my back stroked.'
THERAPIST: 'Was Sally's pressure right?'
DAVID: 'Yes, it was a bit too light to start with but I told her to put more pressure on me and that turned out better.'

THERAPIST: 'Which area did you enjoy being massaged, Sally?'
SALLY: 'My back; David touched just right.'

At this stage there was a long pause and Diana and John did not volunteer information. Tamara aggressively broke the silence:

TAMARA: 'How about you, Diana? Did you break the rules, John?'
JOHN: 'No.'
THERAPIST: 'Was everything all right, Diana?'
JOHN: 'No.'
THERAPIST: 'Would you like to tell us what happened, John?'
JOHN: 'Diana said I made her sore.'
THERAPIST: 'What do you mean?'
DIANA: 'He pressed so hard on my shoulders that he made my skin feel raw, it was awful.'

At this stage Tamara started laughing.

THERAPIST: 'Stop laughing, Tamara. Pain is not an amusing thing. Obviously you were pressing too hard, John.'
DIANA: 'I told him so but he went on doing it hard.'
JOHN: 'Well I'd had that sort of pressure when I have been massaged before football.'
THERAPIST: 'But that's a remedial massage.'
DIANA: 'We did it twice and it was just as bad the second time round.'
THERAPIST: 'John, have you ever massaged anyone else before?'
JOHN: 'No.'
THERAPIST: 'I would like to do an exercise so that each woman here massages the arm of her partner for five minutes, then I shall ask you to reverse the order.'

The group set out to do the task watched by the therapist who had deliberately not asked John to massage Diana with everyone else watching. When it came to John's turn to massage Diana he was unbelievably rough.

THERAPIST: 'Now each of the men try to be very gentle indeed; just lightly stroke your partner's arm now.'

John continued his heavy pressure.

THERAPIST: 'Just gently tickle your partner's arm. That's better. Now do some stroking. John, can you be very careful to do this gently with

a much lighter pressure, more like when you were tickling. How is that, Diana?'
DIANA: 'That's nice.'
JOHN: 'Really? Good.'

Sometimes the therapist needs to observe exactly what is going on, but it is more difficult in a group situation. Some therapists might have shown John how to massage Diana's arm or asked another person in the group to show John, but this could be interpreted as invading a couple's territory. If the partners manage to shape their behaviour so that the desired response is achieved then this is preferable.

THERAPIST: 'Are there any other comments?'
BEN: 'Yes. You suggested that we should take turns over initiating the massage. Tamara did not invite me once for a massage, I had to do all the initiating.'
TAMARA: 'I didn't refuse you. How do you know I really wanted to invite you to do a massage?'
BEN: 'You agreed to in the last session of the group.'
DIANA: 'Yes we did, that's true.'
TAMARA: 'I bet you didn't initiate the massage too much with your heavy-handed husband.'
JOHN: 'No. I did the inviting, I would have liked you to have asked me once, Diana.'
SALLY: 'That's probably because Diana did not enjoy it. Now that you touch better things will improve.'
DAVID: 'I wish you practised what you preach, Sally. You did not initiate the massage at all, either. What's wrong with you women?'
TAMARA: 'Well, I still associate the message with sex and I don't totally trust Ben, especially as he got erect on two occasions.'
BEN: 'That probably did not please you, eh?'
TAMARA: 'The sight of your erection did not thrill me, I must admit. Nothing was going to be done with it – that's what I meant last week when I talked about prick teasing.'
THERAPIST: 'Does any other woman here have any ideas to offer on why initiation did not take place?'
SALLY: 'I suppose it's because we have a low sex interest and we subconsciously connect touch with sex and that puts us off. I don't know.'
THERAPIST: 'That's quite a good interpretation. It could also be that women are conditioned to be passive and not take the initiative as it's not considered lady-like to do so.'
TAMARA: 'That's quite a good one! I am not like that.'

BEN: 'I am sure you consciously connect touch with sex and are bloody negative.'
DIANA: 'I know I do.'
JOHN: 'You always say I'm rough when we have sex.'
SALLY: 'One thing I did not mention is that I feel fine when I massage David but feel awkward when he massages me.'

Sally had interrupted at the right time in the discussion as the situation between Ben and Tamara was becoming aggressive, and that of Diana and John too personal. One rather embarrassing point was that John was not quite as bright as the other men; he tended also to be rather inarticulate which did not help matters. It was also fortuitous that they did not discuss occupations as Ben and David were professional businessmen whereas John worked on the railways, mending the tracks. The others probably realised he did rougher work than they did but John was protected by the rules of the group and did not have to disclose what he did for a living. Diana worked in a shop and was much more upwardly mobile socially than her partner.

THERAPIST: 'Sometimes people do feel awkward when they receive a massage, so perhaps you could relax more. Today I would like to continue with the contract therapy we worked on last week and see how that went and how things could be improved. Sally and David, how did your contract go? Can you remind me what your tasks were?'
SALLY: 'David said he would help in the house if I coped with the children when he came in from work as they bother him.'
DIANA: 'Yes, I like to relax and enjoy some television. I do like telling them bed-time stories later so it worked out well. I can't stand demanding children as soon as I open the front door.'
SALLY: 'David helped me with the washing-up each night and did the repair jobs at the weekend.'
THERAPIST: 'What would you like the contract to be this week, Sally?'
SALLY: 'I would like David to do some small repairs after dinner, instead of washing-up.'
THERAPIST: 'Fine. Do you agree with that, David, and if so what would you like Sally to do in exchange?'
DAVID: 'I would like her to take her share of the initiative over the massage, as I think you said we had to do it throughout the course.'
THERAPIST: 'That's right. But the contract lasts a week only, and is up for renewal each week. Do you agree to take the initiative half the time over the massage, Sally.'
SALLY: 'Yes, I do if he does those repair jobs.'

Significantly, all the men chose the same contract as David.
This type of contract was originally designed for non-sexual activities but the therapist saw no reason why it should not be used in the way the clients wanted, provided that they both agreed.

The two-way physical examination

This two-way physical examination took place for each couple during the second session of therapy. the therapist explained its purpose:

THERAPIST: 'Right at the beginning of therapy I mentioned the fact that you would be physically examined by each other in my presence. I will be there to check out that you know the names of your genitals and can identify sexually arousing parts on each other's genitals. As I said before, each couple will be examined in total privacy. I think we shall start in alphabetical order and I'll ask Diana and John to undress in the room across the corridor.'

During these physical examinations most of them got the names right apart from the clitoris. Several men did not know about the clitoris, and surprisingly enough four of the fourteen women in the four groups at Rochford General Hospital did not know about it either.

As was expected, John was rough when he examined Diana. Neither of them knew about the clitoris, so it was quite a good opportunity for them to get some sex education and for John to learn how to touch her gently.

The other couples were more sophisticated in their knowledge but Sally showed a certain reluctance to touch and identify David's sexual parts.

THERAPIST: 'Yes, you identified David's foreskin but you don't seem too clever at pulling it back a little.'
SALLY: 'I'm not very good at that, I must admit.'
DAVID: 'That's true.'
THERAPIST: 'David, can you show her how to do it?'
DAVID: 'Yes, like this. Look.'
THERAPIST: 'Can you have another try, Sally? Yes, that's it; that's much better.'
SALLY: 'I know why I feel embarrassed. It's because I associate the whole thing with sex and I'm not much good at that.'
THERAPIST: 'You are changing already and you will get more confident as the course progresses.'
SALLY: 'Do you really think so?'

A more relaxed Sally returned to the group; a little encouragement goes a long way.

One wonders what the others talked about when Tamara and Ben had their turn. They both knew exactly how to touch one another. Admittedly, Ben was circumcised and this made touching easier, but Tamara was very skilled for someone who appeared to dislike sex so much. It was easy to start wondering why these two had such a bad sexual relationship and were so aggressive, when they both examined one another in such a gentle and considerate manner. It would have been out of turn, however, to start asking them questions in private because of the experimental nature of the groups.

When each partner had been examined a discussion took place about self-stimulation or masturbation. The difference in attitudes between the women was quite revealing:

TAMARA: 'Yes, I used to masturbate regularly. I got a good climax then compared with sex with Ben, but it became boring. I gave it up.'
SALLY: 'I occasionally masturbate but it's very infrequent now.'
THERAPIST: 'Have you ever tried it, Diana?'
DIANA: 'No, I don't really know much about it.'
TAMARA: 'It's stimulating your clitoris. Do you know about that?'
DIANA: 'Yes, I do, but I would only do that if I had to.'
THERAPIST: 'Yes, it would be helpful as far as your sexual interest goes for all of you to masturbate every other day before we meet next week. I would like you to masturbate on your own and use any method to get excited, but to switch to an image of your partner as you climax during masturbation, and to imagine your partner earlier on in subsequent sessions. We are running out of time for this meeting so I shall briefly explain that I want you to continue your massages on the alternate days before we next meet. I am giving you all homework sheets in any case and now I would like to talk about the Kegel PC exercises [see Appendix]. One last thing, I would like each of you when you go home to tell your partner three things which please you about the other.

Session 3

Homework was discussed initially, as usual. There was good news from Diana; she had enjoyed her massage with John and he was much gentler. She had also enjoyed masturbating. Ben and Tamara had enjoyed their massage and she had initiated it twice and was rather less aggressive than usual. It came to Sally's turn:

SALLY: 'Yes, I also initiated it twice. David said that I should start to ask him for a massage as he had done the inviting previously.'
DAVID: 'Yes, it was nice to be asked. I also liked being told the three nice things Sally liked about me.'
THERAPIST: 'Would you like to share with the group one of the things Sally said about you?'
DAVID: 'Yes, she said I was very considerate.'
THERAPIST: 'That's nice. Sally, would you like to share with the group one of the things that David said about you?'
SALLY: 'Yes, he liked the way I was always responsible. The only disappointing thing is that he said he liked the way I was so sexy but I can't say I feel sexy myself.'
THERAPIST: 'Did you feel more sexy when you masturbated?'
SALLY: 'Not really, it helped relieve tension.'
TAMARA: 'Funny you should say that – I found that too.'
THERAPIST: 'Well, that's positive for you both. Today I would like you to share the masturbation for your homework and make it mutual. I would always like you to start the homework sessions massaging one another, and to take it in turns over the initiative.'

It is a pity that these sessions have to be so abbreviated, but the really amusing part of the session should not be left out. Tamara and Ben reported back on one of the things they liked about one another:

TAMARA: 'He liked my *hutzpah*, that's a kind of quality associated with having courage, being daring or outspoken or bold.'
BEN: 'Tamara liked my predictability.'

One wonders whether these two made up these items for the benefit of the group, as they appeared to be real tongue-in-cheek, sarcastic remarks.

Session 4

Oral sex was the new topic for the fourth session. Usually this aroused most suspicion and hostility, especially fellatio. Most women in the groups did not want to try this and needed to be reassured that they need not swallow sperm if they did not want to. All the women in the present group were unanimous over condemning fellatio but were willing to discuss the art of cunnilingus.

TAMARA: 'Ben did that to me several times. It was quite pleasant but he was not too keen – were you, dear?'

BEN: 'No, because it was one-sided; you would not kiss me down below.'
SALLY: 'I am not sure if I would like to be kissed there, but it sounds quite nice the way you say it, Tamara. What do you think, Diana?'
DIANA: 'I don't think John would like it.'
JOHN: 'I'd try it if you did it to me like Ben said.'
THERAPIST: 'You all seem to be against the idea of fellatio but I don't object to it if cunnilingus is given in return. Why don't you all try both activities and find out for yourselves?'
TAMARA: 'Well, I have done that and I wouldn't do it again if I was paid. It turned me off.'
THERAPIST: 'Well, bear in mind that oral sex is a good bridging point between manual stimulation and sexual intercourse. Let's do some desensitisation over oral sex when we relax and imagine doing it.'

This was rarely a good session for any of the groups as oral sex seemed to inhibit people, but usually when they returned for the next session at least one couple reported having enjoyed experimenting with oral sex.

The session ended with looking at and swapping some sex magazines couples had been recommended to buy in the last session. Then followed some fantasy guidance in which the clients were asked to imagine some sexual scenes as observers, and to choose a day in the love life of some historical character.

Session 5

As predicted, two couples returned with some good news over oral sex. Diana and John had tried and enjoyed pleasuring and kissing one another especially as John had learned to be gentle. Tamara and Ben had not ventured into this activity, but Sally and David had experimented with cunnilingus.

SALLY: 'We tried the cunnilingus and I must say it was nice. David did to me on two occasions.'
DAVID: 'I was pleased that you enjoyed yourself.'
SALLY: 'But I felt guilty I was not kissing you down below.'
DAVID: 'I am not pressing for that. It's nice to see you enjoying yourself.'

David usually managed to say the right thing. In fact, he had found time to write a very amusing account of a day in the life of King Henry VIII which he read to the group.

The group on the whole had reacted quite well to recommended magazines like *Forum* and *Knave*. They had quite enjoyed reading *Fanny Hill* and other books like *The Joy of Sex*[9] from the recommended erotic book-list. Then a clever projective technique was used, showing a book of photographs that looked like genitalia and people had to guess what was shown. Tamara and Ben were the ones who guessed that only fingers had been photographed and the group was surprised to learn this; they were also shocked to hear that a certain disciplinary body had asked the artist to withdraw such obscene pictures from an end-of-year art exhibition, but had to change their minds and accept the pictures when they learnt that the supposedly indecent display consisted only of fingers after all. This provided an excellent opportunity to discuss attitudes and people's 'set' towards sex and erotica, and how authoritarianism can be linked with sexual disapproval. After the showing of the finger book, some pictures of women masturbating and oral sex pictures were passed around and attitudes and techniques were discussed.

SALLY: 'Having tried the cunnilingus I don't find the pictures of it disgusting, but I don't like the pictures of women doing it to men.'
DIANA: 'Well, I've tried both and I don't really like the pictures of any of them, it's like looking at models or something.'
TAMARA: 'I consider they are vulgar. It's like men want women to be and I don't like it.'
BEN: 'Well, I must admit I'm not turned on by this type of picture.'
DAVID: 'Well, I'm not turned off.'
JOHN: 'Neither am I.'

The talk about erotica continued and then sexual intercourse was discussed and the 'woman above position' was recommended for homework. Members of the group had no objection to this position, although in some other groups some of the men thought this position unfeminine.

Session 6

All the couples had tried the 'woman above position' but Diana preferred foreplay as John came too quickly, although he had been given instructions on the 'stop start' technique. Sally and David were quite happy with this position, but Tamara was bored. The subject of other positions was brought up and Tamara thought she would like the 'feel free' position with some direct clitoral stimulation.

During this last session a history of erotica was covered and this included Japanese and Indian prints and early heterosexual pornography obtainable in the UK in the 1950s, showing rather crude monochrome pictures of tarts and studs, the effect of which was humorous. This led to more homely and artistic 1960s and 1970s couples, in colour, with a background of tasteful antiques. Reactions were discussed and any necessary reassurances given, with instructions to go home and fantasise.

All clients were given this carefully graded approach to erotica and encouraged to enjoy it. If one couple seemed prudish someone else in the group enthused, so the therapist never had to 'push' it. The atmosphere could be described as permissive and warm.

All the couples in this particular group improved in communication and in their relationship. All the women increased their sexual interest. Even Tamara admitted that sex was better at follow-up. Sally summed it up:

SALLY: 'I now have more desire. We decided to experiment and I also have good fantasies now. We are happier.'

The group had been successful according to each client. This Rochford study showed that stimulation therapy was the significant factor in sex therapy for women with low sexual interest. The stimulation therapy devised for such groups consisted of erotic pictures, books and magazines, presented in a gradual manner. The method was initially to show and read magazines like *Viva* and *Forum*, discussing bodies and the way men can look erotic. The magazines were usually lent to the clients so that they could look at and read them at home with their partners. By the next session some of the women might have developed fantasies about such material and some were willing to discuss this. A slide show was provided of both male and female 'pin-ups' and this usually led to a discussion about erotic preferences and fantasies. At this stage clients were asked to write their fantasies as homework.

Later sessions were usually devoted to some fantasy guidance in which couples were asked to imagine some sexual scenes as observers, and then choose a day in the love life of some historical character. Clients usually were happy to share such fantasies and good discussions took place with humour. During these sessions Nancy Friday's books *My Secret Garden*[10] and *Forbidden Flowers*[11] were discussed and also Alex Comfort's *The Joy of Sex*[9].

During session 5 the viewing of Irene Kai's[12] photographs of fingers that look like genitalia is a good projective test and group members usually respond well to this exercise. It is a good lead into showing pictures of masturbation and oral sex which usually provoke plenty of negative comments. On the whole women are much more tolerant of pictures or films of other women masturbating than men who are disapproving when they see masturbation pictures of males. Both sexes are permissive of pictures of members of the opposite sex masturbating. English findings confirm those of Schmidt and Sigusch in Germany[13]. Oral sex pictures produce considerable hostility and aggression in groups. This sort of disapproval was found only in Tamara's comments in the present group as she found the pictures of cunnilingus vulgar, but the others were less dismissive. The present group was not very hostile towards the pictures of fellatio, but the other group which received stimulation therapy intensely disliked these pictures although one couple showed approval and recommended the pictures plus the actual activity to the others.

The last stimulation therapy task of a history of erotica is a good note for therapy to end on. It is in good taste and few clients can object to the exquisite prints of Indian and Japanese sex. Although the fifties pictures are cruder they do produce a laugh which helps to lighten the atmosphere. Pornography of the sixties and seventies is more natural and less clinical. Some of the people look real as opposed to the contrived tarts and studs of the fifties.

Stimulation therapy is strongly recommended for women with low sexual interest. It should be stressed that this was combined in the Rochford group study with Masters and Johnson-type sex tasks. The interesting point about this study is that the experimental design included controlling for the Masters and Johnson-type tasks.

One stimulation therapy group combined stimulation therapy with discussing and carrying out Masters and Johnson-type tasks in a graded manner, starting with massage and finishing with sexual intercourse (as illustrated by the description of therapy for the present group discussed in this chapter). The other stimulation therapy group was given the Masters and Johnson-type tasks in reverse, starting with intercourse and finishing with massage, as though they were being flooded. Both groups received stimulation therapy and there was no difference in results between the two groups. So in this context desensitisation, as opposed to flooding, for the Masters and Johnson-type tasks made no difference to therapy results. In the Rochford General Hospital study the essential ingredient for women with low sexual interest was the stimulation therapy, as the women in the two groups who did not receive stimulation therapy fared less well.

More emphasis could be placed on stimulation therapy for men or women with low sexual interest. Most therapists tend to stick to more conventional therapy based on Masters and Johnson techniques and do not venture outside this rather traditional model, but now that experimental evidence demonstrating the efficacy of stimulation therapy is available perhaps more therapists will consider using this method.

Later, two general sex therapy groups were carried out at The Maudsley Hospital by Crowe and Gillan, based on a modified Masters and Johnson model of desensitisation, without stimulation therapy. These were not as successful, however, probably because the couples had mixed problems rather than just low sexual interest and were more heterogeneous. There had been more integration in the Rochford study as all the women suffered from low sexual interest. It would appear that groups for couples are worthwhile and that future group therapy could be provided in more clinics.

References

1. Gillan, Patricia. (1979) 'Group therapy for sexual dysfunction'. *Journal of Sex Education and Therapy.* 27–30.
2. Gillan, Patricia. (1979) 'Increasing the sexual interest of female patients and their partners'. In *Love and Attraction* eds. Mark Cook and Glenn Wilson. Pergamon Press.
3. O'Gorman, E.C. 'The treatment of frigidity by group desensitisation'. In *Progress in Behaviour Therapy,* pages 105–7. Springer-Verlag.
4. Leiblum, S., Rosen, R.C. and Pierce, D. (1976) 'Group treatment format: mixed sexual dysfunctions'. *Arch.Sexual Behav.* Vol.5. No.4
5. Leiblum, S. and Ersner-Hershfield, R. (1977) 'Sexual enhancement groups for dysfunctional women: an evaluation.' *Jnl.Sex and Marital Ther.* 3. 139–152.
6. Kayata, Lisa and Szydlo, David. (1986) 'The treatment of psychosexual dysfunction in a mixed sex group: a new approach.' *Sexual and Marital Therapy.* Vol.1. No.1.
7. Kaplan, H.S., Kohn, R.N., Pomeroy, W.B., Offit, A.K., and Hogan, B. (1978) 'Group treatment of premature ejaculation.' *Archives of Sexual Behaviour.* 3. 443–452.
8. Duddle, C.M. and Ingram,A. (1980) 'Treating sexual dysfunction in couples groups'. In *Medical Sexology* (ed. R.Forleo and W.Pasini) pp. 598–605. Elsevier North Holland.
9. Comfort, Alex. (1972) *The Joy of Sex.* Simon & Schuster.
10. Friday, Nancy. (1973) *My Secret Garden.* Virago.
11. Friday, Nancy. (1975) *Forbidden Flowers.* Pocket Books. New York.
12. Irene Kai. (1973) 'Collection of Photographs' Royal College of Art, London.
13. Schmidt, G. and Sigusch, V. (1970) 'Sex difference in response to psychosexual stimulation by film slides.' *Jrnl. of Sex Research.* 6. 268–283.

Chapter 12

Therapy for Sexual Offenders

What is a sexual offence? It is a sexual act that breaks the law. Probably Walmsley and White[1] provide the most comprehensive list of possible conditions which are classified as a sexual offence:

(1) Sexual behaviour that takes place without the consent of the other party (and he or she is not married to the other party).
(2) Sexual behaviour that takes place with a person under the age of consent (16 for heterosexual, 21 for homosexual behaviour).
(3) The sexual behaviour itself is prohibited by law (i.e. incest, bestiality, buggery with a female or intercourse with a mental defective).
(4) Homosexual behaviour between males not committed in private.
(5) Homosexual behaviour by a male himself under the age of consent.

There are various inconsistencies in the above classifications. It seems strange that it is illegal for a consenting man and woman to have anal sex, yet it is legal for a consenting men to have anal sex. Why should a girl of 16 have reached the age of consent for heterosexual intercourse, whereas a male has to wait until he is 21 before he can have anal sex?

Different countries vary over the precise categories of the above. In England and Wales most categories of sexual offences are tried in a Crown Court before a jury, as opposed to a Magistrate's Court, and are classified as indictable. The classification of sexual offences varies more in the USA where one sexual act may be legal in one state and illegal in another.

The other category of non-indictable offences are mainly clustered around prostitution and include living on a prostitute's earnings, brothel-keeping, soliciting and male importuning. Indecent exposure seems like the odd man out of the classification.

Paraphilias

Some people do not get their sexual satisfaction from conventional sexual behaviour which involves foreplay and sexual intercourse. They prefer some alternative type of sex and maybe have an orgasm when dressed in rubber or being whipped. Sometimes such people who want to vary their sexual behaviour are called perverts or sexual deviants but these terms are like a condemnation and are no longer appropriate. To some extent, modern thinking considers that people are not wholly responsible for their style of behaviour and thus should not be blamed for what they do. Equally, many now believe that others should be allowed to indulge in whatever activities they please, unless they are seriously harmful either to themselves or others. The favoured alternative word nowadays is paraphiliac.

Nowadays, the idea behind a 'paraphilia' is this. The majority of people will behave in a certain manner, for example, the majority prefer heterosexual intercourse in the man above position. However, in any large group there will always be a number of people who behave in unusual ways, deviating from the norm.

Usually paraphilias are classified as harmless; it is when other people who are upset or shocked by such behaviour become involved that problems start. Most fetishists mean no harm, and it is only when the occasional one goes in pursuit of a pair of knickers or a handbag that they become a nuisance. An exhibitionist also means no offence, he only wants to shock slightly the person to whom he exposes himself but unwittingly he can upset people, although he would almost never dream of physically touching them.

These paraphilias are usually considered to be due to some quite fundamental personality disorders which often reach back into childhood. Probably the majority of paraphiliacs have no desire to change their behaviour and would never think of consulting a therapist. This usually only happens when some non-consenting person is involved.

As far as the therapist is concerned paraphilias are important for three reasons:

(1) The paraphiliacs may want to increase their sexual options: for

instance, they may want to try heterosexual intercourse and marry.

(2) Minor degrees of sexual interest bordering on paraphilias are common among people who call themselves 'normal'. This behaviour may be a source of shame and conflict. It may be concealed from the partner and may divert sexual energy from the relationship. Where the other partner can accept the paraphilia the problem usually disappears, as do many unnecessary worries when brought out into the open.

(3) The paraphilia may be difficult to displace as the preferred mode of sexual expression.

Where a paraphilia is found in one of the marital partners the therapist does not usually attempt to eradicate it. Most therapists now prefer to increase the satisfaction derived from alternative and more cooperative sexual behaviour. Where this is accomplished the paraphilia may fade. The therapist will attempt to teach the client a new manner of behaviour and to teach it in such a way as to establish it as the main source of satisfaction, or at least a pleasurable alternative.

Orgasmic reconditioning is quite an effective form of therapy. The client masturbates to his paraphilia imagery and switches to an image or photograph of the partner at orgasm. This switch to the desired stimulus takes place earlier and earlier in the masturbation until hopefully the socially acceptable image will turn the client on. Many paraphiliacs do not have partners and need to work with an image of a potential partner.

Exhibitionism

Exhibitionists are usually men for whom genital display to members of the opposite sex is an end in itself. It usually leads to an erect penis and masturbation rather than sexual contact with the victim. The majority of exhibitionists hope that the reaction of the victim will be that of fear and disgust rather than indifference.

Eric: the exhibitionist

Eric was referred for therapy by the court as he had become a recidivist.

He looked quite young for his 43 years with a full head of rather striking straight blond hair and ruddy complexion. He was rather overweight and this spoilt his appearance. He attended the clinic with a shrew of a wife, Pauline, aged 42 but looking about 50, with a disapproving and aggressive manner. She was the sort of woman who would antagonise any therapist by complaining that she had been kept waiting.

It was hardly surprising that they failed to get on well together. She complained before the assessment interviews had taken place:

PAULINE: 'He takes no responsibility. He has never paid a bill in his life. I have to do everything at home.'
ERIC: 'Yes, you do.'
THERAPIST: 'Would you like to pay the bills?'
ERIC: 'I don't mind.'
PAULINE: 'I could not trust you with money. Nor can I trust you to go in the street and behave like a gentleman.'
ERIC: 'I try.'
PAULINE: 'How many times have you done it now? It's a good thing your Mum is dead – she would turn in her grave.'
THERAPIST: 'That's quite a tough thing to say, Pauline.'
PAULINE: 'He makes me angry. Some of the time he behaves like an animal. I've been to the zoo and seen some of those monkeys showing themselves. It's disgusting.'
ERIC: 'It makes me laugh.'
PAULINE: 'The thing is that those monkeys can do it but Eric can't. We have not had sex for 17 years now.'
ERIC: 'Yes, I'm sorry about it.'
THERAPIST: 'What goes wrong?'
PAULINE: 'He is impotent. He manages to get hard when he exposes himself to young women but not when I'm around.'

This dominant woman and Eric made an ill-assorted pair and he was almost like a caricature of the hen-pecked husband. It was not as though he made bad money working as a labourer. During the evening he did quite a lot of voluntary work for a political group and his wife resented that, although she belonged to the same political party. She preferred to spend her spare time and energy in the chapel around the corner from their home. It turned out that she was quite religious and thwarted by the fact that praying had not saved her Eric.

Eric's mother had been very similar in personality and his father had taken to drink. Pauline strongly disapproved of drinking and remarked that Eric had first lost his erection when he was drunk at Christmas and that he was turning out to be just like his Dad.

One therapy goal was to try to do some work on their relationship to make it more positive. The therapist asked what they would both like of one another for the marital contracts:

PAULINE: 'I would really like Eric to take some responsibility.'
THERAPIST: 'In what way?'
PAULINE: 'He organises the bills for the party but not here.'
THERAPIST: 'Would you be prepared to deal with some bills at home, Eric, if Pauline did something nice for you?
ERIC: 'Yes, I would, whatever she likes.'
THERAPIST: 'Yes but what would you like in return?'
ERIC: 'That she won't be nasty all the time.'
THERAPIST: 'That's worded in a rather negative way.'
PAULINE: 'Why don't you say just stop nagging and have done?'
ERIC: 'Yes, if you like.'
THERAPIST: 'No, it would be better to phrase it positively. Maybe you could ask for more praise.'
ERIC: 'Yes, all right.'
PAULINE: 'What for?'
ERIC: 'For doing the bills.'

At least at this stage Eric had not been passive and humble, he had answered Pauline. The therapist wondered how this would affect her and sat silently.

PAULINE: 'That's all the praise you are going to get from me and then only if you do the job properly.'
ERIC: 'I'll try.'
PAULINE: 'You better had.'

The therapist realised that Eric needed some assertion training to be more effective with Pauline. When he had an individual session with the therapist and enquiries were made about his social skills he appeared to function well in all his other communications apart from with Pauline. It was difficult at the time to imagine him getting sexually aroused in her presence. He talked about what did actually excite him sexually.

ERIC: 'You see these young schoolgirls in the park. There they are fresh and innocent as daises. I wouldn't hurt them for anything in the world.'
THERAPIST: 'Do you talk with them?'
ERIC: 'Yes, a little bit and then I flash it.'
THERAPIST: 'How does that feel?'

ERIC: 'Good. Some of them blush and giggle and they look hard. It's not that they don't look, I'm telling you. They want to see what I've got.'
THERAPIST: 'But then you get caught.'
ERIC: 'Not always. Sometimes I run to the gents and relieve myself. I can get quite a hard on when I see those girls.'
THERAPIST: 'How old do they have to be?'
ERIC: 'Girls developing their sex. I like to see a bit of bosom, that's nice. I like a nice smile, too.'
THERAPIST: 'What about boys?'
ERIC: 'No. I would not get excited by a boy or a man.'
THERAPIST: 'Does Pauline excite you?'
ERIC: 'Not at all. She is more like a man in her ways although she does not look like one.'
THERAPIST: 'Do you ask her to wear special clothes for sex?'
ERIC: 'No, she would refuse.'
THERAPIST: 'What would you like her to wear?'
ERIC: 'A black lace bra.'
THERAPIST: 'Perhaps during your reconditioning therapy which I will explain to you in a minute you could imagine Pauline wearing such a bra, enjoying sex with you.'

The reconditioning therapy was not at all successful. Pauline's image was too aggressive for Eric to handle, even wearing a black lace bra. He succeeded in being assertive with her, but this altered the balance of their relationship and annoyed her.

By the fourteenth session the therapist was ready to give up but Eric asked for an individual session and announced that he was thinking about leaving Pauline as he had fallen in love with the clerk at Party Headquarters and had enjoyed sex with her. The new lady was not that young but had rather a shy personality and obviously Eric felt good with her. He had not exposed himself for two weeks since he had got to know her better.

Sometimes the therapist is asked about decisions over a client leaving his or her partner, and the client would really like the therapist to make the decision. It is good to give the client advice but essential to let the client take full responsibility for the decision.

Eric did leave Pauline and live with his shy lady. The therapist spent several sessions picking up the pieces with Pauline who did not seem greatly disturbed when she rationalised the separation at the end of her individual therapy:

PAULINE: 'I must say that I am glad to be rid of him. He became too aggressive; he changed.'

Although reconditioning therapy did not work with Eric the principle of being sexually aroused by another stimulus like his new lady worked and he stopped exposing himself. At follow-up, a year later, he had settled down and had not exposed himself in the park again.

Some therapists suggest a change of job to stop a client exhibiting himself in a convenient environment which he could not easily avoid because of his occupation. But exhibitionists find a way of finding a suitable onlooker even if they have to go out of their way. One other client used to spend the evening on the tube and flash in and out of the trains as the automatic doors were closing. He judged the timing perfectly until one day he got stuck between the doors.

Voyeurism

This is not as common as exhibitionism according to statistics, but perhaps fewer people get reported for this type of offence.

It would be considered quite normal for an individual to look at interesting sexual scenes and there are outlets nowadays, in Soho and other red light districts, where glass booths contain masturbating women on display. This type of voyeurism is legal and safe and provides a good outlet for such characters as they usually masturbate while viewing.

It is the midnight prowler type or traditional Peeping Tom who is more threatening. Sometimes such a person will put on a burglar's disguise which makes the whole offence worse if he is caught. These voyeurs masturbate as they watch their 'turn on'.

Not many women appear to go in for exhibitionism or voyeurism, perhaps because they have more opportunities to display themselves legitimately, for instance as strippers in strip tease clubs, if they want to.

The nightingale case: profile of a voyeur

Nick was a 29-year-old Scotsman who appeared very respectable and rather staid for a young man. He worked as a civil servant, adapting well to the Establishment and reaching a good grade. He was not successful with women; he had been strictly brought up as a Presbyterian and lacked much experience with women. He had tried sexual intercourse with a high class prostitute which he did not enjoy, as he was worried about hygiene and the money he was spending on the experience.

The sexual activity he did enjoy was watching young women undress when they were unaware of his presence. He could get a good erection and ejaculation under these circumstances.

He had not been prosecuted for his voyeuring because he was clever. His alibi was birdwatching, with a particular interest in recording the nightingale's song. This gave him the perfect excuse to roam the countryside on his motorcycle at twilight, ostensibly in search of the nightingale but in reality in search of a window without drawn curtains and the silhouette of a young woman removing her bra. He was quite particular about firm breasts.

Nick referred himself for therapy as the Civil Service had asked him some searching questions about his sexual orientation. He suspected that they really thought he was gay and that this would stop his progress in upgrading. Also he had actually been caught and interviewed by the police when he had been found in the grounds of a certain stately home with his binoculars trained on the window of the Hon. X, waiting for her nightly strip tease. Fortunately his obsessional behaviour had saved him as his tape recorder was already turned on. He was able to justify training his binoculars on the house by saying the nightingale flew up on the roof. The police swallowed this story and he was in the clear.

Therapy consisted of sex education and social skills training. He made good progress during therapy and found a girlfriend who was also a civil servant. It turned out that Nick had a phobia of vaginal secretion, mainly based on disliking such odours. He needed some systematic desensitisation to get used to such aromas and learned to relax deeply and imagine events like removing his girlfriend's knickers and smelling her pheromones. Fortunately, he always got sexually aroused when he saw her undressing and removing her bra.

Nick was able to channel his sexual drive into a socially acceptable pattern. The therapist relied on his subjective accounts of his sexual success since Nick did not want his girlfriend to attend for therapy and know about his problems.

Most voyeurs do not refer themselves for therapy as they see no point in denying themselves their positive reinforcement. It is usually only when they are in trouble with the law that they agree to have therapy, so Nick's case is unusual. One man treated by the author remarked if only he could transfer his voyeurism to his domestic life to get sexually aroused, but this activity would alienate his wife. Eventually his wife consented to allow him to peep through the keyhole whilst she got undressed and he has not been reconvicted since then.

Incest

Incest has been a taboo subject for a long time. In the past ten years workshops have been arranged to discuss this subject and to try to bring it out in the open. Coinciding with this attempt to get therapists to discuss methods to deal with incest there have been several television programmes in which a phone-in service to discuss incest was provided. Many victims have used this service.

Cultures vary in their approach to incest. It certainly was not taboo for the high nobility in Peru during the days of the Incas. Breeding had taken place between brothers and sisters for fourteen generations and there were no accounts of any biological deformity.

The environment can be an influential factor, affecting the sexual availability of close relatives. In many lower socio-economic groups there is a shortage of bedroom space and overcrowding can lead to incest. Most working class families in the UK, however, are very strict in insisting that the boys share one bed and the girls share another. In certain areas of South America, however, some mothers who are single parents encourage their sons to have sex with them so as to help support and provide for a large number of younger siblings. The son will therefore stay at home for a longer period and his income will be available to help out.

The most common type of relationship in incest cases is between father and daughter with sibling incest second on the list. In family studies of incest the sexual relationship of the parents is often unsatisfactory. Violence rarely occurs; it is more a psychological violation of a young person's privacy, trust and rights. It is relatively easy for an adult to take advantage of a child in the same house when the 'control factor' operates. Sibling incest seems much more natural as often the adolescents are roughly the same age. Sometimes incest can be the result of natural experimentation where youngsters are exploring sex differences and this leads to intercourse. The need for sex education in these cases is obvious.

Sometimes the mother finds it a relief for her husband to have sex with their daughter and might even encourage her daughter to submit; sometimes a daughter might enjoy such experiences. Incest can, of course, take place between father and son, but this is much more unusual.

Incest can affect other members of the family as family dynamics alter and the whole family can be disrupted. Both the offender and the victim may experience intense guilt and other strong emotions that they do not know how to deal with.

The long-term effect on the victim can be damaging especially in a father-daughter relationship where she has unwillingly submitted. She might develop a guilt complex about sex. She could be put off sex for many years, if not forever. She might become afraid of men. Katz and Mazur[2] reported that a high incidence of incest has been found in studies of delinquent girls and in one study 75 per cent of prostitutes were found to have been the victims of incest.

Therapy for the victim usually occurs much later on in life. Desensitisation to the event is the preferred therapy with self-stimulation tasks and joint masturbation for clients with partners.

It is preferable to provide therapy for victims immediately incest has been discovered but this is, of course, difficult as many cases go unreported. It is extremely upsetting for a victim to have to go to court to report the case and see a family member punished by going to prison. Obviously, supportive therapy is necessary then. Family therapy is a good way of dealing with incest as the delicate interactions and relationships can be discussed in a relaxed and caring manner with a sympathetic outsider.

Recently techniques have been developed using dolls so that young children can communicate that they have been interfered with or violated by a member of their own family. Play techniques can reveal a lot about young children and it was surprising to learn how young some of the children were who had been sexually assaulted. Some such cases in South America have been particularly horrific, expecially the case of a 5-year-old boy who had been fellated by his father and choked to death.

Hyacinth: an incest victim

Hyacinth came to the clinic for help as she was referred by a gynaecologist who had noticed that she had a mild form of vaginismus when examined. Her problem had been that she had very irregular periods and that she was losing weight rapidly. It was suggested that she was anorexic, although she denied this.

She was frightened of having sexual intercourse with her boyfriend as he might find out she was not a virgin and in any case she was frightened of sex because of bad associations. When taking her case history it turned out that her father had molested her during the school holidays throughout her adolescence. He had forced her to have sexual intercourse with him when her mother was out working in the afternoons. He was on shift work so he was at home during the day and always stopped her from going out to play with her friends. She was terrified of him and equally frightened of reporting him to her mother. Her younger sister was allowed to go out and play and Hyacinth had been very protective towards her, dreading that it would be the 10-year-old's turn next if she did not cooperate.

Therapy consisted of reassuring her that it was not her fault that incest had occurred as she had been an unwilling victim. Some cognitive therapy took place in which she pictured her father touching her breasts and taking out his penis and making her stroke him and lie down so that he could enter her. Throughout the visual tasks she expressed her feelings and told him what a lout he was. She actually no longer saw her father or visited her family and was fully independent as a shop assistant.

Hyacinth was taught to relax and imagine her boyfriend kissing and indulging in foreplay, leading to mutual masturbation and sexual intercourse. Later she carried out some of this activity and gradually came to terms with the horror of her incestuous father.

Sexual assault and rape

According to Bancroft[3] these offences are usually associated with violence and a recent overall rape report showed that 80 per cent of cases involve violence. In about 20 per cent of cases the violence is extreme. Physical violence is most common with adult women and least common with children, although it is worrying that there has been an increase in the number of reports of missing young children who have later been found sexually violated and/or strangled.

Rape is usually a heterosexual assault. There have been reported cases of men who have been buggered and this type of rape happens in many male prisons. Weaker prisoners are the victims and the pattern is that of a power game. The same system of homosexual rape can take place also in women's prisons.

There has been an increase in the number of women raped by gangs, both in the UK and the USA, especially in the large cities. Men who rape in gangs are usually more violent and this could have a modelling effect in a group – if one man is violent the others think this is acceptable for them too. Katz and Mazur[2] showed that men who were impotent during an assault became violent. Sexual intercourse usually takes place but other acts, like fellatio or urination, can occur.

The relationship between the offender and the victim has been reported by Holmstrom and Burgess[4]. In the USA adults are usually raped by complete strangers, whereas in the UK half the adult victims already know the offender. American children and adolescents usually know the offender, and this also applies to the UK.

Several research studies have been carried out on the sexual offender. Holmstrom and Burgess[4] concluded that there are four principal 'meanings' of sexual assault:

(1) the experience of power and control over the victim;
(2) the expression of anger or hatred;
(3) with group or pair rape, the male camaraderie experienced by the rapists,
(4) the sexual experience which in Holmstrom and Burgess' view is never the dominant theme.

Other studies show that the convicted rapist is predominantly a young man and probably from the lower socio-economic groups. There is a definite link between rape and the consumption of alcohol.

Profile of a rapist

One fallacy associated with rape is that usually the rapist is a shy, socially inadequate man who rapes to get some sexual satisfaction. The majority of rapists are not like that.

John was a bold, aggressive man who did not care about the publicity.

JOHN: 'I don't mind what people write about me. If there's money in it, I want my cut, though.'
THERAPIST: 'What sort of work did you do before you went to prison?'
JOHN: 'Construction work – you know, building and that sort of thing.'
THERAPIST: 'Did you work for yourself?'
JOHN: 'No. I used to go round building sites and get hired. Look, I'm a strong man.'
THERAPIST: 'Yes, you are. Do you think if you had not been so strong the injuries to the woman you raped would not have been so bad?'
JOHN: 'No. That bitch started to stop me so I let her have it.'
THERAPIST: 'What happened? Were you making sexual advances that she resisted?'
JOHN: 'Yes you could put it like that. In any case, that bitch is a prostitute so she'd expect sex, wouldn't she?'
THERAPIST: 'I am getting confused. I am not sure what happened. Could you tell me, John?'

In fact, the therapist knew exactly what had happened, according to the court report. The victim was indeed a prostitute but she refused to go with him as she thought he looked kinky. She had walked away from him and he had seen her go off with another customer. This had so annoyed him that later he coldly plotted to get her. The next night he carried a knife and managed to abduct her to a car he had stolen for the night. His previous criminal record consisted of petty offences and he had never been convicted of rape before.

JOHN: 'She went with me for a ride in my car and when we got by the river she started saying she wanted more money than she'd said at first. She thought I only wanted a blow job but I'd said the works to her, so she knew what it was I was after.'
THERAPIST: 'So what did you do?'
JOHN: 'I said she could do it for the money she said before.'
THERAPIST: 'Did she agree?'
JOHN: 'No, she started arguing and saying she would only give me the blow job. My dick was quite big by this time and I wanted it bad.'
THERAPIST: 'So I suppose you lost your erection?'
JOHN: 'No, because I knew I could get what she had promised by making her fuck.'
THERAPIST: 'You mean by forcing her to have sex with you?'
JOHN: 'Yes, because that's what she had promised at first.'
THERAPIST: 'Yes, but even if there had been a misunderstanding you were not justified in using violence like you did.'
JOHN: 'Who says? You women are all the same. You all really want it and pretend you don't. I know you.'

At this stage of discussing the offence John was becoming aggressive in his manner towards the female therapist. When a client becomes aggressive during therapy there are several ways for the therapist to handle the situation: another topic of conversation can be chosen to distract the client; the therapist can go along in a passive state, agreeing with the client; or the session can be terminated. In many ways, passively going along with what the client is saying is rather like not offering any resistance during rape, and reinforcing the client. It is very difficult also for a therapist, whether male or female, to remain detached and objective whilst listening to a client's account of rape. It requires a lot of emotional control to try to be reasonable and non-judgmental. In this instance the therapist decided to distract the client.

THERAPIST: 'How old did you say you were?'
JOHN: 'What's that got to do with it?'
THERAPIST: 'You look quite young, but you also look as though you have had a lot of sexual experience as you seem very confident.'

JOHN: 'I am 24. I have always been confident with women, they like me. I've got good money and I can take them out to the pub and give them a good time.'
THERAPIST: 'Do you have a steady woman friend, or are you married?
JOHN: 'No. I don't want a regular girlfriend yet or to get married.'
THERAPIST: 'One of the things our therapy programme covers is what we call 'social skills training' and I would like to discuss with you what this involves.'

A discussion of John's social life ensued. It appeared that his only social contacts were made in pubs. He and his friend were quite skilled at picking women up.

JOHN: 'I can get sex quite easily. All I need do is pay for it.'
THERAPIST: 'Do you have sex with any women for free?'
JOHN: 'No, I prefer to pay and get what I want. That's why I go to whores.'

Obviously there was something going wrong with John's relationships with women if he always had to pay for sex and never developed a friendship. The therapist intuitively felt that John disliked women but it was difficult to approach John directly with this.

THERAPIST: 'A lot of men who pay for sex don't really like women. Are you like that, John?'
JOHN: 'I like women all right; it's feminists I don't like. Dykes, like you get at Greenham Common. They don't give anything away, they don't. After all, women are the weaker sex.'
THERAPIST: 'You are very strong. Have you forced women to have sex before?'
JOHN: 'Yes, my first girlfriend led me on. She was a prick tease – she started feeling my cock and laughing at me. I got a hard on and she would go no further so I held her down and did to her hard.'
THERAPIST: 'Did you ever see her again?'
JOHN: 'Yes, she went regularly with me for a time. She really liked a good fuck, but she went back to Belfast. So I didn't see her any more.'

From then on John had gone with prostitutes. He had no respect for women and needed to change his attitude. Some of the role playing activities were heavy going but he understood that he had to make an effort to change. He knew that it made sense to try to get into a friendship in which sex occurred naturally. It was not that he wanted kinky sexual activity; he was happy to have sexual intercourse in the man above position and he had no sexual problems.

John knew that the alternative therapy was a course of a drug called Androcur which would lower his sexual interest. In spite of his efforts he still retained a negative attitude towards women and the choice of drug therapy was made by his assessors six months after he had pursued a course of social skills and supportive therapy.

Profile of a victim of sexual assualt

Maria was a Venezuelan broadcaster who went over to Trinidad to cover the carnival for the national radio station she worked for. She had been sexually assaulted by a taxi driver. Unlike John the rapist who got caught, the taxi driver is still at large.

MARIA: 'He was very thin and tall. I still have nightmares about him.'
THERAPIST: 'What happened?'
MARIA: 'I had been recording the panorama finals. In Trinidad the steel bands compete yearly for a prize at carnival. It was fun and I felt good but tired. It had got to 10 pm and my friends wanted to stay and listen to the other bands.'
THERAPIST: 'So you decided to leave on your own.'
MARIA: 'That's right. I thought nothing of it. I was carrying my recording equipment and it was heavy. This tall thin man appeared and told me it was late for a European to be walking around alone and it was safer to take a taxi. I said I was actually looking for a taxi. That was the coincidence, so he said that he was a taxi driver and he had been to hear the steel bands but wanted to get back to work.'
THERAPIST: 'Were you suspicious?'
MARIA: 'No he seemed *bona fide*. The taxi had an H number registration and that's legal.'
THERAPIST: 'So what happened then?'
MARIA: 'Instead of going straight on he took a turn up the hill by the savannah. I said he was going in the wrong direction but he said it was a short cut.'
THERAPIST: 'Did you believe him?'
MARIA: 'I had a sinking feeling in my stomach, knowing he would make trouble. He stopped the car and I jumped out but he ran after me. He hit me on the head, holding me down and telling me to shut up.'
THERAPIST: 'Did he sexually assault you then?'
MARIA: 'He started ripping my blouse and knickers, scratching my breasts and legs, then telling me what he was going to do. He said he

would rape me first and then murder me. I felt as though I was frozen. He said that he had already done this to other tourists. He would then take my money and equipment. I said I had very little money on me as I had travellers' cheques and was staying with friends in any case. He said I was lying, but he didn't want me to talk when he was telling me about himself. He lit a cigarette. As he did this I suddenly knew I could act fast and I kicked him in the balls with my knee. He winced with pain and I got up and jumped off the cliff.'
THERAPIST: 'You got away, but you could have died jumping.'
MARIA: 'I managed to cling on to some grass all night. He had gone by the morning and I went to the police.'

This event had scarred Maria; although rape had not taken place she had been assaulted and humiliated. She became phobic of going abroad. When she heard about a women's sex therapy group that was being run in Caracas she joined it but did not want the others to know her full story. She said that she had gone off sex for three years and had not been able to relate to men.

Here was an independent, capable woman, not the expected inadequate lower socio-economic group victim. Fortunately, she did not come from a Muslim culture where she would be ostracised and shamed for an event she had no control over. Some desensitisation tasks – like imagining the rapist, having her clothes torn, her breasts touched, kicking him in the testicles, and winning – were given to her before the group started and during the group she did well with these tasks. At follow-up she had found a man friend who was sympathetic towards her and wanted marriage, which she was considering.

Paedophilia

Once this was a taboo subject. People continue to be very disapproving of sexual relationships between adults and children because they appear to be an abuse of trust and exploit a child's comparative weakness. In prison this type of offender needs special protection.

These offenders are not usually violent, in fact the offences are often carried out with the full permission of the child, although it could be said that a child has not reached sexual maturity and could have been misled or exploited by the offender. Gebhard[5] reported that some children encouraged the offender. Although various groups have canvassed for 'the sexual rights of the child' this has been ineffective.

Most people are very sexist in their attitudes towards this offence. Men bear the brunt of the blame but probably women get away with it more easily and go unreported. Very occasionally during a case history taking session a female client will reveal that she has sexually fondled children.

Research on such offenders shows them to be older than the average age of most sexual offenders; they are usually in their thirties. Most of them prefer either boys or girls, but a few of them like both. They usually have a good cover up as most of them get married. Most of them appear to be quite caring, and many are involved in providing social welfare for the boys or girls they befriend.

There is a stigma attached to paedophilia which implies that the victims are buggered, but this is not so. The most common activity is mutual genital touching. For many of these men this type of sex with a child is less threatening and demanding than with an adult. They usually are not interested in sexual intercourse with their regular partners.

George: a case of paedophilia

George came to the clinic, referred by his psychiatrist who thought behaviour therapy might solve some of the grave problems associated with this very inadequate and unemployed 32-year-old man. He admitted to fondling and touching the genitals of several young boys aged between 13 and 15. They were all willing participants and sometimes they had requested to masturbate George. The offence came to light when George was on holiday at his grandmother's house. The elder brother of one of the boys had discovered George's activities and had attempted to blackmail him. George was on the dole and had no money to pay up so the brother went to the police who treated George badly. Paedophiliacs are often victimised and, if imprisoned, are usually the lowest in the pecking order of prisoners.

George looked about ten years younger than his real age. He had a smooth youthful skin although he shaved daily. At the first interview he only answered when he was spoken to and it took several sessions to get him to communicate effectively, with eye contact. He had little contact with people, living at home with his mother whom he described as 'a bossy nosey parker'. He liked his grandmother who sounded a very active 76-year-old, helping to organise church fetes and outings. Unfortunately this was the perfect scene that was so convenient for George to find co-operative and lonely young boys who were pleased to be singled out and helped by him. George only felt confident and mature in the presence of such boys. George had been a carpenter and he provided some tuition for the younger boys who also got some apprenticeship in male sexuality. He was very popular and the boys liked and admired him, requesting to join his holiday classes.

One of the first things covered in therapy was sex education, which was mainly about female sexuality. George was inexperienced and almost phobic of women. He was very friendly at therapy sessions and eager to change his habits, mainly on account of his grandmother who had been very upset over his offence. In fact, poor George had not been on holiday since his offence and his mother was getting increasingly irritated by him and nagging him more than ever. He remarked several times that he felt depressed over the whole business and guilty that he had done things to young boys. From talking with him it appeared that the boys had been quite encouraging and cooperative.

The first part of the therapy went well and he reached a stage where social skills helped and he could chat up older women. He was particularly nervous about meeting young, attractive women whom he found more threatening, although they were sexually more attractive. He liked slim, boyish-looking women but they did not seem to want to bother with George.

The breakthrough in therapy came when he started the 'orgasmic reconditioning'. He did his homework and initially imagined young boys when he masturbated and then switched to a photograph of an attractive woman when he was about to ejaculate. After the fourth session of his therapy he met an older woman of 43 who had just got a divorce. She had two daughters of nine and twelve who accepted George as their mother's new boyfriend. She was extremely relaxing and kind but George was not sexually attracted to her although she liked him and wanted to make love. He was instructed by the therapist to change his final image and imagine this particular woman friend when he ejaculated at home. This worked well and he was already thinking of her earlier when he masturbated.

After five more sessions of therapy George was able to tell his woman friend about his problems and she was supportive and understanding. George had been afraid that she would reject him as his paedophilia might endanger her two daughters. When he had confessed he was able to suggest a massage and this was successful. They continued with genital sensate focussing and he was confident over this, but informed the therapist later that he still relied on his original fantasies involving paedophilia to get excited. He wondered whether he should tell his woman friend about his fantasies but the therapist advised against this.

Eventually George's relationship flourished and he moved into his friend's house and they decided to marry. Sexual intercourse was successful but at the six-monthly follow-up he reported that he still needed his original paedophilia fantasies to get sexually aroused. The therapist emphasised that this was perfectly all right and he was not to worry about this, as his therapy was successful in that he had achieved his goal of a relationship with a woman and had enjoyed sex as a therapy bonus. Follow-up also confirmed that George had not been involved in further paedophilia.

Orgasmic reconditioning is not always so successful for paedophiliacs. It is always preferable for such a man to have a relationship with an adult, hopefully ensuring an available sexual partner. Obviously a real partner who is sexually arousing is better than relying on the image of a fantasy woman in a sex magazine. Of course, some paedophiliacs might have negative relationships with available partners and marital or relationship therapy should be given to improve the situation, but this is difficult and often unrewarding therapy.

Types of therapy for sexual offenders

(1) Conjoint therapy

The presence of a co-operative and sympathetic partner who is willing to improve the sexual relationship with the offender obviously enhances the prognosis. Sometimes a partner who has previously been kept in the dark over the offence can be sympathetic and co-operative once involved; in the past he or she might have thought the partner was being unfaithful because of such an apparently low sex drive. Therapy can clear up many misunderstandings.

Relationship or marital therapy on a contractual basis can help a couple. For example, sometimes a partner can behave in an undesirable way and a contract can be arranged for such a partner to sit down and watch the client's favourite television programme instead of washing the dishes and making a noise. In return the client might be asked to dress in a more acceptable manner, wearing a clean sweater instead of one which is frayed and food-stained.

The sexual relationship can often be improved by sex therapy. The couple often needs to be taught that a non-sexual massage leading to genital stimulation can be an affective alternative to sexual intercourse. They need to learn to avoid the pressure of sexual intercourse. Sometimes when the pressure of sexual intercourse is lowered and the relationship is worked on the sexual relationship can be enhanced. Both partners need to put a lot of work into such therapy.

(2) Individual therapy

Sometimes the problem is based on low self-esteem and the client needs supportive therapy and social skills training to be more effective as a person. Peter Mark and Anita Sydow[6] have pointed out that paedophiles have a low self-esteem with adults and they feel safer forming friendships with children as this helps them feel good.

Other offenders may lack self-control and need to be taught how to acquire this and learn to discipline themselves sexually.

Orgasmic reconditioning plays an important part in individual therapy and this appears to be one of the most hopeful therapies to help an offender change his or her sexual arousal towards a more acceptable sexual stimulus, like a suitable partner. Admittedly, the client needs to be highly motivated to do this. This type of therapy should be assessed from time to time in a laboratory by getting the client to view slides of stimuli associated with his or her offence and then to switch to the photograph used in orgasmic reconditioning therapy. Penile plethysmography can be used to assess male clients' responses and vaginal blood flow for female clients' responses, although it is rare for women to be charged with sexual offences.

(3) Group therapy

Advances have been made in group therapy for sex offenders. Crawford and Allen[7] show promising results for the treatment of such offenders at Broadmoor. Methods included sex education, orgasmic reconditioning and social skills training. Obviously social skills training is more suitable for group than individual therapy, as the individual can identify with peers and get their feedback.

Such groups are even better in a non-institutional setting where the offenders learn to cope with their own home environment. Gunn[8] pointed out that a probation order as a condition of treatment is an almost ideal disposal for the majority of sex offenders.

One of the best known studies of group therapy is the Berkeley group in Bristol in which Fox and Weaver[9] mixed paedophiles and exhibitionists. This was a highly structured group in which participants carried out pencil and paper exercises introduced by the leaders who also led discussions. Success of this type of group therapy was measured by the low reconviction rate. They developed their ideas from the work of Mathis and Collins [10] in the USA, who recommended male and female co-therapists, mandatory attendance, and that symptoms and goals should be held in common.

The Kensington High Street 'location' groups run by Peter Mark and Anita Sydow also provided group therapy based on discussions for paedophiles and exhibitionists but were less structured than previous groups. The group participants themselves were given responsibility for introducing themes and taking space for themselves, with the leaders concentrating more on group dynamics.

The initial difficulty encountered in the first group was for the members to reveal their offence to the others, and this was cleverly done by getting each member to write a story anonymously about his offence, then pool these accounts and read them back to the group, whereupon members discussed them.

Important ingredients of the group therapy appeared to be: expressing feelings and taking the risks associated with this; getting feedback from fellow members and the two group leaders; and being able to discuss female sexuality informally with the female leader, Anita Sydow. Results were good in terms of reconviction rates and attendance.

(4) Drug therapy

When it is impossible to get the offender to change his sexual stimuli to more acceptable alternatives, hormonal drug therapy is available if he is labelled dangerous. This kind of drug therapy lowers the offender's sexual interest and makes it less likely that he will commit another sexual offence. The problem with drug therapy is checking whether the client has taken the drug, if he is living out in the community.

Although these drugs are administered with the offender's consent there are the problems of side effects. Originally, the side effects of oestrogen were associated with feminisation, testicular atrophy, reduced sperm counts and even cancer. This led to alternative anti-libidinal drugs being developed. Tennent *et al.*[11] have discussed drugs like benperidol, which in clinical trials showed fewer side effects but with little effect on sexual behaviour, and Cyproterone Acetate, which again has feminisation side effects but the advantage of wearing off quickly when discontinued. Mark and Sydow have mentioned the fact that there is no simple correlation between human chemical levels and degree and type of sexual response. They stressed the potential abuse of 'chemical castration' and its effects on the already vulnerable and insecure masculinity most sex offenders experience. They recommend group therapy.

(5) Psychosurgery

Sometimes psychosurgery or castration have been recommended as a last resort. This type of operation is irreversible, however, and ethically unacceptable to the medical profession in most countries.

The above facts show how important it is to encourage research on psychological therapy for sexual disorders. Sex therapy has gone a long way in the last twenty years and, hopefully, with the help of media cooperation and well applied research more advances will be made.

References

1. Walmsley, R. and White, K. (1979) 'Sexual offence, consent and sentencing.' *Home Office Research Study, No. 54*. HMSO, London.
2. Katz, S. and Mazur, M.A. (1979) *Understanding Rape Victims: a Synthesis of Research Findings*. Wiley.
3. Bancroft, John. (1983) *Human Sexuality and its Problems*. Churchill Livingstone.
4. Holmstrom, L.L. and Burgess, A.W. (1980) 'Sexual behavior of assailants during reported rapes'. *Archives Sexual Behavior*, 9. 427–446.
5. Gebhard, P., Gagnon, J., Pomeroy, N, Christenson, C. (1965) *Sex Offenders*. Harper and Row.
6. Mark, Peter and Sydow, Anita. (1985) *A Study of Sex Offenders*. Inner London Probation and After-care Service Benevolent and Educational Trust.
7. Crawford, D.A. and Allen, J.V. (1979) 'A social skills training programme for sex offenders – a symposium'. Gunn, J. (ed.) *Special Hospital Research Report. No 14*.
8. Gunn, J. (1976) 'Sexual offenders'. *Brit. J. Hosp. Med.* 15, 1, 57–65.
9. Fox, C. and Weaver, C. (1978) 'Group work with sexual offenders'. *Probation Journal*. Sept.
10. Mathis, J. and Collins, M. (1970) 'Mandatory group for exhibitionists'. *American. Jrnl. Psychiat.* Feb.
11. Tennent, G., Bancroft, J., Cass, J. 'The control of deviant sexual behaviour by drugs: a double blind controlled study of benperidol, chlorpromazine and placebo'. *Archives of Sexual Behavior*. 3. 261–271.

Appendix 1

Therapist's Instructions

PHYSICAL EXAMINATION

This routine procedure is based on Masters and Johnson's approach to treatment of sexual problems. It involves the presence of the co-therapist and both partners. Complete privacy should be assured.

The physical examination must be carried out by the medical co-therapist first and followed by the client's partner. The therapist wears surgical gloves, but this is not necessary for the partner. The non-examining co-therapist should remain in the room, looking relaxed and friendly.

The general anatomy of the sexual organs must be pointed out and understood. Partners are asked to name each other's sexual organs, both in technical and colloquial terms.

Other causes of sexual dysfunction, including lassitude, etc. should be ruled out by appropriate physical, urine and blood examinations.

Clients' attitudes to the examination are important and should be observed. This could be described as a 'modelling procedure' as the clients touch each other's genitalia, after the therapist has shown them how to do this. The therapists should be relaxed and calm throughout. It is essential for them to take time over this task and not to appear to be rushed or hurried. Another factor in this procedure is 'desensitisation' – some clients might be afraid of touching each other genitally and this is a step in desensitising them.

Female examination

The woman is asked to remove her clothes from the waist down and then requested to lie down on her back. Initially she can be covered with a blanket.

She should then draw up her legs, keeping her feet together on the bed. The therapist should ask her to relax her thighs and allow them to fall apart. If the woman seems tense it is advisable to instruct her to take a few deep breaths and allow her mouth to open – usually this helps to relax her.

A vaginal examination can now take place, the therapist first inserting the index finger and then the index and middle fingers. The cervix is felt for and used as a base from which to palpate the other pelvic organs. Any pathology, e.g. fibroids, prolapse, deep tenderness, discharge, painful scars, must be assessed.

The woman is then instructed to constrict her pubococcygeal muscle. If she is not familiar with this she is asked:

(a) to squeeze the vaginal muscle on the examiner's fingers;
(b) to pretend she is stopping a flow of urine.

Her partner can now try inserting his index finger and then his index and middle fingers. When his fingers are in position she should be asked to demonstrate her PC muscle. Her labia minora and clitoris should then be identified by her partner. She should then show him her sensitive areas, if she is aware of them. If not, the female therapist should show the couple the female erogenous zones, pointing these out on the female patient.

Male examination

The man is asked to remove his clothing from the waist down, and requested to lie on his back and relax. He can initially be covered with a blanket.

His scrotum and penis are palpated and inspected. Again, pathology must be excluded, e.g. urethral discharge, any sores, infections, severe varicocoeles, herniae, associated lymphadenopathy, etc. The female partner should then touch his testicles gently and the penis as she identifies and points out his complete sex anatomy. The man should then show her the sensitive areas of his genitalia, especially his frenulum and coronal ridge. If these are unfamiliar they can be pointed out by the male therapist.

Appendix 2

Client's Instructions

HOMEWORK CONTRACT

Name ______________________ Date of contract ______________________

What task? ____

____

Where? ______________________ With whom? ______________________

For how long each time? ____

Starting when? ______________________ How often? ______________________

I have decided to do this task because, even if it upsets me, it will help me get better.

Signed ______________________ Date ______________________

Witness ______________________ Date ______________________

No.	Date	Distress score at start	Distress score near end	Comment and praise

RELAXATION INSTRUCTIONS

Relaxation is a useful technique whenever you feel tense.

Preparation

Sit in a comfortable chair or, better still, lie down. Choose a quiet, warm room, when you are not too tired and where you will not be interrupted.

If you are sitting, take off your shoes, uncross your legs and rest your arms along the arms of the chair.

If you are lying down, lie on your back, with your arms at your sides.

Close your eyes, and be aware of your body: notice how you are breathing, and where the muscular tensions in your body are. Make sure you are comfortable.

Breathing

Start to breathe slowly and deeply, expanding your abdomen as you breathe IN, then raising your rib cage to let more air in, till your lungs are filled right to the top. Hold your breath for a couple of seconds and then breathe OUT slowly, allowing your rib cage and stomach to relax, and empty your lungs completely.

Do not strain; with practice it will become much easier.

Keep this slow, deep rhythmic breathing going throughout your relaxation session.

Relaxation

After you have got your breathing pattern established, start the following sequence:

(1) Curl your toes hard and press your feet down:
Tense up on an IN breath, hold your breath for 10 seconds while you keep your muscles tense, then relax and breathe OUT at the same time.

(2) Now press your heels down and bend your feet up:
Tense up on an IN breath, hold your breath for 10 seconds; relax on an OUT breath.

(3) Now tense your calf muscles:
Tense up on an IN breath, hold for 10 seconds, relax on an OUT breath.

(4) Now tense your thigh muscles, straightening your knees and making your legs stiff:

Tense up on an IN breath; hold for 10 seconds; relax on an OUT breath.

(5) Now make your buttocks tight:
Tense up on an IN breath; hold for 10 seconds; relax on an OUT breath.

(6) Now tense your stomach as if to receive a punch:
Tense up on an IN breath; hold for 10 seconds; relax on an OUT breath.

(7) Now bend your elbows and tense the muscles of your arms:
Tense up on an IN breath; hold for 10 seconds; relax on an OUT breath.

(8) Now hunch your shoulders and press your head back into the cushion:
Tense up on an IN breath; hold for 10 seconds; relax on an OUT breath.

(9) Now clench your jaws, frown, and screw up your eyes really tight:
Tense up on an IN breath; hold for 10 seconds; relax on an OUT breath.

(10) Now tense all your muscles together:
Tense up on an IN breath; hold for 10 seconds; relax on an OUT breath.

Remember to breathe deeply, and be aware when you relax of the feeling of physical well-being and heaviness spreading through your body.
After you have done the whole sequences from 1 – 10, still breathing slowly and deeply, imagine a white rose on a black background.
Try to 'see' the rose as clearly as possible, concentrating your attention on it for 30 seconds. Do *not* hold your breath during this time, continue to breathe as you have been doing.
After this, go on to visualise anything else your therapist may have suggested, or give yourself the instruction that when you open your eyes you will be perfectly relaxed but alert.
Count to 3 and then open your eyes.

When you have become familiar with this technique, if you want to relax at any time when you have a few minutes only, do the sequence in shortened form, leaving out some muscle groups, but always working from your feet upwards. For example, you might do Nos. 1, 4, 6, 8 and 10 if you did not have time to do the complete sequence.

INSTRUCTIONS FOR A MASSAGE

(1) Make sure that the place you choose for your massage (what Masters and Johnson refer to as 'sensate focussing') is warm and comfortable. If the bedroom is cold, try the sitting room in front of a fire. Some couples find it helpful to have a hot bath first. The vital thing is that you are being given another chance to get together physically and to explore areas of your bodies you never knew you could respond to and enjoy. You are being given an opportunity to please each other and to get to know each other better by making a completely fresh start in your love life.

(2) No sexual intercourse should take place during these early stages, and no touching of breasts, nipples, penis, testicles, vagina or clitoris. But you can kiss and cuddle as much as you like.

(3) The idea is to learn to 'give to get', that is, to enjoy providing pleasure when you touch your partner.

(4) During the sessions you should use a lotion to rub each other's bodies with. We recommend 'Johnson's Baby Lotion' in that it helps to provide a smooth texture and it is not too sticky. You should both undress completely.

(5) Your therapist will suggest who should take the 'active role' initially. One of you should approach the other partner who should be lying comfortably. Use the lotion to massage, fondle and trade the outlines of your partner's body. Try to discover the degree of pressure that is most enjoyable. Some women report that their partner has too heavy a touch, and some men complain that they do not feel very much, as the female touch is too light and gentle. Try to get some 'feedback' on how your partner likes to be massaged by talking about it, or by placing your hand under your partner's hand so you can be guided by your partner. Then change places, and this time the one who has been massaging can lie down and enjoy some new sensations.

(6) Instructions for massaging different parts of the body are given below. We find it preferable for partners to take the massaging of different parts of the body in turns, in stages, rather than having one partner spending a whole 20 minutes massaging the whole body.

(a) A lies on tummy; B massages A's back, neck, arms, buttocks, legs. (About ten minutes.)

(b) B lies on tummy; A massages B's back, neck, arms, buttocks, legs. (About ten minutes.)

(c) A lies on back. B massages A's neck, chest, stomach, shoulders, arms, legs. (About ten minutes.)
(d) B lies on back. A massages B's neck, chest, stomach, shoulders, arms, legs. (About ten minutes.)

(7) Try to repeat the above sessions with your own imaginative variations, on several different occasions, making the whole thing into a 'fun session'. Try to be relaxed and not to 'strain' to experience sensations; these should come easily enough when you are relaxed.

SELF-FOCUSSING: INSTRUCTIONS FOR WOMEN

Pubococcygeal muscle exercises

The purpose of this brief training programme is to help you tone up your vaginal or PC muscles. The use of this muscle increases your pleasure during sexual intercourse. Both you and your partner will benefit from the new sensitivity from your vagina.

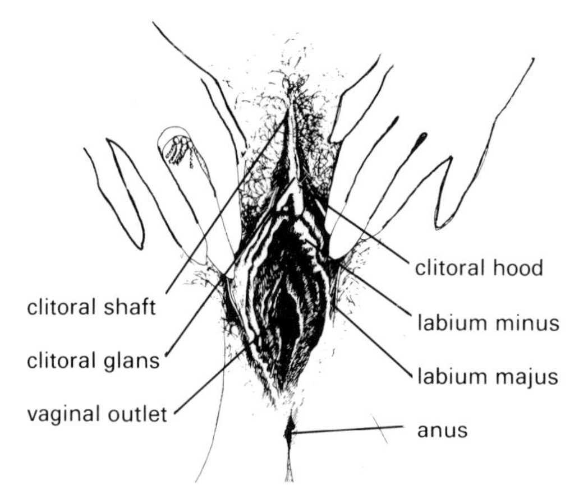

(1) *First week.* Locate the PC muscle by pretending to stop a flow of urine. If this is difficult then actually try this when you are urinating. Do this several times. Each time you urinate start and stop the flow of urine, and during urination only pass a teaspoon of urine at a time, stopping the stream by using the PC muscle.
(2) Lie down and put your finger in your vagina and contract the PC muscle. Feel the contraction around your finger.
(3) Practise 10 contractions on 6 different occasions each day. Each timed you have a drink you could do this. No-one else knows you are doing this, so you can do it anytime, e.g. when you answer the telephone at work or at home. Try to make each contraction last 3 seconds.
(4) *Second week.* Contract the PC muscle but release it quickly. This called *twitching* or *fluttering*. Try to rapidly contract and release the PC muscle 6 times a day, increasing the number of contractions from 10 to 20.
(5) The next stage is to imagine you have a tampon at the opening of your vagina and that you use these muscles to suck it into your vagina. Continue the twitching 10 times a session and try to have

6 sessions a day. Continue with the ordinary paced contractions and increase these to 50 a session. When you are doing this try to enjoy some sexual fantasies and also try to picture your partner.

(6) The last exercise is to bear down, as if you were making a bowel movement, but with the emphasis more on the vagina than the anal area. Try holding this for about 3 seconds and practise it 10 times.

Clitoral stimulation

(1) Look at your genitalia in the mirror. Try to locate the sensitive parts of your genitalia by touching yourself and looking at that area.
(2) Concentrate on stimulating that area. Vary the stimulation you use. Try making circular or up and down movements of your finger on your clitoris. Vary the speed of movement and pressure. You can lubricate yourself by placing the tip of your finger in your vagina, but if this is not yet moist enough try a little KY jelly on your finger.
(3) Try to imagine some of the fantasies you like and stimulate yourself with your finger until something happens or you get tired. If you do not climax you could get a hand-held vibrator and try this. If you climax, immediately switch to the image of your partner.
(4) As you practise the self-stimulation exercises try to make the switch to the image of your partner earlier on, before you climax.
(5) Lastly, try a couple of sessions stimulating yourself in front of your partner. If it's difficult, try again the next day and do not worry.
(6) Remember, there is no 'set way' of masturbation; the idea is to have fun and *please yourself*.

SELF-FOCUSSING: INSTRUCTIONS FOR MEN

(1) Ensure that you have complete privacy and explore your genitalia by looking at yourself in a hand mirror.

(2) Try touching your scrotum gently. Then run your hand up and down your penile shaft. Touch your *frenulum*.

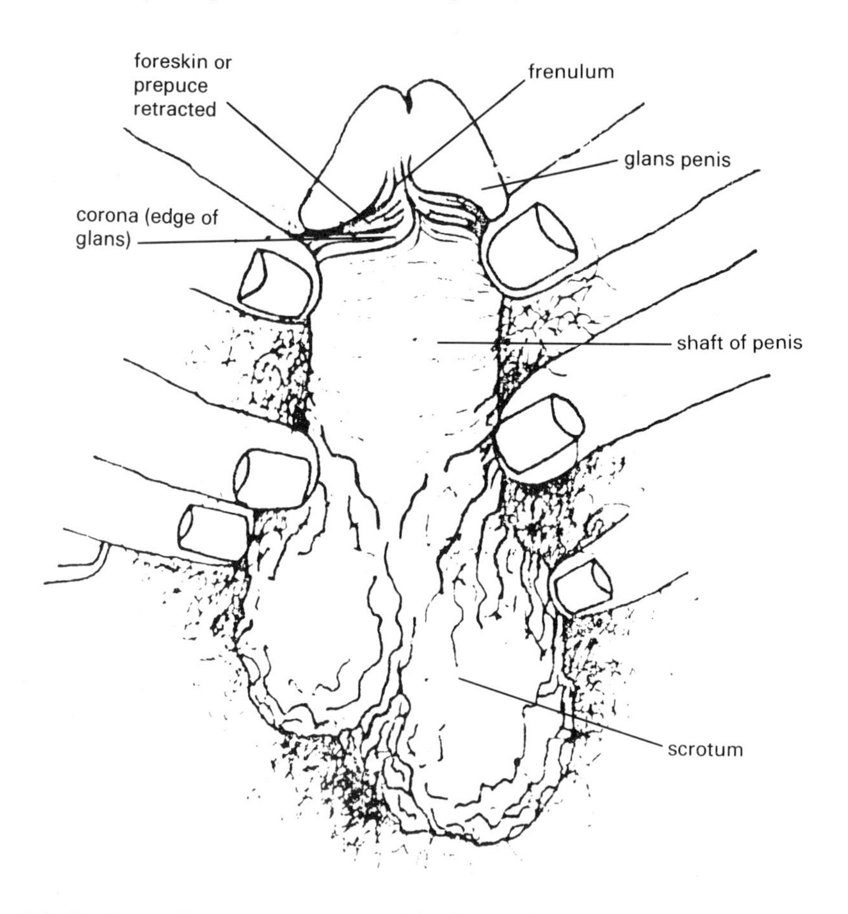

(3) Explore the sensations you like best. If you are uncircumcised try drawing back your foreskin very slightly and then pull it up again to cover your glans. Your glans can be very sensitive, but explore this area getting some feedback over your sensations. If you are circumcised, move the skin covering your penis, squeezing and releasing it to induce accumulated tensions in your glans.

(4) Vary the pressure of your touch. Maybe you will enjoy grasping yourself firmly but maybe you enjoy stroking various areas of your penis very gently. Try varying the speed of your movements.

Some men like a slow downwards movement and a rapid upwards movement, others the other way round. It is up to you to choose what you personally like.

(5) At this stage try to imagine some of the fantasies you have been asked to picture. Try to imagine them as vividly as possible.

(6) As you get more excited and stimulate your penis more quickly and feel you are going to 'come' or climax, switch to a mental or actual picture of your partner in the nude and imagine you are making love with her, at the same time as you have your orgasm.

(7) The next occasion you try this programme you will know which areas you like to stimulate. If you are already familiar with masturbation techniques try numbers 5 and 6 and practise shaping your fantasies but switch to your partner's image during orgasm. Then try to switch to the image or fantasies of your partner at earlier points in time, until eventually just the thought of your partner will turn you on.

(8) The last step here is to invite your partner to watch you stimulating yourself. Do not feel embarrassed or shy about this as this will more than likely turn her on and you will both enjoy this step.

(9) If you are not getting a climax or if you are not getting excited we suggest that you try using a hand-held vibrator to help you, but continue your fantasy-shaping at the same time. If you feel anxious about these sessions we will have discussed this with you and will have instructed you on how to relax. Don't forget to do your relaxation exercises before you attempt any of the sessions. The relaxation will help you to overcome your anxiety.

(10) We would like you to try contracting the muscles you use when you want to move your penis about without using your hands. If this is difficult try to pretend you are stopping a flow of urine. Try this next time you urinate. Practise this muscular contraction 10 times on 6 occasions. These movements will help you tone your muscles and get pleasurable sensations.

INSTRUCTIONS FOR GENITAL SENSATE FOCUSSING

(1) Carry out previous instructions (a) to (d) for massage again (see previous sheet) with any variations you may both have enjoyed.
(2) Follow this by the next step:

(e) A gently massages B's breasts and nipples using lotion. (About five minutes.)
(f) B gently massages A's breasts and nipples using lotion. (About five minutes.)

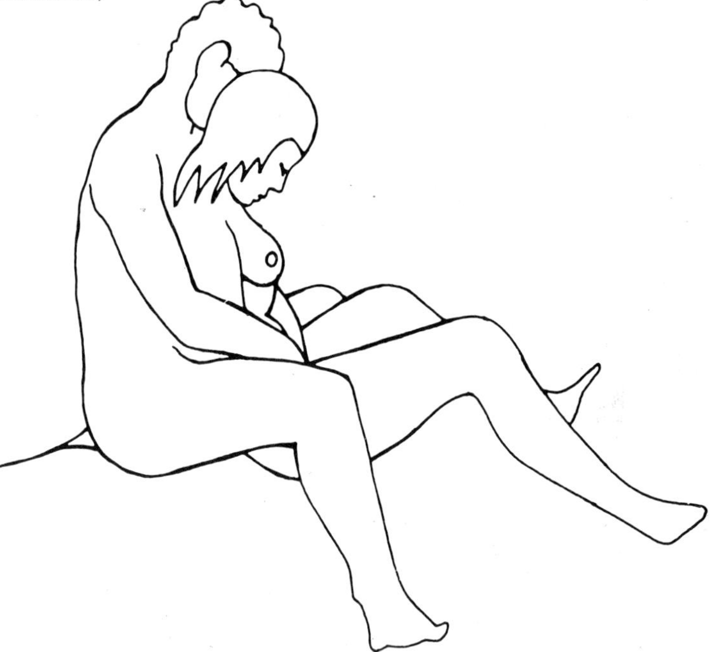

(3) Carry on the next step slowly, in a 'non-demanding' way, with a lubricant such as KY jelly if you feel it is necessary. An orgasm is not required at this stage. If you do get so excited that you do have a climax it does not matter, but the aim of the exercises given below is to get used to touching and being touched genitally and to enjoy this:

(g) The man gently touches the woman's clitoral shaft. (About five minutes.)
(h) The woman gently touches the man's testicles. (About five minutes.)
(i) The man gently touches the woman's clitoris glans and entrance to vagina. (About five minutes.)

(j) The woman gently touches the man's penis; shaft and glans. (About five minutes.)

(4) For the next step, get into the recommended 'comfortable position for female stimulation' illustrated here, with the man leaning against the pillows or other support. She should then be stimulated according to her wishes, using her 'hand guidance' if necessary. Stimulate her outer vagina and clitoris very gently at first, and then increase the speed of stimulation. Take a rest for a few minutes, then do the same again. This is called a 'teasing technique'. If she wants, she can then have a 'manual clitoral climax', but this is not part of the plan at this point. Introduce variations (for instance stimulating other parts of the body) if you both want to.

(5) The equivalent 'male comfortable' or 'training' position is shown here, in which the woman leans back on the pillows or other support. He can show her how to rub his penis (in particular his frenulum), testicles or thighs, to help the development of an erection: the erection can then be lost, by stopping the activity, and regained (another 'teasing technique'). The exercise can be repeated several times and the vigour and speed of the stimulation can be varied. If he gets very excited he can be given a 'manual climax', but remember that after an ejaculation it is very difficult to obtain another erection for some hours. The important thing is for him to enjoy being touched.

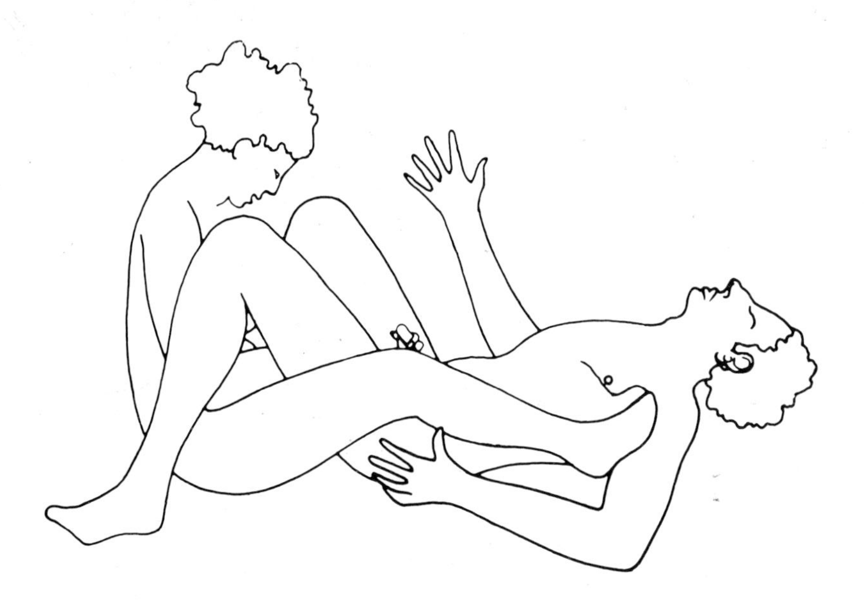

(6) Your therapist might suggest other things for you to do when you are being stimulated and these instructions might include relaxing deeply or concentrating on some fantasies. If erections or orgasms do not occur imediately do not worry; there is always another day. These will come eventually as you relax and enjoy your sessions together.

Oral sex

(1) Try the above positions several times and then you could attempt some oral lovemaking.
(i) *Male*: you can use your tongue to kiss and lick your partner's clitoral shaft and glans. Be gentle and see how she responds before increasing tongue pressure and speed.
(ii) *Female*: you can lick and kiss your partner's penile shaft and tip of his penis, gently taking it into your mouth and sucking.

(2) One of the best ways of obtaining mutual satisfaction is to try a position called *soixante-neuf* or 'position 69,' which is illustrated below. Try lying down together so that your heads are placed by your partner's genitals and you can both suck and kiss each other simultaneously in this position. Many couples try this position with one partner lying above the other. Some couples prefer to try this in a 'sideways position'. Try both methods and choose which you prefer. Try to relax and enjoy the sensations when you are exploring each other. If one of you feels shy initially you do not have to try this simultaneously; only one partner needs to stimulate the other – it is up to you what you do. If you happen to have a climax at this stage you are allowed to, but this is not part of the plan at this point.

These oral techniques can excite both partners – enjoy yourselves.

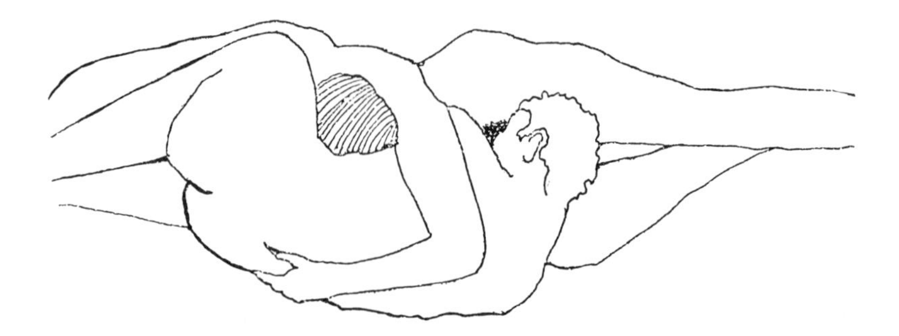

THE WOMAN ABOVE POSITION

(1) This position is an important one in almost all kinds of sexual problems. It gets away from the anxiety associated with intercourse in the traditional, or man above position. It allows the man with a problem of potency or ejaculatory control to relax and achieve a degree of penetration without having to manoeuvre into position. For the woman with difficulty in allowing penetration or achieving orgasm, it gives the opportunity to move towards these goals at her own pace. The purpose of this exercise is not, however, erection, orgasm or penetration: try to enjoy the sensation of genital contact for its own sake, even without erection or penetration, and relax.

(2) Follow the instructions for genital sensate focussing. Then practise getting into the position illustrated here but do not attempt insertion.

(3) (a) *Male*: You lie on your back. Just relax and enjoy your partner's attentions and do not try to have an erection.

(b) *Female*: You kneel astride and face to face with your partner. Move around until you feel comfortable, but do not attempt insertion. Tease and stroke your partner's genitals. Take your time – there is no time limit. When you are both excited rub his penis against your clitoris and vagina. When you feel pleasure tell him. As he becomes more excited guide his penis into your vagina (remember it is not necessary for his penis to be fully erect at this stage).

Keep still, pause and relax and enjoy the feeling of contact between penis and vagina. As you become more familiar with this position move around gently backwards and forwards on the penis for a few minutes. Try to think of the penis as yours to play with, feel, explore and enjoy. Remember that you need not be afraid of too deep penetration as this can be controlled by you. When you sit upright it is at its deepest and when you lean right forward it is at its shallowest. You can easily reduce penetration by leaning forward. If you like clitoral stimulation this is an especially good position, as the base of the penis often rubs against your clitoris in this particular position – so you can enjoy clitoral and vaginal sensations. Ask your partner to move more when you both feel ready for this. If you would like some more manual stimulation of the clitoris ask him to touch you there, or do this yourself whilst his penis is inside you.

(4) Repeat this several times and alternate this position with lying side

by side, letting feelings subside. Then tease each other and try the position again. Remember that mutual enjoyment is most important in this exercise.

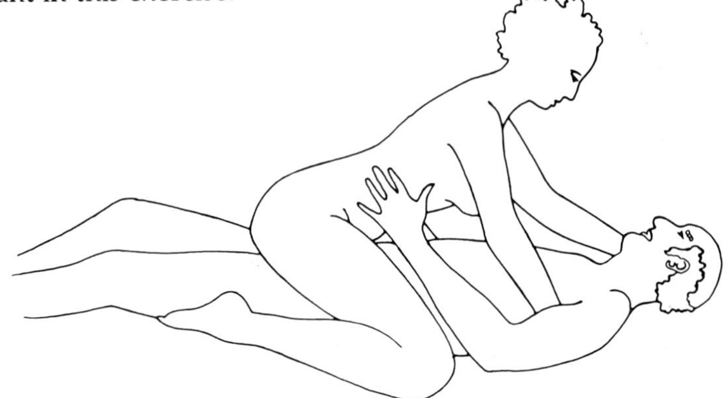

THE FEEL FREE POSITION

Many women can achieve an orgasm by manually stimulating the clitoris, either themselves or with the help of their partner. However, it is often difficult for them to progress from this to full intercourse, with a climax produced by the movement of the penis. There are two possible ways to achieve this, both of which involve a gradual progression from manual to penile stimulation.

It is a good idea to start these exercises by relaxation and massage, before proceeding to clitoral stimulation.

(1) Start with manual stimulation, in the 'feel free' position (see below). Just before the climax is reached, insert the penis and continue stimulating until the climax. Next, the insertion is timed to take place a little earlier and the manual stimulation is stopped a little earlier, the orgasm being achieved by movement of the penis. By stopping the manual stimulation earlier and earlier, the woman can eventually allow orgasm to occur with penile movement alone.

(2) Alternatively, the penis is inserted early on, with the partners in the 'feel free' position. The clitoris is stimulated manually by either the woman or the man. In the earlier session, this stimulation continues to orgasm. Next, the stimulation stops short a little earlier, and orgasm is allowed to occur by penile thrusting. Manual stimulation is gradually faded out, until orgasm can be achieved with penile movement alone. Different positions can then be used, with or without manual stimulation first.

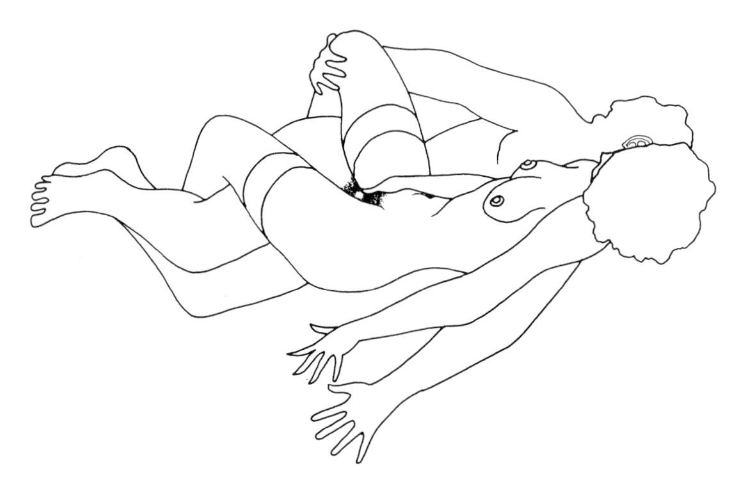

REAR ENTRY POSITIONS

Lateral rear entry

This position is easy to get into and offers freedom of movement. The woman lies on her side, facing away from her partner. The man lies on his side facing her from behind with one of his legs in between hers.

She can guide his penis into her vagina whilst she bends her knees.

Penetration is good and there is a certain amount of clitoral stimulation. If this is inadequate either partner can manually stimulate the clitoris.

It is possible to go to sleep in this position with the genitals in contact after orgasm.

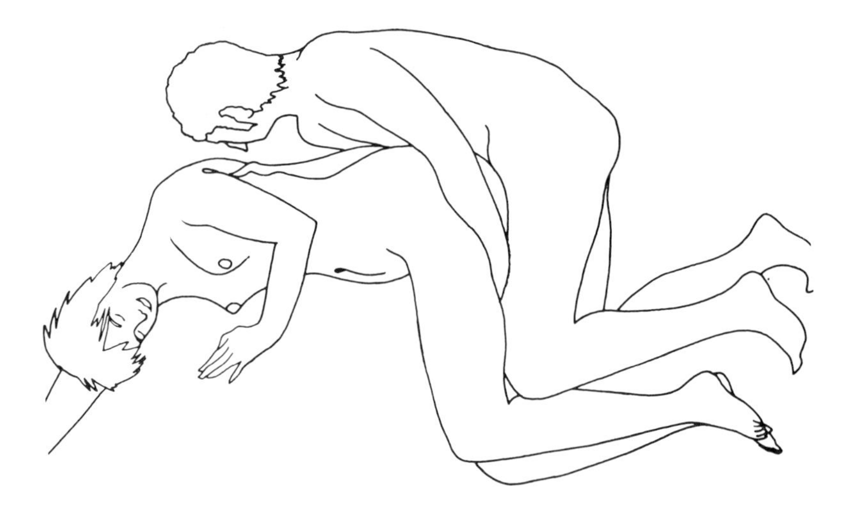

Upright rear entry

This is a very natural and normal position which many couples enjoy, but some do not know about. Both the man and the woman kneel.

The depth of penetration can be controlled by the man, taking care to see how deep his thrusts are in his partner's vagina.

If clitoral stimulation provided by the penis is not very satisfactory this can be helped by the man kneeling upright and the woman kneeling with her head resting on the pillows, or by manual stimulation of the clitoris applied by either the man or the woman.

In general this is a good position and the man can easily stroke the woman's breasts and thighs.

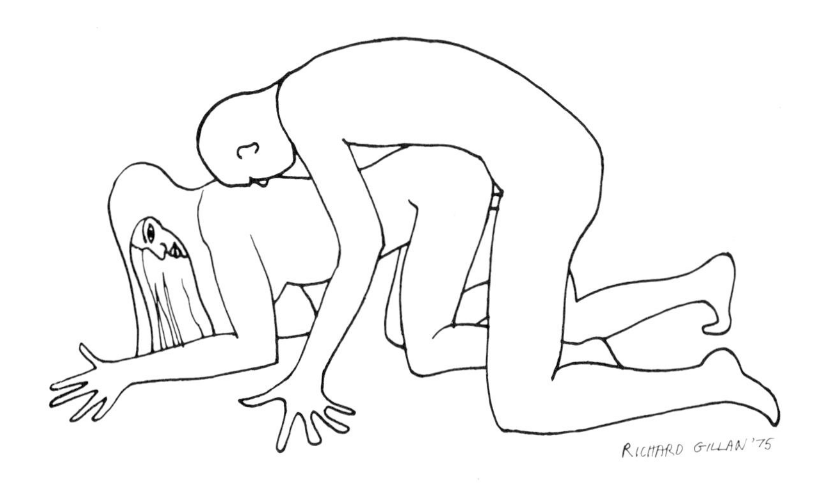

THE MAN ABOVE POSITION

This is usually the final position your therapist will recommend, due to bad associations and failure you might have experienced with it in the past. You are now ready to try it with confidence. The advantages with this position are that it is intimate. You may kiss, bite or nibble one another and talk intimately. The disadvantages are connected with the man who has a weight problem and is too heavy for the woman, or for the woman who prefers manual stimulation to take place simultaneously with penile thrusting.

Many couples make love in this position with their legs straight, maybe aided by a couple of pillows being placed under the woman's buttocks. Some women prefer to bend their knees and keep their feet on the bed.

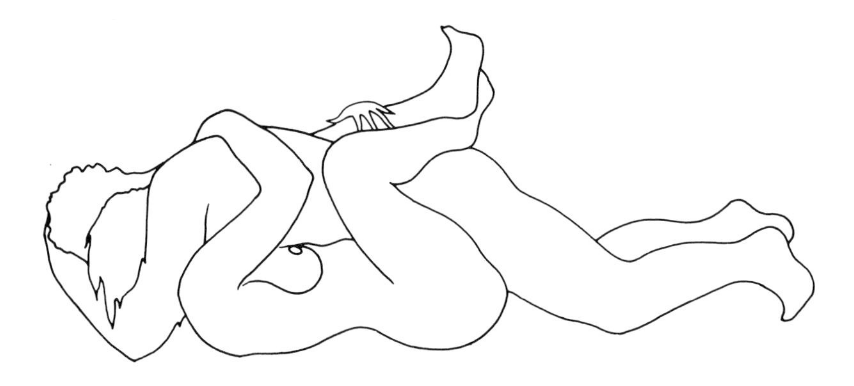

(1) The woman's knees drawn up

Here penetration is deep and clitoral stimulation is good, provided by the pushing and rubbing of the penis against the clitoris.

This position is said to be the best for securing pregnancy.

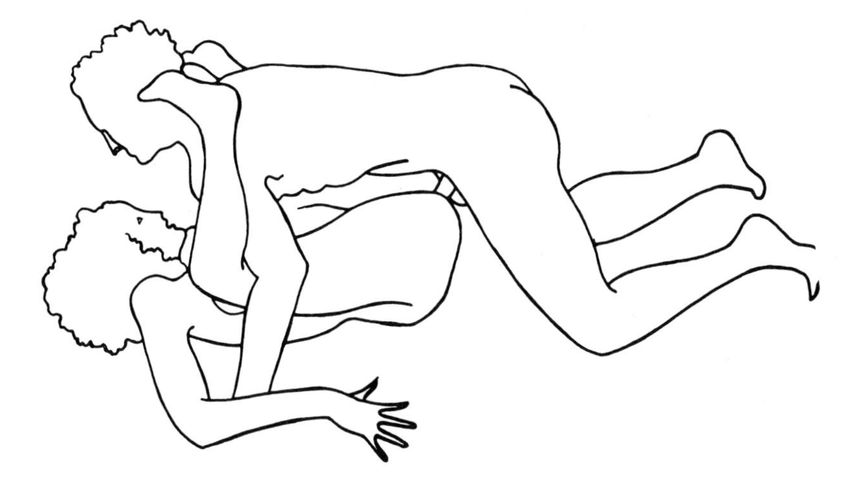

(2) The woman's knees drawn right up with her feet in the air or crossed over the man's back

This position is somewhat more acrobatic but has the advantage of the deepest penetration.

ORGASMIC DYSFUNCTION

(1) This is easy to cure, provided that you forget the way in which society has conditioned you to be the 'passive partner' who does not seek to obtain her own pleasure during lovemaking. Try to ignore cultural brainwashing like – 'only do what is proper for a girl' or 'women do not initiate sex and get pleasure'.

(2) To start off, we suggest you read *The Sensuous Woman* by J. We would also like you to experiment, on your own, with some masturbation techniques. You will have seen pictures and a model of the clitoris, so when you are alone look at your own clitoris. You can feel it, then look at it, by using a hand mirror. Explore yourself by touching the shaft of your clitoris and then gently rub and later apply more pressure to your clitoral glans. Try and relax when you do this and try to 'let yourself go'. Then, during the treatment you can go ahead and express your need for full sexual experience with your partner, during lovemaking.

(3) Try the massage exercises with your partner. This will help you to discover, maybe for the first time, what is sexually arousing for you. Enjoy this technique several times.

(4) The next step is 'genital sensate focussing'. During this session try to encourage and show your partner what you want him to do. He will have been instructed not to make a direct 'attack' on your clitoral glans and not to insert his fingers deep into your vagina, so you can enjoy the way he touches and stimulates you. We recommend 'the comfortable position for female stimulation' for this technique to be tried out. Later you don't have to stick to this position, but try it out and see how you like it. Both of you should enjoy the 'teasing technique' when he plays with your clitoris and you can feel it swelling, and then he stops and you lose the feelings of pleasure, which return when he touches you again. Remember to show your partner exactly what you want, rather than just letting him do what he thinks you want. Tell him, if you enjoy it, to stroke the insides of your thighs and the lips of your vagina. This latter movement can help lubricate the stroking of the clitoris, as it's not as pleasurable when it is dry. The purpose of all this is for you to enjoy the feelings you get. If you happen to have a climax when your partner is stimulating you, that's a 'bonus', but it's not an essential part of the session. Remember that you must not attempt to break our rules of 'no internal sex', and start to ask for insertion at this stage. Please remember to stick to the rules as it's much better to wait and build up confidence before insertion.

(5) Try the above position on several occasions and on each occasion you can enjoy some clitoral stimulation and maybe follow this with touching your partner's penis and teasing him, enjoying seeing him erect. Then you could try some oral sex. We will instruct you both how to do this. Before you start a session you could look at some of the books and magazines we have recommended. We might also ask you to see the occasional film and you can practise your tasks when you return home. You are allowed to have an orgasm manually or orally, but only if it comes naturally. You are not obliged to experience this.

(6) Try the woman above position. You kneel or sit astride your partner and mount him in this kneeling position, with your knees placed approximately in line with his nipples and parallel to his trunk. Your partner lies flat on his back and you can use the 'teasing technique' to help him become erect. You can then guide his penis into you and insert it at your own pace, according to how well lubricated and excited you feel. Then keep still and explore and enjoy your vaginal sensations. As you feel pleasure increasing, move slowly backwards and forwards on the penis for a few minutes. Think of the penis as yours to play with, to feel and to enjoy. After you have repeated this several days and are enjoying the sensations, you can then ask your partner to try some pelvic thrusting in a non-demanding manner, at your preferred pace. If you happen to get a climax at this stage, enjoy it, and on a later occasion repeat the above instructions during your next session. Maybe you both prefer external ejaculatory relief at this stage, rather than an internal orgasm – if so you can masturbate each other to a climax or try having a climax orally (that is position '69' which we have explained to you).

Perhaps you do not want to experiment with an orgasm yourself at this stage, but bear in mind that it's often frustrating for your partner to control himself and hold back from thrusting and climaxing internally, when you feel you are not yet up to it. If this is the case, help him to come manually. Even if you do not feel like having your clitoris stimulated you can stimulate him and manipulate him to ejaculation. Otherwise he is having to cope with too much tension. On later occasions your partner will be instructed to help you use a 'teasing technique' during insertion – that is, both of you enjoy insertion and slow thrusting, then separate from each other and have a cuddle, then reinsert.

(7) Convert the female superior position to the feel free position.

(8) Experiment with and enjoy some of the other positions your therapists recommend.

(9) Don't forget that the whole procedure is intended to be enjoyable – treat it more as a fun session than an exercise.

VAGINISMUS

(1) This is the easiest of the 'female sexual disorders' to cure. We shall first explain this problem in detail, by showing you diagrams and then physically demonstrating the condition to you and your partner. We will examine you and then ask your partner to put on a rubber glove and feel the spasm for himself. We will then show you some dilators, in graduated sizes, and explain to you how we want you to use them at home.
(2) On a suitable occasion at home, in the bedroom, try relaxing and then ask your partner to insert the smallest dilator into you, guiding him by the hand. Then as you feel more confident and the spasm lessens you can ask him to insert the next smallest dilator and guide his hand again. You can try the next size dilator in this manner and after you have the largest size dilator inserted keep it inside you for several hours (just before you go to sleep), lying comfortably and relaxed on the bed. We suggest that you keep the largest dilator inserted for two hours on two separate nights.
(3) We recommend instructions for 'orgasmic dysfunction' next. You can try playing with your clitoris and experimenting with yourself when you are alone. Then you can try out some massage with your partner. The next step is to repeat the dilation procedure and then progress to the instructions for genital sensate focussing, enjoying stimulation and maybe trying out some oral sex.
(4) Continue with the instructions for the woman above position but use your dilators (your partner can insert the two largest ones – inserting the smaller one first, then removing it and inserting the largest one, then removing it), and then you can insert his penis into you, at your own pace.
(5) Go on to the lateral position and repeat the dilation before inserting your partner's penis.
(6) Try the other positions – you don't have to continue the dilation procedure unless it makes you feel more confident – otherwise, forget about it and enjoy your partner's penis inside you and experiment with any position we recommend.

IMPOTENCE

(1) This is a fairly easy problem to cure and we can assure you that this condition can be easily reversed.
(2) Carry out the recommendations for massage and then continue with genital sensate focussing up to number (3). Then both of you can get into the 'comfortable position for female stimulation' and follow number (4) instructions, remembering to stimulate your partner's clitoris very gently initially – you will probably find this quite exciting and enjoyable yourself, seeing how your partner's clitoris swells slightly and providing her with pleasure. It is not essential that she reaches a climax at this stage. Then you could both look at some of the books we have recommended and go on to the next stage.
(3) Get into the position we recommend in number (5), the male comfortable training position. Male: relax as much as you can and enjoy your partner stroking your penis – you are not required to have an erection at this stage – the important thing is that you can enjoy being stroked and fondled. Then your partner will stop touching your penis and you will lose the exciting sensations you were experiencing but they will return when your partner stimulates you again. This teasing technique will be repeated several times. If you do get quite hard and erect when your partner teases you and you want to go on to orgasm, you are encouraged to try this at this stage, either being rubbed by her or stimulating yourself. Sometimes people get quite a stiff erection at this stage and are very excited and attempt to break our rules of 'no internal sex'. Please remember to stick to the rules at this stage. It is much better to wait and build up confidence before inserting.
(4) Repeat the above on several occasions. We might recommend the occasional film for you both to go along and see, recommending that you do your exercises and tasks when you return home.
(5) Try the oral lovemaking tasks described on the separate sheet. Then look at your pictures again. You are allowed to have an orgasm orally or manually if you want to.
(6) Try the woman above position, and then continue with the recommended positions your therapist has suggested. If you lose your erection during a session it does not matter; you can always have a rest, maybe look at the 'fun books', and have a cuddle and stimulate each other again, or maybe try again another day. The important thing is to give yourself an opportunity to feel pleasure and relax sufficiently to enjoy feelings. There should never be any

concern for ejaculation. The idea of the sessions is to learn to enjoy feelings of sexiness and to give your partner pleasure, either manually, orally or internally. You can both have fun once again, and your programme is arranged so that you gradually get back your confidence to try new things.

EJACULATORY CONTROL

A premature ejaculator is a man who wants to last longer but can't for a number of reasons. It is a relatively easy problem to treat if the instructions are carefully followed.

Your therapist will have asked you to practise some relaxation exercises and these will teach you how to reduce tension in your body and mind. If you have a partner you will also have been asked to try some sensate focussing or massaging together. You will have found favourite areas you enjoy being massaged.

Stage 1

The first stage of ejaculatory control is finding some time on you own and stimulating your penis with a *dry hand* (without any body lotion) for 15 minutes without ejaculating. If you feel you are getting over-excited or are near to ejaculation, stop and relax for a few minutes and then continue touching your penis. If you like, after 15 minutes of avoiding ejaculation, let yourself go and enjoy 'coming'. If you have 'come' before the target of 15 minutes, try the task again. Many men with this problem can get another erection quite quickly after ejaculating. If not, there is always another day to practise. Do this on three occasions.

Stage 2

After succeeding three times with the above method, lasting 15 minutes on each occasion, use the same technique again, but this time with a *wet hand* (use a cream like KY jelly or body oil). Again 15 minutes on three occasions is your goal.

Stage 3

You will now have built up confidence over controlling your ejaculation. The next stage is to try stage 1 with your partner. Let her stimulate your penis with a *dry hand*. This obviously is more difficult for you to control, but you can succeed by telling her to stop if you feel too excited – relax for a minute or two before continuing. Try and do this for 15 minutes on three occasions.

Stage 4

Again your partner is involved in a repeat of stage 2, with her stimulating your penis with a *wet hand* (KY jelly or body oil). Again, aim for 15 minutes before ejaculatin on three occasions.

Stage 5

If your therapist recommends *oral* sex, let your partner stimulate your penis in this way. Again your goal is to last 15 minutes without ejaculating.

Stage 6

Try the *woman above position* when you are not too erect – even if your penis is fairly flaccid you can try 'stuffing'. Let your partner kneel over you and stuff your limp penis into her vagina: both of you should remain still for 5 minutes. Then she can move gently and you will probably get an erection, but you yourself should remain still for a further 10 minutes while your partner moves. If you feel any urge to ejaculate, ask your partner to stop for a few minutes while you relax. Next try doing this with a stiffer penis.

Stage 7

The next stage is to last for 15 minutes on two occasions when your partner is in the woman above position and you are moving your erect penis inside her.

Stage 8

The above stage can be repeated in different positions. We recommend the *rear* position and last of all the *man above position*.

Remember if you fail at any stage go back a step and practise some of the earlier stages. Even if you do not have a partner for therapy you can get confident with stages 1 and 2 and if you meet a suitable temporary partner you could try stage 3 by asking her to touch you and even do some massage together.

PREMATURE EJACULATION AND THE 'SQUEEZE TECHNIQUE'

(1) Premature ejaculation is one of the easiest of the 'sexual problems' to cure and we can assure you that this condition can be reversed quite easily.

(2) Carry out the instructions recommended for massage and then continue with the instructions for genital sensate focussing up to number 4. (Remember to stimulate the clitoris gently, perhaps through a fold of skin.) Then get into the 'training position':

(a) Male: Relax and enjoy your partner touching and playing with the penis.
(b) Female: Stimulate the penis manually until it becomes erect, and then use the *squeeze technique*. Hold the penis firmly between

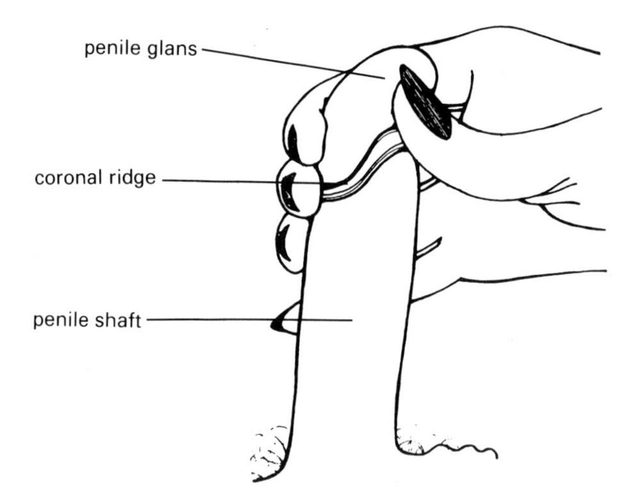

your thumb and two fingers – some women find they cannot exert enough pressure with one hand, and have to use both hands (thumb on top of thumb and fingers on top of fingers). The thumb should be placed on the frenulum, and the two fingers either side of the ridge where the glans meets the shaft of the penis, opposite to the thumb. Squeeze really hard for a few seconds – do not be afraid that this will cause pain. The squeezing will make him lose the urge to ejaculate, and lose part of his erection. Then, after 15 – 30 seconds, you can stimulate the penis again, and once again apply the squeeze technique. You can repeat this procedure several times, and enjoy 15 – 20 minutes of sex play without ejaculation. This can be an extraordinarily reassuring experience for a couple whose sex life has been marred by premature ejaculation.

(3) You can vary the squeeze techniques by stimulating the penis orally, using fingers and thumb to squeeze as before.

(4) Next session try getting into the woman above position.

(a) Female: kneel or sit astride your partner and mount him in this kneeling position, with your knees placed approximately in line with his nipples and parallel to his trunk.
(b) Male: lie flat on your back and allow your partner to come down on you and insert your penis inside her; she will do this for you, so you don't have to fumble about looking for her vagina.

Neither of you should move after penetration. You should let her know in good time when you think you are going to have an orgasm and then she can raise herself, slowly and gently, and apply the 'squeeze technique' and then remount. This can be repeated several times. This stage is often quite tricky, as ejaculation can occur when the female partner raises herself. The secret is practice and good communication.

(5) (a) Male: You are now learning to control your sexual excitement when you are inside your partner and the next step is that you are allowed to thrust a little to maintain your erection. If you feel you might lose control at any time you can ask your partner to squeeze you.
(b) Female: Be ready at this stage, when your partner is gently thrusting, to pull out gently and squeeze hard. Then try making some slow pelvic thrusts yourself, still being alert for signs of his becoming over-aroused; if he does, apply the squeeze technique.

(6) The next recommended practice position is the 'feel free' position. Initially enjoy some foreplay, then:
(a) Female: use the 'squeeze' two or three times before trying the 'feel free' position. Try not to thrust too much when penetration does take place.
(b) Male: Do not thrust too much either.

(7) Practice the squeeze technique each time you have intercourse, at least two or three times before penetration. You can go on to try the 'rear' position, followed by the 'missionary position'. When you

have finished your treatment, continue to employ the squeeze technique at least once a week for the six months which follow treatment. During the time of menstruation, advantage could be taken to have a session of 15 – 20 minutes devoted specifically to manual stimulation of the male with the squeeze technique applied several times.

Appendix 3

Women's Sex Therapy Group Homework

Step 1: Your body (Week 1)

Your body exercise involves taking a warm bath and relaxing as much as you can and enjoy soaping the different areas of your body. Close your eyes and concentrate on touching your arms and hands – how do they feel? Try varying the speed and type of pressure. Then look at your hands and arms, soap your feet and legs, try to be aware of your skin and the feel of your hands on your legs. Does it feel nice? Next, kneel and feel your thighs and buttocks – do they feel soft, strong, flabby? Stand up in the bath and look down at your body, do you like or dislike what you see? Try to appreciate the look of your skin and then using some soap or body lotion run your hands down your body feeling your breasts, tummy, thighs – then pretend you are someone else feeling your body. How do you think someone else would feel about the areas you like or dislike? Maybe it feels nice to touch your breasts – this is perfectly normal. Experiment a bit further to see how you feel when you increase your pressure and maybe stroke or tug your nipples.

The idea of exploring your body is to discover which areas are responsive to touch. It's a good idea to find out what sort of touch you like – some of you might like a very gentle stroking, others prefer a much firmer touch. Some of you might like a slow and gentle massage but others might like a faster, more superficial stroking. Try to experiment several times with this type of bath until you feel confident over and enjoy touching your body.

Looking

If you can look at your genitals and learn about each area and feel comfortable you will have taken a most important step.

One way of looking at your genitals is to lie down on the bed. Do make sure you will not be disturbed; it might be a good idea to lock the bedroom door. Spread you legs apart with your feet resting on the bed and your knees up and hold a mirror at an angle to observe your genitals. You probably are very familiar with the pubic hair which covers the mons, or soft mound at the front of your body. But the parts illustrated by the diagram below will probably not be so familiar.

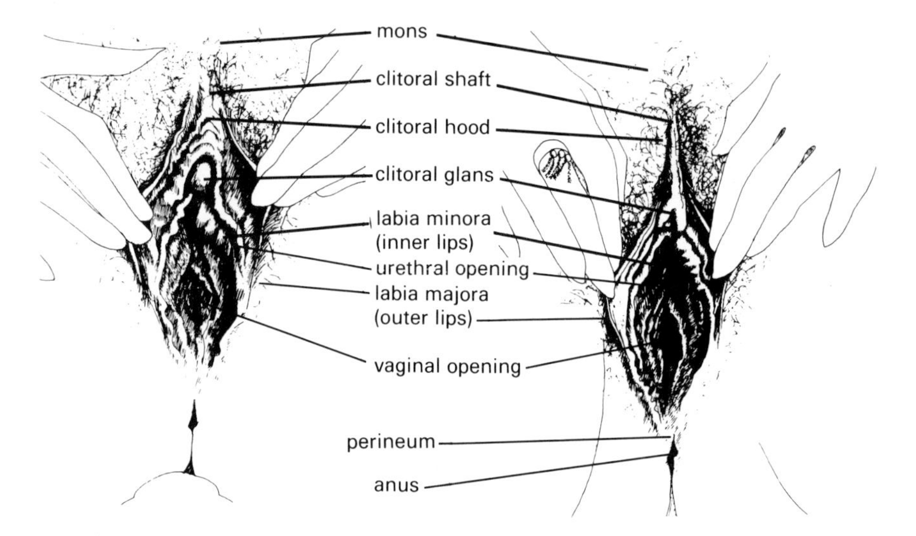

Initially explore the labia minor or inner lips by placing a finger on each lip in turn. Then pull both lips apart with your hand and look at the shaft of your clitoris. It is rather like a tube and runs in an up and down sort of direction. The next part to observe is the clitoral hood lying between the shaft and the labia minora, and this can be moved upwards to reveal the clitoral glans. The picture on the right shows a woman looking at her glans after she has moved the hood. The clitoral glans is similar to the male's penile glans; the function of both male and female glans is to experience sensation. The colour varies from pale plum to a rich burgundy.

Below the clitoris is your vaginal opening. The urethra or urinary opening is also in this area between the labia minora. It's hard to see the urethra as it is very small. The perineum is the area between the vaginal opening and the anus.

Try repeating the above instructions on three days. If you feel at all anxious at any stage just stop and relax and then return to the exercise. Some women have said how embarrassed they felt doing such a thing initially, but later their new confidence was enjoyed and this first stage in the 'self-help' programme is considered to be particularly useful.

Homework checklist: Week 1

Name: ______________________________

Dates: ____________through____________

Please keep a daily record of how many times you engaged in the following behaviours. Indicate the number of times you engaged in any of the activities by putting the number under the day to the right. Mark '0' if you did not engage in the activity.

	Day						
	1	2	3	4	5	6	7
Number of times: (1) I took a warm bath							
(2) I felt my breasts in the tub							
(3) I felt my genitals in the tub							
(4) I felt the rest of my body (legs, arms face, etc.) in the tub							
(5) I explored my mouth with my tongue							
(6) I patted myself dry							
Using the diagram and mirror, I located my: (7) inner lips							
(8) outer lips							
(9) clitoris							
(10) clitoral hood							
(11) urethra							
(12) vaginal opening							
(13) mons							

(14) Did you spend at least one hour on your homework?							
(15) Approximately how much time did you spend on your homework today?							
(16) How was your mood today? 1 2 3 4 5 6 7 Not very happy → happy → perfectly happy							
(17) Did you experience an orgasm today?							
(18) If yes, how many?							
(19) I engaged in a sexual or sensual activity not listed. Describe:							

____

____

____

Step 2: Touching your genitals (Week 2)

Often people talk about the guilt they feel when enjoying self-stimulation. This is very sad, as it spoils maximum pleasure. If you are afraid that you might be disturbed whilst attempting this step this could lead to guilt feelings and worry that can only be overcome by locking the door. Do try and choose a room in which no one, including children, will disturb you. First, privacy is essential for this step and secondly, time is important – give yourself a good hour for the exercises. Enjoy your room and maybe burn some incense or pour some of your favourite perfume on your pillow.

Vary the time of day or evening you try the touching sessions. Initially it's a good idea to take a bath and enjoy using a body lotion afterwards and massage your body and enjoy the sensations, experimenting with touching yourself in different ways, varying the pressure on your breasts and arms and then stroking your outer then your inner thighs. Try using some sort of cream or body lotion. Johnson's Baby Lotion or Oil is a safe ingredient and a non-irritant for most people. It's a good idea to use some sort of lotion to lubricate the genitals and reduce friction. If you have not got any oil, don't worry, try some saliva or put your finger in your vagina and try some vaginal secretions. Never use vaginal deodorants or any substance that contains alcohol in your genital area as these will cause irritation.

By now you will know where to find your inner lips. Stroke these lightly and then increase the pressure. Most women prefer to use the index or middle finger or both for this type of touching. Using your favourite body lotion, try massaging your clitoral shaft and hood, moving your fingers up and down, maybe holding the hood back with your left hand and touching the clitoral glans. Alternatively, you might prefer to rub this area using a circular movement with the pads of your fingers. You will soon discover the method you prefer. There is no set way to touch your genitals nor is there a 'set position' in which to enjoy it. Many women choose to lie down with their feet on the bed and their knees in the air or spread out. Other women like to kneel down or lie on their stomach, whilst others prefer to stand up or sit on a chair. It's up to you to choose the most comfortable position you prefer.

It's a good idea to be experimental and vary pressure on the clitoris, alternating a light touch with a firmer touch and maybe applying even more pressure. Similarly, at this stage you can rub slowly or more quickly. Try stopping all movement and see what that feels like and see what it's like when you touch again.

Try also touching your perineum (the area between the anus and your genitals). This is a much neglected area and many women enjoy touching here.

You will probably have noticed that if you started thinking about how you looked or whether you felt awkward or self-conscious, you ceased to want to touch yourself. This is the biggest 'turn-off' as it is almost impossible to feel sexually confident if you are embarrassed. If you feel anxious or awkward, stop touching and try having some relaxation and then return to touching.

The goal of the above exercise is to become confident and relaxed over touching your clitoris. Try doing the above exercises several times during the week until you feel comfortable and confident. Perhaps next time you might prefer to spend 15 minutes or maybe more time, it's up to you.

Homework checklist: Week 2

Name: ______________________________

Dates: ____________through____________

Please keep a daily record of how many times you engaged in the following behaviours. Indicate the number of times you engaged in any of the activities by putting the number under the day to the right. Mark '0' if you did not engage in the activity.

	Day						
	1	2	3	4	5	6	7
Number of times: (1) I took a warm bath							
(2) I felt my breasts in the tub							
(3) I felt my genitals in the tub							
(4) I felt the rest of my body (legs, arms face, etc.) in the tub							
(5) I explored my mouth with my tongue							
(6) I patted myself dry							
Using the diagram and mirror, I located my: (7) inner lips							
(8) outer lips							
(9) clitoris							
(10) clitoral hood							
(11) urethra							
(12) vaginal opening							
(13) mons							

(14) Did you spend at least one hour on your homework?							
(15) Approximately how much time did you spend on your homework today?							
(16) How was your mood today? 1 2 3 4 5 6 7 Not very happy → happy → perfectly happy							
(17) Did you experience an orgasm today?							
(18) If yes, how many?							
(19) I engaged in a sexual or sensual activity not listed. Describe:							

____

____

____

Step 3: Self-focussing (Week 3)

You will now have become familiar with touching and will have developed a preference for certain genital areas.

By this time it probably is not necessary to take a bath first and you will feel more relaxed about touching yourself all over. If you feel tense or 'not in the mood' for the exercises, have the warm bath and then relax before the next step, which might last for 30 minutes to an hour.

Concentrate on touching areas of your body you enjoy most. What do you feel today? Sometimes people say they feel the exercises are rather clinical or mechanical as they have been told to do these and there is little pleasure gained. New ways of discovering pleasure take time, especially if you have previously associated touching with guilt.

First of all focus on your mood. How do you feel? Try sitting down with your eyes open and focus on one particular spot in the room. Observe this carefully, then close your eyes and concentrate on a particular sound in the room or your own breathing if it's quiet in the room. Then concentrate on a white rose against the black background. After this, become aware of each area of your body, starting with your hands and arms, legs and feet, upper body, lower body, your genitals. Try to feel warmth into the centre of your body, trying to feel warmth in your genitals.

You probably feel good now. Using some body lotion, slowly touch your genitals a little and then focus on the area around the clitoris. Experiment with touching the shaft, which is usually not very sensitive, and continue the movement of your fingers to the glans.

Try various rhythms and varieties of touching. Try using your entire hand in a circular motion. When you have tried this, roll your clitoris between your fingers. It is said that women do not like the direct stimulation of the glans but this has not been the case in laboratory tests so see what you prefer and try some direct glans touching after you have pulled up the hood. If you find this is over-sensitive, stimulate the glans with the foreskin above. Try to develop a regular rhythm. Concentrate solely on the sensations you enjoy and you will probably feel warmth and tingling; carry on touching. Try squeezing your PC muscle at this stage whilst you are rubbing your clitoris. Then continue touching your clitoris. You might have a sort of fluttering feeling or a series of vaginal contractions; if so, continue touching your clitoris until these flutterings have stopped. This might be an orgasm, which is a bonus at this stage. The idea of the exercise is to focus on the exciting feelings and let them build up without trying to stop them. Try doing this exercise daily for about half an hour until you feel really good and can enjoy sensations without tension or guilt.

If you do not feel this build-up of contractions, do not worry - sometimes it takes time to achieve this. Instead, carry on improving you PC muscle movement whilst you are touching your clitoris.

PC fluttering

This week contract your PC muscle but release it quickly. This is called *twitching* or *fluttering*. Try to rapidly contract and release your PC muscle six times a day, increasing the number of contractions from 10–20. Practise this daily.

Homework checklist: Week 3

Name: ______________________________

Dates: ____________through____________

Please keep a daily record of how many times you engaged in the following behaviours. Indicate the number of times you engaged in any of the activities by putting the number under the day to the right. Mark '0' if you did not engage in the activity.

	Day 1	2	3	4	5	6	7
Number of times: (1) I took a warm bath							
(2) I felt my breasts in the tub							
(3) I felt my genitals in the tub							
(4) I felt the rest of my body (legs, arms face, etc.) in the tub							
(5) I explored my mouth with my tongue							
(6) I patted myself dry							
I began masturbating and: (7) used one finger to rub clitoris							
(8) used entire hand in circular motion							
(9) rolled clitoris between two fingers							
(10) squeezed PC muscle while rubbing clitoris							
(11) 'flutter' PC, 10 times, 3 times a day							
(12) 10 3-second PC squeezes, 3 times a day							
(13) created a sensuous environment							

(14) Did you spend at least one hour on your homework?							
(15) Approximately how much time did you spend on your homework today?							
(16) How was your mood today? 1 2 3 4 5 6 7 Not very happy → happy → perfectly happy							
(17) Did you experience an orgasm today?							
(18) If yes, how many?							
(19) I engaged in a sexual or sensual activity not listed. Describe:							

___

___

___

Step 4: Enjoying your fantasies (Week 4)

Many people think that women do not have sexual fantacies. This maybe is due to the Kinsey Report which revealed that women do not respond as much as men to erotic visual material and prefer romantic stories. This is a fallacy and nowadays research has been undertaken to explore both male and female sexual responses under properly controlled laboratory conditions.

Julia Heiman is the pioneer of the measurement of female sexual responses to arousing stories. When men's erections were measured by a penile cuff which is sensitive to stretching, she found that the best responses were produced by stories in which women initiated sex play.

She measured female responses by inserting a probe into the vagina which detects the increased blood flow and engorgement of the vaginal walls. By doing this she reported that women also responded most to the stories in which women initiated sex. However, many women when asked to rate their arousal underestimated the degree of their sexual response. This shows how important it is to provide some 'feedback' as to how a woman is actually responding rather than relying, as Kinsey did, on self-report.

What is a fantasy? A fantasy is an imaginary situation, scene or sequence. It could be defined as a 'day dream' as a dream is a form of fantasy. We can control our fantasies when we day dream and conjure up images at will. Fantasies can vary and some fantasies can lead to sexual feeling. The more one practises fantasies the better they become. People's capacity to fantasise varies tremendously and this ability is useful if a person wants to get turned on sexually.

Many people feel bored with sex and need some additional stimulation. Fantasies can provide extra pleasure. If you feel embarrassed by your fantasies, try to relax. Fantasies are private and need only be shared if you want them to be. Inventing sexual stories for a loved partner can be pleasant and arousing for both partners.

Some people say that their fantasies worry them and what would happen if they lost control and acted out such ideas? This rarely happens so you can feel reassured by this fact. If you feel guilty and that it is wrong for you to fantasise you are bearing the burden that society has imposed on us – 'it's wrong to enjoy ourselves'. Many women are taught as children to repress any sexual feeling and fantasies and consequently find it very difficult to fantasise.

Fantasies are often enjoyed during masturbation. Several sex therapists, including Helen Kaplan, have stated that erotic fantasies are an invaluable tool for overcoming inhibition over orgasm. She mentioned that if people feel guilty about masturbation it is up to the therapist to encourage and reassure them so they can be free to enjoy their fantasies.

How do people go about learning how to fantasise if they have spent years repressing such thoughts? One way is to read about other people's fantasies. Recently two excellent anthologies of women's fantasies have been edited by Nancy Friday. They are in two books: *My Secret Garden* and *Forbidden Flowers*. Many women who have read these books have been surprised that these are women's fantasies. It's a good idea to dip into these books and not to read them from cover to cover but to read one or two stories and then savour them.

We have recommended some books and films for you to enjoy and to help you with your fantasies. Also we have included a fantasy checklist to give you an idea of the range of fantasies available. Choose a fantasy and imagine you yourself are involved in it. Concentrate on this or another fantasy every day for a week until you feel excited just thinking of it.

You could buy a magazine like *Forum* to give you other ideas about the range of fantasies available. Remember, it is not perverted or repulsive to have fantasies, it is normal. Some of the fantasies you might read about might disgust, excite, amuse or arouse you.

Homework checklist: Week 4

Name: ______________________________

Dates: ____________through____________

Please keep a daily record of how many times you engaged in the following behaviours. Indicate the number of times you engaged in any of the activities by putting the number under the day to the right. Mark '0' if you did not engage in the activity.

	Day						
	1	2	3	4	5	6	7
Number of times: (1) I took a warm bath							
(2) I felt my breasts in the tub							
(3) I felt my genitals in the tub							
(4) I felt the rest of my body (legs, arms face, etc.) in the tub							
(5) Rubbed clitoris with hand (out of tub)							
(6) Squeezed PC muscle while rubbing clitoris							
(7) I tried exaggerating a fear(s) about masturbation.							
(8) 10 3-second squeezes, 3 times a day							
(9) 'Flutter' PC 10 times, 3 times a day							
(10) New 'suck in' PC 10 times, 3 times a day							
(11) Massaged breasts							
(12) Massaged thighs							
(13) Massaged genitals (goal: 45 minutes)							

(14) Did you spend at least one hour on your homework?							
(15) Approximately how much time did you spend on your homework today?							
(16) How was your mood today? 1 2 3 4 5 6 7 Not very happy → happy → perfectly happy							
(17) Did you experience an orgasm today?							
(18) If yes, how many?							
(19) I engaged in a sexual or sensual activity not listed. Describe:							
(20) I thought of a fantasy							
(21) I read *Viva, Forum* or another sexy mag.							
(22) I read Nancy Friday's *My Secret Garden* or *Forbidden Flowers* or *Fanny Hill* by John Cleland							

Step 5: Role playing orgasm (Week 5)

During some of the sessions so far you probably have experienced the responses which occur during the 'excitement and plateau phase' but you are still not 'tipping over' into the 'orgasmic phase'. Do not worry; there are ways to overcome this.

Julie Heiman and Leslie and Joseph LoPiccolo have made some films in which a woman role plays orgasm. They recommend setting aside about half an hour to one hour. Then, before become extremely aroused they suggest role playing an orgasm at the beginning of self-pleasuring. You can also try this by simulating ecstasy; groan and moan and cry out, sigh and shudder, make jerking or arching movements of the body then let your body become rigid with sexual tension and make fast fluttering movements with your PC muscles. Even if you feel this exercise is unnecessary for you, try it, and the more you exaggerate the better it will be.

In the USA there is a couple called the Grabers who have written an excellent book on woman's orgasm. They recommend an additional exercise of escalating your breathing and sighing into a full-blown noise of an 'ah', varying the tone and the pitch so that the sound wavers and goes up and down. Breathe slowly and deeply.

This next session could last 30–45 minutes. Start by thinking of a fantasy and then masturbate and try a teasing technique of stopping touching the area you are enjoying stimulating and feeling some frustration and desire to return to that area and then doing so. Do this several times then begin breathing deeply and slowly and make the 'ah' sound. Then try some fluttering of your PC muscles and then role play an orgasm, not worrying about exaggerating and grimacing, clenching your hands, tensing your legs, pointing your toes. Do not be afraid to make a noise, scream or shout erotic words, let yourself go and lose control.

If you do not feel you are able to completely let go, just continue touching your clitoris until something happens or you get tired..

By the way, some women in previous groups remarked that one of their basic fears of having climax is that they might lose control of their bladder and urinate. So what? There is nothing wrong with a little urine. Lie on a towel and relax.

Step 6: The PC muscle – bearing down

Bearing down with the PC muscles is quite a difficult task. Pretend to bear down, as though you are forcing something out of your vagina or making a bowel movement. Try holding this for about 3 seconds and practise it 10 times.

Homework checklist: Week 5

Name: ______________________________

Dates: ____________through____________

Please keep a daily record of how many times you engaged in the following behaviours. Indicate the number of times you engaged in any of the activities by putting the number under the day to the right. Mark '0' if you did not engage in the activity.

Number of times:	Day 1	2	3	4	5	6	7
(1) I took a warm bath							
(2) I felt my breasts in the tub							
(3) I felt my genitals in the tub							
(4) I felt the rest of my body (legs, arms face, etc.) in the tub							
(5) I rubbed clitoris with hand (out of tub)							
(6) I squeezed PC muscle while rubbing clitoris							
(7) I spent up to an hour a day masturbating with my vibrator							
(8) I 'role played' an orgasm							
(9) I fantasised while masturbating							
(10) 10 3-second squeezes, 3 times a day							
(11) 'Flutter' PC 10 times, 3 times a day							
(12) 'Suck in' PC 10 times, 3 times a day							
(13) 'Bear down' 3 seconds, 3 times a day							

(14) Did you spend at least one hour on your homework?							
(15) Approximately how much time did you spend on your homework today?							
(16) How was your mood today? 1 2 3 4 5 6 7 Not very happy → happy → perfectly happy							
(17) Did you experience an orgasm today?							
(18) If yes, how many?							
(19) I engaged in a sexual or sensual activity not listed. Describe:							

Suggested reading:
Circle any you have read this week. *My Secret Garden* by Nancy Friday. *Forbidden Flowers* by Nancy Friday. *Lolita* by Vladimir Nabokov. *The Pearl: A Journal of Voluptuous Reading* (Grove Press). *Fanny Hill* by John Cleland. *The Story of O* by Pauline Reage. *Forum*. *Viva*.

Step 7: Sharing a massage (Week 6)

All the previous exercises have been recommended for you to carry out in privacy. However, many of you will have a partner you would like to share your new experiences with. Some of you might not have a present partner but would like to be prepared for sharing with a future partner.

The first sharing step could be taking a bath together and soaping each other, telling one another how you like to be touched and giving one another pleasure, although you should avoid the genital areas at this stage. This helps to improve communication and is relaxing and natural.

The next stage is to touch, caress or massage each other in a warm room using some body oil or lotion. Start by taking it in turns to pleasure one another with a back, arms and legs massage. When you do this, communicate what sort of stroking and pressure and speed you enjoy. Continue with giving each other 'frontal' massage, avoiding touching the genital areas, and again communicate what you enjoy. If you feel tense at any stage, stop and relax. Remember, it's good experience to take turns being the giver and the receiver; it is necessary to share taking turns to massage as one person would get rather tired doing a back followed by a frontal massage all in one session. At the end of the session it's nice to have a cuddle but avoid further genital touching or sexual intercourse even if you feel very aroused. If you feel you need to climax it is better to do this without your partner present as this is another stage to develop.

Step 8: Sharing masturbation

Clitoral stimulation is something you probably want to share with your partner. You could invite him to watch you masturbating when you feel ready to share this with him. He will probably find this experience very exciting, especially when he sees you reaching a climax. You might like to invite him to show you how he masturbates.

After this experience you probably will not feel shy about the next step of inviting your partner to touch your genitals. Several decades ago, Helena Wright described how useful partner participation could be and how the woman could show the man the exact way she enjoyed stimulation. Masters and Johnson also include this stage in their therapy programme. You can sit between your partner's legs while he supports you by leaning against the pillows. You can guide his hand (placing your hand above or below his) and show him how you like to be touched and what pressure to apply. If you get an orgasm, that's nice, it's a bonus. Do not strive for this, but if you do not get an orgasm there is always tomorrow.

Step 9: Losing control with your partner

Some of you will find the next step unnecessary, but perhaps you still feel embarrassed about becoming aroused and 'letting yourself go' in your partner's presence. Remember the work you did in allowing yourself to lose control and make a fool of yourself when alone? There are stages of simulating this with your partner, by 'role playing' movement and sound. LoPiccolo said pre-orgasmic women reported good results in achieving orgasm with the help of these graded exercises. The Grabers suggest some of the programme below.

You can initially lie down side by side and breathe in and then exhale slowly and loudly as though you are both sighing. If this embarrassing, keep your clothes on and do this in the dark and at the same time as listening to some music on the radio or a tape recorder. The next stage is to practise making the 'ah' sound at the same time as exaggerating your movements. You can then ask your partner to touch your clitoris at the same time as making the 'ah' sound and breathing heavily and writhing. By this time you should have forgotten your inhibitions.

Step 10: Making love with your partner

At this stage you might like to continue with mutual masturbation or oral sex. Most women want to try sexual intercourse and the instructions on pages 272–8 are applicable.

Homework checklist: Week 6

Name: ______________________________

Dates: ______________through______________

Please keep a daily record of how many times you engaged in the following behaviours. Indicate the number of times you engaged in any of the activities by putting the number under the day to the right. Mark '0' if you did not engage in the activity.

Number of times:	Day 1	2	3	4	5	6	7
(1) I took a warm bath							
(2) I felt my breasts in the tub							
(3) I felt my genitals in the tub							
(4) I felt the rest of my body (legs, arms face, etc.) in the tub							
(5) Rubbed clitoris with hand (out of tub)							
(6) I masturbated with vibrator for up to an hour							
(7) I used fantasies while masturbating							
(8) I squeezed my PC muscle while masturbating							
(9) I tried intercourse with me on top							
(10) I tried intercourse 'side to side'							
(11) I tried intercourse with partner entering vagina from behind							
(12) I continued my PC exercises							
(13) I showed my PC power to my partner							

(14) Did you spend at least one hour on your homework?							
(15) Approximately how much time did you spend on your homework today?							
(16) How was your mood today? 1 2 3 4 5 6 7 Not very happy → happy → perfectly happy							
(17) Did you experience an orgasm today?							
(18) If yes, how many?							
(19) I engaged in a sexual or sensual activity not listed. Describe:							
(20) If I have a partner: I masturbated to orgasm in front of him							
(21) My partner masturbated me to orgasm							
(22) I had orgasm with my partner's penis in my vagina							

Appendix 4

Men's Sex Therapy Group Homework

These homework sheets are devised by Dr Maurice Yaffé, following the techniques recommended by Bernie Zilbergeld, and are reproduced with permission.

1. Client's initials: ________ Sex: M F Date: __________

Between session: ________ and ________

Activity (Be specific – one item per line	Duration	Pleasant 1 = least 10 = most		Arousing 1 = least 10 = most		Comments (Positive or negative reactions, problems thoughts, bodily response, etc.)
		You		You		
Choose ten objects of different textures, temperatures, etc. Touch all parts of body except genitals, focussing on the different sensations with different types of touch. List all ten items below and put your comments and rating of each.						

2. Client's initials: ________ Sex: M F Date: __________

Between session: ________ and ________

Activity (Be specific - one item per line	Duration	Pleasant 1 = least 10 = most		Arousing 1 = least 10 = most		Comments (Positive or negative reactions, problems thoughts, bodily response, etc.)
		You		You		
Continue the sensate focus exercises. Use your originality to make them more interesting for yourself. You may want to select various times of the day, locations, fantasies, etc. Do this as many times as you feel comfortable.						

3. Client's initials: ________ Sex: M F Date: __________

Between session: ________ and ________

Activity (Be specific - one item per line	Duration	Pleasant 1 = least 10 = most		Arousing 1 = least 10 = most		Comments (Positive or negative reactions, problems thoughts, bodily response, etc.)
		You		You		
Stand in front of the mirror and do a total body visual exploration for 15 minutes. Then spend the remaining 15 minutes examining your genitals and identifying and saying aloud the different parts.						

4. Client's initials: ________ Sex: M F Date: __________

Between session: ________ and ________

Activity (Be specific – one item per line	Duration	Pleasant 1 = least 10 = most		Arousing 1 = least 10 = most		Comments (Positive or negative reactions, problems thoughts, bodily response, etc.)
		You		You		
Tactile exploration (1) Spend 30 minutes exploring your body except for your genitals. Identify particular locations and types of touching (for example, speed, direction, pressure, etc.) that feel pleasant or un-pleasant. *Do not concern yourself with arousal,* but rather, focus on what feels good, where, and how.						

5. Client's initials: ________ Sex: M F Date: __________

Between session: ________ and ________

Activity (Be specific – one item per line	Duration	Pleasant 1 = least 10 = most		Arousing 1 = least 10 = most		Comments (Positive or negative reactions, problems thoughts, bodily response, etc.)
		You		You		
Tactile exploration (2) Spend 30 minutes exploring your body and the genital area, identifying particular locations and types of touching (for example, speed, direction, pressure, etc.) that feel pleasant or unpleasant. *Do not concern yourself with arousal*, but rather, focus on what feels good, where, and how.						

6. Client's initials: ________ Sex: M F Date: __________

Between session: ________ and ________

Activity (Be specific – one item per line	Duration	Pleasant 1 = least 10 = most		Arousing 1 = least 10 = most		Comments (Positive or negative reactions, problems thoughts, bodily response, etc.)
		You		You		
Tactile exploration (3) Do this exercise at least twice during the week, for a period of 20–30 minutes each time. Continue the exploration of your whole body and genitals, focussing on the different sensations you experience. You may proceed to orgasm if you wish.						

7. Client's initials: ________ Sex: M F Date: __________

Between session: ________ and ________

Activity (Be specific – one item per line	Duration	Pleasant 1 = least 10 = most		Arousing 1 = least 10 = most		Comments (Positive or negative reactions, problems thoughts, bodily response, etc.)
		You		You		
Explore your whole body and genitals, touching yourself using different strokes, pressures, etc. Stimulate yourself in a way that is erotic to you. The purpose of this exercise is to try and touch yourself in a pleasurable way – not to try and get an erection. Even if you begin to get an erection, stop the stimulation, and let the erection go down. When the erection is down, try touching again and letting it go down two or three times at most. You may stimulate yourself to orgasm after stopping a couple of times. Repeat this exercise three times during the next week. Plan on spending a minimum of 30 minutes on this exercise.						

8. Client's initials: ________ Sex: M F Date: __________

Between session: ________ and ________

Activity (Be specific – one item per line	Duration	Pleasant 1 = least 10 = most		Arousing 1 = least 10 = most		Comments (Positive or negative reactions, problems thoughts, bodily response, etc.)
		You		You		
Explore your whole body and genitals, touching yourself using different strokes, pressures, etc. Stimulate yourself in a way that is erotic to you. The purpose of this exercise is to try to touch yourself in a pleasurable way – not to try to get an erection. Even if you begin to get an erection, stop the stimulation, and let the erection go down. When the erection is down, try touching again and letting it go down 2–3 times at most. While you are doing this, think of a situation where you are giving or receiving a massage. It can be like what you saw in the film, or be something completely different that you find more interesting. You may stimulate yourself to orgasm after stopping a couple of times. Repeat this exercise three times during the next week. Plan on spending a minimum of 30 minutes on this exercise.						

9. Client's initials: ________ Sex: M F Date: __________

Between session: ________ and ________

Activity (Be specific – one item per line	Duration	Pleasant 1 = least 10 = most		Arousing 1 = least 10 = most		Comments (Positive or negative reactions, problems thoughts, bodily response, etc.)
		You		You		
Write down, *for your own use, not on this paper*, a sexual fantasy that you find arousing or pleasing. Your fantasy is for your own use and you will not be asked to discuss the fantasy with the group. The fantasy can be brief and can be about *any* topic or scene that you feel would be pleasing.						

10. Client's initials: ________ Sex: M F Date: __________

Between session: ________ and ________

Activity (Be specific – one item per line	Duration	Pleasant 1 = least 10 = most		Arousing 1 = least 10 = most		Comments (Positive or negative reactions, problems thoughts, bodily response, etc.)
		You		You		
Meet at least two new people this week. This may just be to say hello to someone. On this sheet, write down your feelings about what it was like each time you met a new person						

11. Client's initials: ______ Sex: M F Date: ______

Between session: ______ and ______

Activity (Be specific – one item per line	Duration	Pleasant 1 = least 10 = most		Arousing 1 = least 10 = most		Comments (Positive or negative reactions, problems thoughts, bodily response, etc.)
		You		You		
Role play, in front of a mirror: (1) 'saying no': to a non-sexual request from a partner or potential partner; (2) 'saying no' to a sexual request made by a partner; (3) discussing your nervousness about new sexual encounters; (4) asking a potential partner to engage in sensate activities, such as a full body massage; asking for sensual contact only for the pleasure of touching; saying you don't want a more sexual encounter.						

12. Client's initials: ________ Sex: M F Date: __________

Between session: ________ and ________

Activity (Be specific – one item per line	Duration	Pleasant 1 = least 10 = most		Arousing 1 = least 10 = most		Comments (Positive or negative reactions, problems thoughts, bodily response, etc.)
		You		You		
Now use what you have practised in role playing in front of a mirror and share that information with another person in whatever way seems right for you. You may be just starting a conversation with another person or talking with someone you already know. Again, gain practice by disclosing some information about your problem or about being in this group or whatever. Share at least three things about yourself with at least two other people.						

13. I. What did you see as the difficulties you had when you came into the programme, both with your own sexuality (behaviour and attitudes) and with your previous partners?	II. What have you learned specifically to overcome each of these? (For example, techniques, attitude change, information.)	III. What new problems do you anticipate arising in the future, and how are you going to handle them?
1.	1.	1.
2.	2.	2.
3.	3.	3.
4.	4.	4.
5.	5.	5.
etc.	etc.	etc.

Appendix 5

Stimulation Therapy

PLEASURE SHEETS

The following list is a selection of poetry, books, audio and videotapes, pictures, magazines and films which have been found in the context of stimulation therapy to be helpful in making it easier for couples to communicate sexually. In some cases there has been an increase in sexual interest and libido. All these recommendations will not appeal to everybody, but there is a wide choice and therapists and their clients can obviously pick and choose.

(1) Literature

1. *Amores.*
   Ovid.
2. *The Arabian Nights.*
   Translated by Sir Richard Burton.
3. *Cage me a Peacock.*
   Noel Langley.
4. *The Decameron.*
   Giovanni Boccaccio.
5. *The Diary of Anais Nin.*
   Anais Nin.
6. *Fear of Flying.*
   Erica Jong.
7. *Forbidden Flowers.*
   Nancy Friday.
8. *The Garden of Tortures.*
   Octave Mirabeau.
9. *The God of the Labyrinth.*
   Colin Wilson.
10. *The Happy Hooker.*
    Xaviera Hollander.
11. *Histoire de l'Oeil.*
    George Bataille.
12. *Inside Linda Lovelace.*
    Linda Lovelace.
13. *The Joy of Sex.*
    Alex Comfort.
14. *Juliette.*
    Marquis de Sade.

15. *Justine.*
    Marquis de Sade.
16. *The Kama Sutra.*
    Vatsayana.
17. *Lady Chatterley's Lover.*
    D.H. Lawrence.
18. *La Motocyclette.*
    André Pierre de Mandiargues.
19. *Lolita.*
    Vladimir Nabokov.
20. *Memoires of Casanova.*
    Casanova.
21. *Fanny Hill.*
    John Cleland.
22. *My Life and Loves.*
    Frank Harris.
23. *My Secret Garden.*
    Nancy Friday.
24. *My Secret Life.*
    Edward Sellon.
25. *Myra Breckenridge.*
    Gore Vidal.
26. *The Other Victorians.*
    Steven Marcus.
27. *The Pearl.*
    Anonymous.
28. *The Sensuous Wife.*
    Robert Chartham.
29. *The Sensuous Woman.*
    By J.
30. *The Story of 'O'.*
    Pauline Reage.
31. *The Surrogate Wife.*
    Valerie X. Scott.
32. *Tropic of Cancer.*
    Henry Miller.
33. *Tropic of Capricorn.*
    Henry Miller.
34. *Venus in Furs.*
    Von Sacher-Masoch.
35. *The Virgin and the Gypsy.*
    D.H. Lawrence.

(2) Magazines

Color Climax. Cupido. Fiesta. Forum. Knave. Mayfair. Men Only. Oui. Penthouse. Playboy. Playgirl.

(3) Sound and tapes

Tapes in the 'Sounds of Sex' Japanese tape series. Indian evening ragas. Ravel's *Bolero.* High Life Music from West and East Africa. Reggae. Soul. Calypsos from Trinidad. Brazilian music: Gilberto Gil, Gal Costa and Candeia. Umbaqanga music from South Africa.

(4) Art

Sculpture

Indian sculpture at Khajarhao and Konarak.
Doug John's genitalia sculpture is most erotic and can be obtained in New York.

Pictures

Prints, paintings, drawings etc. by Francis Bacon, Aubrey Beardsley, Bosch, Botticelli, Edward Burra, Sir Richard Burton, Salvador Dali, Betty Dodson, Eisen, Fuseli, Richard Gillan, Goya, Hogarth, David Hockney, Hokusai, Alan Jones, Gustav Klimt, L.S. Lowry, Michelangelo, Picasso, Patrick Proctor, Rodin, Rowlandson, Rubens, Egon Schiele, Stanley Spencer, Titian, Keith Vaughan.

Japanese and erotic prints including Hokusai and Eiser can be viewed at the British Museum. The Royal Asiatic Society houses Sir Richard Burton's illustrations –the ones saved from Lady Isabel Burton's arson. Indian miniatures: usually fakes are on sale at tourist shops in Bombay and the customers should ask for 'something rude'. Some erotic decorations can be found on Greek vases. Some Ancient Egyptian and Roman examples of erotica also can be found.

(5) Films and videos

Young love

Daddy. Debbie Does Dallas. Don't Deliver Us From Evil. Lolita. Miss Mary. My Dearest Love. Seventeen.

Heterosexuality

Barbarella. The Bed. Behind the Green Door. Blow Up. Castaway. Claire's Knee. Danish Blue. The Devil in Miss Jones. Diary of a Shinjuku Thief. Don't Look Now. El. Emmanuelle. Erotikon. Free. Fuses. The Harrad Experiment. Immoral Tales. Jubiaba. Kontacte. La Collectioneuse. La Mano en La Trampa. The Language of Love. Last Tango in Paris. Les Amants. The Lickerish Quartet. The Light Across the Street. Love in the Afternoon. Love Making. Men. Misty Beethoven. My Little Chickadee. Painted Lips. Pandora's Box. Partie de Campagne. Quiet Days in Clichy. The Round Up. Secrets of Sex. She Done Him Wrong. She Gotta Have it. The Switchboard Operator. Tom Jones. Tristana. The Witching Hour. Woman of the Dunes. Women in Love. W.R. Mysteries of the Human Organism.Zabriskie Point.

Female homosexuality

Anima. The Conformists. Les Biches. The Fox. The Lickerish Quartet. Persona. The Silence. Terese and Isabel.

Male homosexuality

A Bigger Splash. Auto-American Dream. Chant d'Amour. Dearest Love. Death in Venice. Dona Herlinda and her Son. Early Morning. Flesh. One on One. Robert Having His Nipples Pierced. Satyricon. Soma Touch. Sunday Bloody Sunday. View From the Top.

Sexual fantasies

The Balcony. Belle de Jour. Blow Out. Deep Throat. Diary of a Chamber-maid. Divine's Films. El Bruto. Girl on a Motorbike. Goto, Isle of Love. Immoral Tales. L'Age d'Or. La Sorcière de Salem. Maitresse. Matador. Morgiana. Sweet Movie. Tristana. The White Sheikh.

Sexual fantasies (not usually recommended):

Blanche. Clockwork Orange. Dynamo. Extremeties. L'Empire des Senses. Eros + Massacre. 101 Days of Sodom. The Night Porter. Nosferatu. The Other Side of Underneath. Peeping Tom. Straw Dogs. Vamp. The Virgin Spring. Viva la Muerte.

Many of the above films can be seen at The National Film Theatre or the ICA (Institute of Contemporary Arts) in London.

SAR films and catalogue from Multi-Media Resource Centre, 1525 Franklin St., San Francisco, CA 94109, USA.

Martin Cole's films from the Institute for Sex Education and Research, 38 School Road, Moseley, Birmingham.

(6) Slides

Therapy slides prepared by Patricia Gillan and covering sex education and stimulation therapy can be obtained from Therapy Slides, Box 4ZB, London W1A 4ZB.

(7) Sex aids

Pifco massagers which can be used as vibrators are obtainable from large chemists like Boots and other large department stores. Do not

purchase machines which are designed for heat therapy. Electric tooth brushes may also be used.
Aroma therapy massage oils from The Body Shop.
KY Jelly from any chemist.

Sensory Impressions Checklist

(1) Tick any of the following you like touching:
Female body. Male body. Silk. Satin. Fur. Rubber. Plastic. Nylon. Marble. Sand. Velvet. Wool. Sculpture. Glass. Sandpaper. Seaweed. Vaseline. Water. Hand cream. Your partner's body.

(2) Tick any of the following you like the odour of:
Outdoor odours: Smoke, cut hay, grass, earth, sea, manure.
Scented products: floral, citrus, spicy, exotic, oriental, mossy, pine.
Foods: fish, vanilla, curry, garlic, gorgonzola, strawberries, beer, wine, cigars.
Leather. Incense. Some body smells. Your partner's body without scent. Soap.

(3) Tick any of the following you like listening to:
Music: Classical, Modern, Pop, Rock, Soul, Reggae, Ragas, Drumming.
The Radio. Sex Sounds. Laughter. Sighing. Groaning. Giggling. Panting. Stories.
Voices: Male, Female. Your partner's voice.

(4) Do you read erotic literature, e.g. *Fanny Hill*? YES/NO

(5) Would you, if you had the chance to do? YES/NO

(6) Do you look at sexy magazines, e.g. *Knave: Men Only; Playgirl; Playboy; Forum*? YES/NO

(7) Would you if you had the chance to do so? YES/NO

(8) Do you get sexual pleasure out of looking at attractive people? YES/NO

(9) Have you ever been to a blue film, e.g. *Emmanuelle*? YES/NO

(10) Would you go to a blue film if you had the opportunity? YES/NO

(11) Do you have sexual fantasies? OFTEN/SOMETIMES/RARELY

(12) How many times have you climaxed without genital stimulation, through either fantasy or erotic material (not counting wet dreams).

(13) Since you were 20 how often have you come more than once (by any means) in a half-hour period? USUALLY/FAIRLY OFTEN/ A FEW TIMES/NEVER

(14) Do you have oral sex? OFTEN/SELDOM/NEVER

(15) Would you like your partner to give you oral sex? YES/NO
(16) Would you like to give oral sex to your partner? YES/NO
(17) How often do you masturbate? OFTEN/SOMETIMES/ NEVER
(18) How many positions have you tried when you make love?
(19) Tick how many places you have made love in. The sea; beach; bath; shower; car; work; field; wood; sitting-room; kitchen.
(20) You are in hospital with two broken arms. You face a long period without sexual satisfaction of any kind. Would this be: almost intolerable; frustrating, but bearable; not too much of a problem at all?

THE VIBRATOR

Advice to clients

Why a vibrator? Mainly because the use of vibrators is now well established to achieve orgasmic release. Lobitz and LoPiccolo in 1972 reported good results for anorgasmic women who found it difficult to experience an orgasm when masturbating with their fingers.

Several women reported they needed just a little extra stimulation to 'tip them over into orgasm' and this was when a vibrator was suggested and found to help.

In 1974 Asizdas and Beech suggested that the anorgasmic women they were helping would benefit from trying a battery-driven vibrator and most of the women reported satisfaction when using a vibrator. American reports by Betty Dodson, Lonnie Barbach and Susan McMullen all agreed that the vibrator was useful for therapy, although these authors did not include a non-vibrator control group in their studies.

Some people think that a vibrator is unnatural but, if the natural way of touching oneself produces no results, surely it would be better to accept some help from a vibrator rather than condemn oneself to a life of no orgasms?

Others have asked what would happen if they got 'hooked on a vibrator' and needed it all the time? There is no evidence that women who use vibrators cannot reach orgasm by manual stimulation and in any case who decides what is right and wrong? You are responsible for what you want. Using a vibrator can be the way to have your first orgasm and perhaps some of you will no longer find the vibrator necessary after the first initial orgasm, especially if the problem has been 'letting yourself go'. Riley and Riley showed in their study of pre-orgasmic women that the women could easily transfer from the vibrator to a finger.

(a) Body massage

You can try your vibrator initially for a body massage, but *never* use it in the bath. Use your favourite oil or body lotion and try your vibrator on shoulders and arms initially, place it on your neck and forehead, then your tummy, lower back, buttocks, legs and feet. Experiment with varying pressure, some people like a light application and others prefer a stronger pressure. Try the different attachments and choose the one you prefer. Take about 20 minutes or longer to experiment with the different attachments. Avoid massaging around the thyroid gland (just below the Adam's Apple).

(b) Genital massage

Initially spread plenty of your favourite lubricant over your genital area. Try holding the vibrator over your outer vaginal area (but do not insert it into your vagina) and then move it towards your clitoris, where it will probably feel more intense. Some women prefer to place some sort of material or towel over their genitals during vibrator stimulations as they are too sensitive to direct contact. Others say they prefer direct stimulation with the vibrator head piece flat on the clitoris and others like a sideways contact with the edge of the vibrator head so that the smallest part of the vibrating surface makes contact with the genital area. Do what you like best, but experiment with light and heavy pressure and vary movement and intensity by the switch. Usually you will get used to the vibrator and enjoy it even if at first it makes you feel over-excited and you feel over-sensitive.

Spend about 20 minutes each time you have a session using your vibrator on your genitals for the first three times, then extend the time to about half an hour, and then for half an hour to an hour. Do not force yourself to have a climax as this defeats the purpose of the exercise. Build up your feelings and allow yourself to enjoy them.

Appendix 6

Recommended Reading List

General sexuality and therapy

1. Annon, Jack. (1975) *The Behavioral Treatment of Sexual Problems.* Kapiolani Health Services, Honolulu.
2. Bancroft, John. (1983) *Human Sexuality and Its Problems.* Churchill Livingstone.
3. Barlow, David. (1981) *Sexually Transmitted Diseases: The Facts.* Oxford University Press.
4. Comfort, Alex. (1972) *The Joy of Sex.* Simon & Schuster.
5. Cooper, Wendy. (1985) *No Change: A Biological Revolution for Women.* Arrow Books.
6. Cousins, Jane. (1980) *Make It Happy.* Fontana.
7. Craft, Michael and Ann. (1985) *Sex and the Mentally Handicapped.* Routledge & Kegan Paul.
8. Crandall, Nelson. (1971) *Sex in the Black-White Marriage.* Academy Press.
9. Ford, C.S. and Beach, F.A. (1951) *Patterns of Sexual Behaviour.* Harper and Row.
10. Gagnon, J.H. and Simon, W. (1974) *Sexual Conduct. The Social Sources of Human Sexuality.* Hutchinson.
11. Gillan, Patricia and Richard. (1976) *Sex Therapy Today.* Open Books.
12. Greenwood, Judy. (1984) *Coping with Sexual Relationships.* MacDonald.
13. Hawton, Keith. (1985) *Sex Therapy. A Practical Guide.* Oxford Medical Publications.
14. Heather, Beryl. (1984) *Sharing.* FPA Publication Unit.
15. Knox. D. (1971) *Marriage Happiness. A Behavioral Approach to Counselling.* Research Press, Illinois.

16. Lee, Carol. (1986) *The Ostrich Position. Sex, Schooling and Mystification.* Allen & Unwin.
17. Littlewood, Roland and Lipsedge, Maurice. (1982) *Aliens and Alienists*. Pelican.
18. Yaffé, Maurice and Fenwick, Elizabeth. (1986) *Sexual Happiness. A Practical Approach.* Dorling Kindersley.

Female sexuality

1. Barbach, Lonnie Garfield. (1975) *For Yourself. The Fulfilment of Female Sexuality*. Doubleday.
2. Dickson, Anne. (1982) *A Woman in Your Own Right. Assertiveness and You*. Quartet.
3. Dickson, Anne. (1985) *The Mirror Within. A New Look at Sexuality.* Quartet Books.
4. Dodson, Betty. (1974) *Liberating Masturbation*. Published and distributed by Betty Dodson, Box 1933, New York, 10001.
5. Friday, Nancy. (1975) *Forbidden Flowers*. Pocket Books, New York.
6. Griffin, Susan. (1984) *Woman and Nature – The Roaring Inside Her.* Women's Press.
7. Heiman, Julia, LoPiccolo, Leslie, and LoPiccolo, Joseph. (1986) *Becoming Orgasmic: A Sexual Growth Program for Women*. Prentice-Hall.
8. Hite, Shere. (1976) *The Hite Report. A Nationwide Study of Female Sexuality*. Dell.
9. Hooper, Anne. (1980) *The Body Electric*. Virago.
10. Hollander, Xaviera. (1975) *The Happy Hooker*. Granada.
11. Martin, Del and Lyon, Phyllis. (1972) *Lesbian Women*. Bantam; New York.
12. Meulenbelt, Anja. (1981) *Four Ourselves*. Sheba.
13. Phillips, Angela and Rakusen, Jill. (1978) *Our Bodies, Ourselves.* Penguin.
14. Rich, Adrienne. (1977) *Of Woman Born: Motherhood an Experience and Institution*. Virago.
15. Patterson, Orlando. (1986) *The Children of Sisyphus*. Longman Caribbean Writers.

Male Sexuality

1. Amis, Kinglsey. (1978) *Jake's Thing*. Hutchinson.
2. Anonymous. (1966) *My Secret Life*. Grove Press.

3. Bailey, Paul. (1982) *An English Madam. The Life and Work of Cynthia Payne*. Johnathan Cape.
4. Hodson, Phillip. (1984) *Men: An Investigation into the Emotional Male*. Ariel Books.
5. Hoffman, Martin. (1968) *The Gay World*. Basic Books.
6. Lewis, Stephen. (1974) *Male Sexual Fantasies*. Ace Books.
7. Lovelace, Earl. (1986) *The Dragon Can't Dance*. Longman Caribbean Writers.
8. Scott, Valerie. X. (1971) *Surrogate Wife*. Dell.
9. Zilbergeld, Bernie. (1980) *Men and Sex*. Fontana.

Appendix 7

Legal Contract for Therapy

Therapists should legally protect themselves against being sued by single clients who have been advised to search for a partner. When it is recommended that such a client should find a sexual partner the question of sexually transmitted diseases comes up. It is a good idea to get such a client to sign a formal contract so that the therapist is covered if the client finds a partner who has such a disease and gives it to the client. e.g. AIDS.

A specimen contract has been outlined below, but therapists should consult their own legal advisors before deciding on a suitable form of words.

Contract

I .... declare that my
Therapist .... has explained to me the dangers of contracting a sexually transmitted disease or diseases from sexual contact with a new partner. The risk of AIDS has been discussed. The precautions necessary in such a contact, e.g. the use of a condom, have been outlined by the therapist. I take full responsibility for my actions and health.

Signed ....

Index